Research Methods in Kinesiology and the Health Sciences

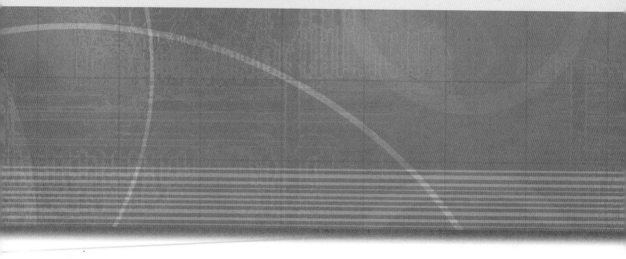

Susan J. Hall, PhD, FACSM
Deputy Dean, College of Health Sciences
University of Delaware
Newark, Delaware

Nancy Getchell, PhD
Associate Professor
Department of Kinesiology and Applied Physiology
University of Delaware
Newark, Delaware

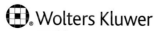 Wolters Kluwer

Health

Philadelphia • Baltimore • New York • London
Buenos Aires • Hong Kong • Sydney • Tokyo

Acquisitions Editor: Emily Lupash
Product Development Editor: Michael Egolf
Marketing Manager: Shauna Kelley
Designer: Joan Wendt
Art Director: Jennifer Clements
Compositor: SPi Global
Printer: RRD Shenzhen

Printed in China

Library of Congress Cataloging-in-Publication Data
Hall, Susan J. (Susan Jean), 1953- author.
 Research methods in kinesiology and the health sciences / Susan Hall, Nancy Getchell. — First edition.
   p. ; cm.
 Includes bibliographical references and index.
 ISBN 978-0-7817-9774-0 (alk. paper)
 I. Getchell, Nancy, 1963- author. II. Title.
 [DNLM: 1. Kinesiology, Applied. 2. Research Design.   WE 103]
 GV361
 613.7072—dc23

                                                                                      2013041074

Contributor

Catherine D. Ennis, PhD
Professor
Department of Kinesiology
University of North Carolina at Greensboro
Greensboro, North Carolina
   Chapter 8: Qualitative Research

Reviewers

Alberto Cordova, PhD
Assistant Professor
College of Education and Human Development
University of Texas at San Antonio
San Antonio, Texas

Jane Crossman, PhD
Professor
School of Kinesiology
Lakehead University
Thunder Bay, Ontario, Canada

Charles Fountaine, PhD
Assistant Professor
Department of Health, Physical Education, and
    Recreation
University of Minnesota Duluth
Duluth, Minnesota

Derek Kivi, PhD
Associate Professor
School of Kinesiology
Lakehead University
Thunder Bay, Ontario, Canada

Jeff Lynn, PhD
Associate Professor
Department of Exercise and Rehabilitative
    Services
Slippery Rock University
Slippery Rock, Pennsylvania

Augusto Rodriquez, PhD
Lecturer
Department of Kinesiology
Rice University
Houston, Texas

Michael Sachs, PhD
Professor
Department of Kinesiology
Temple University
Philadelphia, Pennsylvania

Sheila Stepp, PhD
Department Chair
Department of Movement Science
SUNY Orange
Middletown, New York

Georgios Stylianides, PhD
Instructor
School of Public Service and Health
American Military University
Manassas, Virginia

Brian Wallace, PhD
Distance Learning Faculty
United States Sports Academy
Daphne, Alabama

Preface

What distinguishes this book from similar ones? Designed for introductory research methods courses at the beginning graduate and undergraduate levels in a broad range of health-related programs, this book includes all major topics conventionally addressed in introductory research methods texts. Unlike other textbooks, we have placed emphasis on topics directly related to development of research proposals, since these topics have great practical relevance for beginning researchers. We also include two full chapters on important topics that are *not* addressed in a meaningful way in similar books: (1) research writing style and (2) matching statistical tools with research protocols.

Research writing is a critically important topic related to research methods. Beyond the obvious fact that research proposals, journal manuscripts, and abstracts for conference presentations must be appropriately written to convey their respective purposes, many programs require students to write a thesis or scholarly project paper as the culminating experience for their academic degree. Yet most kinesiology or related health sciences programs virtually ignore the topic, with few curricula including a course in research or technical writing. The research methods course is a logical place to include some focused instruction on research writing style because course assignments typically include writing some components of research proposals and/or reports (real or mock). Logically, teaching students *how* to write about research should occur at the same time they learn how to develop and organize appropriate content for research documents. An understanding of what constitutes good research writing style will be invaluable for many students, not only in their required courses, but in their subsequent education and careers.

The issue of how to infuse topics related to statistics into a course or textbook on research methods is somewhat complicated. Statistics and research methods are inexorably linked in a "chicken and egg" kind of way. Depending on the prevailing philosophy, students may or may not have had a statistics course prior to taking research methods. Keeping this in mind, we have taken the approach of including descriptions and examples of commonly used statistical procedures. Beyond this, however, we also specifically devote a chapter to the relationships between statistical tools and research designs, with practical advice on how to select the appropriate statistical test for a given research problem. Even students with a reasonably good command of basic statistics often struggle with the decision as to which statistical approach is most appropriately used in conjunction with a given research protocol. Our chapter on matching experimental designs with statistical methods should help to alleviate some of the confusion and guess work on the part of novice researchers.

APPROACH

Our treatment of the topics included in the book emphasizes practical relevance for beginning students of research methods. We designed this approach to foster understanding rather than require memorization. To stimulate both interest and understanding, the text is liberally peppered with examples, applications, and related anecdotes. We incorporate examples from a broad range of fields of inquiry in kinesiology and the health sciences. Given that some undergraduate kinesiology students are preparing for careers in physical therapy and other health care professions, examples and applications also include treatment and rehabilitation protocols. With respect for the expansive field of qualitative research, we also include a full chapter on this topical area contributed by internationally respected qualitative researcher Cathy Ennis.

PEDAGOGICAL FEATURES

To enhance student understanding, we include chapter objectives, marginal definitions of key terms, marginal tips (key points of emphasis), highlighted text boxes containing related material of special interest, and chapter summaries, as well as original photographs, line drawings, and tables. At the end of each section within chapters, "Check Your Understanding" questions serve as a review of the preceding content and draw students' attention to the key points.

At the end of each chapter, we include "Related Assignments" and "In-Class Group Exercises." Instructors can utilize the related assignments for class discussion or use them as homework assignments. The group exercises are designed for small group discussion in a problem-based learning format in the classroom. We have found that students benefit from and enjoy collaborative discussion and solution of these exercises to ensure understanding and appropriate applications of course content.

ADDITIONAL RESOURCES

Research Methods in Kinesiology and the Health Sciences includes additional resources for instructors that are available on the book's companion Web site at http://thepoint. lww.com/Hall1e.

Instructors

Approved adopting instructors will be given access to the following additional resources:
- Brownstone test generator
- PowerPoint presentations
- Answers to *Check Your Understanding* questions
- Image bank
- WebCT and Blackboard Ready Cartridge

In addition, instructors can access the searchable Full Text On-line by going to the *Research Methods in Kinesiology and the Health Sciences* Web site at http://thePoint. lww.com. See the inside front cover of this text for more details, including the passcode you will need to gain access to the Web site.

Acknowledgments

We greatly appreciate the opportunity given us by acquisitions editor Emily Lupash to work on this book. The editorial and production teams, including Michael Egolf, Shauna Kelley, Joan Wendt, and Jennifer Clements, have been a pleasure to work with, and we thank them for their work on this project. We also sincerely appreciate the helpful feedback from the reviewers, including Alberto Cordova, Jane Crossman, Charles Fountaine, Derek Kivi, Jeff Lynn, Augusto Rodriguez, Michael Sachs, Sheila Stepp, Georgios Stylianides, and Brian Wallace. Finally, we are most appreciative of the excellent chapter on qualitative research contributed by Cathy Ennis.

Contents

Understanding
the Research Process

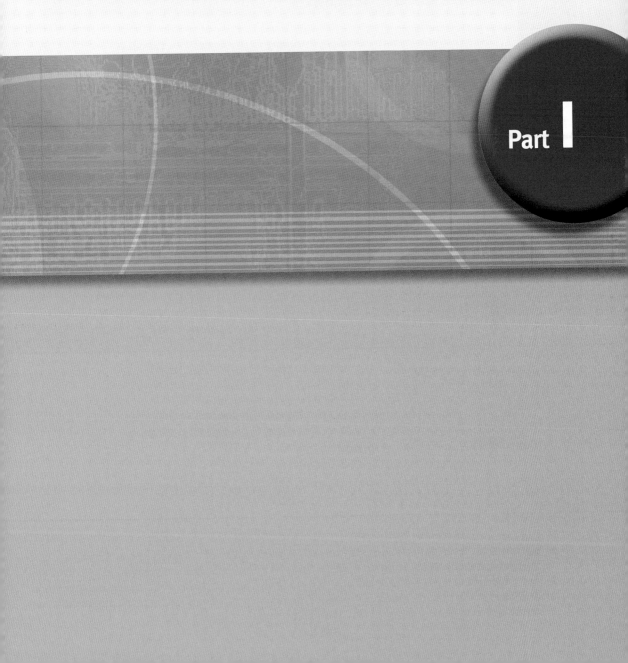

Part I

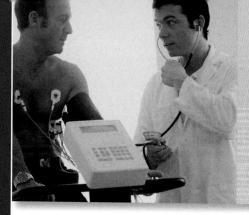

Introduction to Research in Kinesiology

"Somewhere, something incredible is waiting to be known."—Dr. Carl Sagan

CHAPTER OBJECTIVES

After studying this chapter, you will be able to:
1. Define research and explain the importance of the research question or problem.
2. Formulate researchable questions including independent and dependent variables.
3. Describe the sequential steps in the scientific method.
4. Explain the concepts of internal and external validity.
5. Differentiate between basic and applied research, quantitative and qualitative research, and experimental and nonexperimental research.

■ WELCOME to the realm of research! Research is the process of discovering new knowledge and understanding new insights. It drives advances in most fields and, ultimately, improves our lives and helps us understand our world and universe. Research also advances ways of thinking and, over time, leads to changes in culture. Discovery through the research process is exciting and stimulating, and researchers tend to be very engaged and passionate about their work.

This book will serve as your road map for learning to navigate within the realm of research. You will discover that some of the things you thought you knew about research are not exactly true and that some of the terminology you have known and used perfectly correctly has a completely different meaning within the context of research. As you come to understand the research process on a meaningful level, you will find that you have a new ability to critically read and understand the papers published in many research journals. You will also be more thoughtful and sometimes skeptical about some of the "research" findings reported by the media. This new level of understanding will be a valuable asset in your life as an educated professional. If you complete a graduate degree in most fields, part of your degree requirements are likely to be a real research project that will become your master's thesis or doctoral dissertation. This is likely to be a challenging and time-consuming process that will result in quite a sense of accomplishment. You may eventually even decide that a career involving research is in your future. Virtually every field requires some understanding of the research process whether you become a researcher or not. For this reason, most graduate programs require a course in research methods.

WHAT IS RESEARCH?

Sometimes, it is helpful when explaining a new concept to make clear first what familiar things that new concept is *not*. When you were in elementary school, your teachers probably gave you "research" paper assignments on different topics that required going to the library or searching online to find information. Technically, looking up known information is *not* research. That is, research is *not* fact finding. You may also have the notion that researchers wear white lab coats and speak only in multisyllabic jargon. Some, in fact, may do these things, but most do not.

Definitions of Research

Given that research is the gateway to new knowledge in all fields of inquiry, including the sciences, social sciences, humanities, business, and politics, just to name a few, it is not surprising that numerous definitions of research have been formulated.

The National Institutes of Health[1] (NIH) provides the following definition: "*Research* means a systematic investigation, including research development, testing, and evaluation, designed to develop or contribute to generalizable knowledge."

Creswell[2] defines research as follows: "*Research* is a process of steps used to collect and analyze information to increase our understanding of a topic or issue. It consists of three steps: Pose a question, collect data to answer the question, and present an answer to the question."

An internationally recognized definition of the term *researchers* is "professionals engaged in the conception or creation of new knowledge, products, processes, methods, and systems, and in the management of the projects concerned."[3]

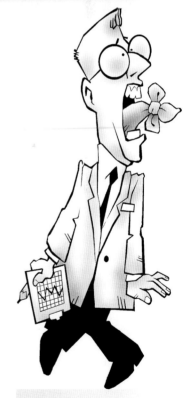

He just explained his theory of relative transgenic multiprolific nonsecreting disestablishmentarianism.

Research A careful, systematic, and structured process for solving problems or answering questions.

Research Question or Problem Important question or obstacle that is the underlying and driving reason for conducting a research study.

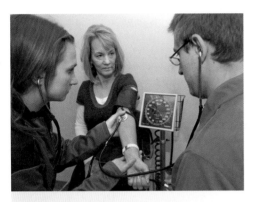

Researchers out of lab coats!

So, what is research? The definitions above clearly indicate that **research** is a process. More specifically, it is a careful, objective, systematic, and structured process for solving problems or answering questions. This means that in the absence of what we call a **research question** or a **research problem**, whatever may be going on is not research. So all research begins with the identification of a specific question for which someone seeks an answer or a problem that someone would like to have solved. Every field of study and every field of work involve numerous questions or problems that, if answered or solved, would advance understanding or improve practice.

There are numerous important questions currently under investigation within kinesiology and the health sciences. What interventions in diet and exercise can best reverse the obesity epidemic? How can individuals prevent and practitioners effectively treat low back pain? How can athletes at all playing levels and across several sports avoid concussions? What lifestyle factors elevate or reduce risks of different cancers and cardiovascular disease? What can motivate people to adhere to an exercise program? What factors distinguish elite from subelite performance in different sports? What approaches work best for teaching children movement skills? How can the elderly decrease their risk of falls? What factors lead to collective violence at soccer games? These are only a few of the challenging question areas of high importance under investigation.

Historical Approaches to Solving Problems

Throughout history, there have been various approaches to solving problems and answering questions. Answers to questions about the unknown have often come from culturally rooted beliefs that at the time people considered "common sense" or "common knowledge." Many were sure that Columbus (1451–1506) would fall off the edge of the earth if he sailed too far, because most people assumed that the earth was flat and "common sense" suggested that it must have edges. Galileo Galilei (1564–1642), the Italian mathematician, physicist, and astronomer who is called the "father of modern science," also refuted some widely held beliefs of his day. During Galileo's time, people still believed the Aristotelian proposition that heavy objects drop at a faster rate than lighter ones. By dropping a variety of objects of different weights off the top of the Leaning Tower of Pisa, Galileo demonstrated that all objects fall at the same rate, regardless of their weights. Based on his astronomical observations through telescopes that he developed, Galileo also advanced the notion that the earth revolves around the sun. However, because most people of the day believed that this contradicted the Bible, Galileo was forced to retract that position. Although we consider ourselves much more sophisticated today, it is likely that a few hundred years from now, people may view some of our commonly held beliefs as rather primitive. (Think about it!)

Questions and problems have also been addressed historically through the proclamations of authority figures. For example, King Henry I of England originally defined the length of a yard as the distance from his nose to the thumb of his extended right arm. Within the United States and the United Kingdom, this system of measurement is still used. Throughout history, people in positions of authority have issued opinions that many have accepted as truth. In reaction to blind acceptance of statements from authority figures, modern-day professor of psychology Timothy Leary famously advocated, "Think for yourself and question authority."

The Birth of Logic

The early Greeks were advanced in that they sought objective ways of viewing the world around them and discovering new knowledge. The concept of applying logical reasoning in solving problems or answering questions appears to have originated with Aristotle. Aristotle's process of **deductive reasoning** employed a logical **syllogism** consisting of two or more premises, or propositions, followed by a conclusion. Here is an example:

> Premise 1: All knee injuries are painful.
>
> Premise 2: Trevor has injured his knee.
>
> Conclusion: Trevor's knee is painful.

Deductive Reasoning Logical thinking that utilizes one or more general assumptions to arrive at a specific answer or solution.

Syllogism Logical argument in which two or more general premises lead to a specific conclusion.

If indeed both premise 1 and premise 2 are true, then it follows logically that the conclusion must also be true. If one of the premises is either false or questionable, however, then the conclusion may also be false or questionable. For example,

> Premise 1: All students are clever.
>
> Premise 2: Buster is a student.
>
> Conclusion: Buster is clever.

Clearly, the utility of the deductive reasoning process is dependent on the truth of the underlying premises.

Whereas deductive reasoning involves starting with general observations and from those general observations deriving a conclusion about a specific case, the process of **inductive reasoning** begins with an observation about one or more specific cases and from that deriving a general conclusion about a larger group of similar cases. For example,

Inductive Reasoning Logical argument in which one or more specific premises lead to a general conclusion.

> Premise: Every bird that I have seen has wings.
>
> Conclusion: All birds have wings.

Considering another example, however, the potential problem with inductive reasoning becomes evident:

> Premise: My dog is cute, smart, and well behaved.
>
> Conclusion: All dogs are cute, smart, and well behaved.

Obviously, in the process of inductive reasoning, a true premise does not guarantee a true conclusion. Instead, there is some level of probability that an inductive conclusion based on a true premise will also be true—or not. The processes of deductive and inductive reasoning are obviously of limited value in isolation for answering questions or solving problems. However, together, they formed the basis for the development of what we now know as the scientific method.

SPECIAL INTEREST BOX 1.1

Inductive Reasoning Meets Science

An artist, an accountant, and a scientist, all from the United States, were traveling by train through New Zealand when they saw a black sheep through the window.

"Look," said the artist, "New Zealand sheep are black."

"Well," said the accountant, "at least some New Zealand sheep are black."

"No," said the scientist, "all we know is that there is at least one sheep in New Zealand and that at least one side of that one sheep is black."

✔ Check Your Understanding

1. Generally, what is the purpose of research?
2. What are the weaknesses of deductive and inductive reasoning when used in isolation?

THE SCIENTIFIC METHOD

The early Greek philosophers apparently understood the limitations of the deductive and inductive reasoning processes. Aristotle advocated that,

> *We must not accept a general principle from logic only, but must prove its application to each fact, for it is in facts that we must seek general principles, and these must always accord with the facts.*[4]

Charles Darwin, who in his developmental work on the theory of evolution was one of the first scientists to integrate deductive and inductive reasoning into a practical and systematic approach

Scientific Method Highly structured, sequential series of steps for conducting a scientific research study.

A thorough understanding of the literature related to an area of research is prerequisite for developing a sound research question.

to answering questions, is often credited with the development of the **scientific method**. The scientific method is a structured, orderly process for conducting a research study. Different authors identify and describe the steps in the scientific method somewhat differently, but a common agreement prevails as to the sequential ordering of these steps.

Why are we talking about the *scientific method* in a book about research in kinesiology and the health sciences? It is because what we are about to describe as the scientific method is the general procedure currently used in countless fields of investigation, including many of the subdisciplines of kinesiology and the health sciences.

Step 1: Understanding the Problem Area

Many research methods textbooks place identifying the research question as the first step in the scientific method. However, this overlooks the fact that the ability to identify a research question or problem is based on knowledge and understanding of the problem area. To understand what questions are relevant or important with respect to a given topic, you must have a thorough understanding of the topic and be aware of the findings other researchers have already published on that topic.

For example, if you are interested in whether participation in elementary physical education classes (PECs) decreases the incidence of obesity among children, you need to understand many surrounding issues. To what extent are the children physically active in PEC? At what exercise intensity do the children work in PEC? On average, how many calories do children burn due to activity in PEC? What percentage of children are obese before starting school? How widely do elementary PECs vary in terms of engaging students in active exercise? Answers to these kinds of questions can be found by reading the research literature. Knowing what researchers have already discovered about the influence of physical activity on childhood obesity will greatly refine your understanding of the topic and better prepare you to conduct a study of your own.

Inventing the wheel. (He neglected to do a literature search...)

Many students will have a research problem for a master's thesis assigned to them by their faculty advisors. If this is the case for you, your advisor will still expect that you will develop a good understanding of the research literature surrounding your topic. You will most likely be expected to give an oral presentation of your thesis proposal to interested faculty and students. Things will go much better if you are prepared to answer questions about the existing research literature related to your topic!

Step 2: Identifying the Research Question or Problem

The research question or research problem is the reason for the study. It is the focal point and the driving force. This means, of course, that the research question or problem is important and that investigating it should be worth an investment of time and effort. A sound research question is also sufficiently specific that it can be investigated through the process of collecting, analyzing, and interpreting data. In other words, it must be a researchable question. Questions such as "What will I do when I graduate?" or "Why can't my team win the pennant?" are unanswerable and do not qualify.

In order for a question or problem to be researchable, you must be able to state it in terms of one or more independent and dependent variables. As you may recall from math classes, a quantitative variable is a symbol, often x or y, that can hold different values. Similarly, a research variable can assume different concepts. The **independent variables** are, in essence, what the researchers want to study. If, for example, the research question is "How does sleep deprivation affect motor performance?" the independent variable is sleep deprivation. One approach to studying sleep deprivation could involve administering a battery of motor performance tests to a group of study participants before and after some period of sleep deprivation. The **dependent variables** are the things the researchers will measure in order to study the effects of the independent variable. In our study of sleep deprivation, the dependent variables are related to motor performance and might include measures of reaction time, movement time, and fine motor ability. Comparison of data collected on the study participants before and after the period of sleep deprivation could provide an indication of the extent to which deprivation of sleep affects each of these three dependent variables. Given this scenario, we could state the research question as, "What are the effects of sleep deprivation on reaction time, movement time, and fine motor ability?" Or we could word it in problem statement format as, "The purpose of this study is to investigate the effects of sleep deprivation on reaction time, movement time, and fine motor ability."

Research questions or problem statements *always* include reference to the independent and dependent variables and sometimes include a description of the characteristics of the study participants. If there are a large number of dependent variables, they may be referred to collectively. For example, if we were measuring 10 dependent variables related to motor performance in our study of sleep deprivation, it would be quite cumbersome to list them all in the purpose statement. Instead, we could say, "The purpose of this study is to investigate the effects of sleep deprivation on motor performance." If a study is focused on a special population, such as people in a certain age group or individuals who have a certain skill, it would also be important to mention the population in the problem statement. For example, "The purpose of this study is to evaluate the effects of caffeine consumption on performance among elite cyclists," or "The purpose of this study is to compare the effects of exercise and nutritional supplementation on bone quality in postmenopausal women."

Independent Variable Variable under study that the researcher manipulates or measures.

Dependent Variable Variable being measured in order to determine the effects of the independent variable.

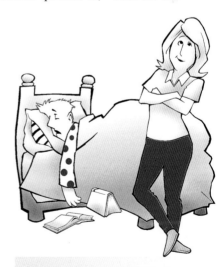

He's studying the effects of sleeping in.

Step 3: Formulating One or More Hypotheses

Research Hypothesis The researcher's informed expectation for the outcome of the study.

A **research hypothesis** is an *educated* guess as to what the outcome of the study will be. It is not merely a hunch or a feeling and certainly not a *wild* guess, but an intelligent expectation based on a thorough understanding of the research problem area. In all cases, the researcher should be able to explain the rationale for the research hypothesis in detail based on the existing literature. An example of a research hypothesis might be, "We hypothesize that reaction time will be significantly longer following 24 hours of sleep deprivation." Notice that this hypothesis can be confirmed (accepted) or not confirmed (rejected) based on the results of the study. This must be the case for all legitimate research hypotheses.

Step 4: Planning the Methodology for the Study

The methodology encompasses all of the organizational aspects of the study. In other words, it includes what the researchers will need to do and what order they will need to do it in order to conduct the study. This includes determining

a. The research design (how many groups participants may be divided into, and how many times they will be tested)
b. The criteria to be used for selection of study participants
c. The number of participants needed
d. The research protocol (or what each subject will be expected to do)
e. The apparatus (equipment) or instruments (surveys) to be used in data collection
f. The statistical tests that will be used to analyze the data. These topics are all described in detail in later chapters.

Internal Validity Extent to which change in the dependent variables can be attributed to manipulation of the independent variables.

In planning a study, researchers must carefully consider two important elements. The first is **internal validity**, or the extent to which any changes measured in the dependent variables can be directly attributed to manipulation of the independent variables. This is also known as the element of control. In order to have "good" internal validity when planning the research design, researchers attempt to control all extraneous factors that might affect the dependent variables. The example in Special Interest Box 1.2 illustrates the concept of experimental control.

External Validity Extent to which the results of the study can be generalized to the sample population.

The second important underlying consideration in designing the methods for a research investigation is **external validity**. External validity is simply the extent to which the results of a study can be generalized to the population represented by the participants in the study. "Good" external validity is primarily based on making sure that the study participants are representative of the population. To a large extent, this relates to ensuring that we study a sufficient number of participants. For example, we would not expect a study performed on two, ten, or even a hundred college students to yield results we could confidently apply to all college students in the United States. It would also be important for those selected as participants to accurately reflect the distribution of characteristics within the population. These concepts related to experimental design are discussed in more detail in Chapter 6.

Step 5: Collecting the Data

Data Observations recorded during the course of a research study.

Data (pronounced *day-tah*), generally speaking, are recorded observations of some sort. Collecting data may involve taking measurements, using computer-linked laboratory apparatus to record data values, distributing

---

SPECIAL INTEREST BOX 1.2

Internal Validity

A researcher wishes to compare the efficacy of two stretching programs on knee range of motion in patients following ACL replacement surgery. She invites a group of 20 post–ACL replacement patients to her clinic to view a demonstration of both stretching programs. She then asks each patient to choose either program A or program B and gives each patient a prepared list of the exercises in the program selected. She then instructs the patients to perform the stretching exercises three times per week and to return in 6 weeks for an assessment of knee range of motion.

What is wrong with this research design? (You will need to make quite a list!) To better appreciate how poor the internal validity is for this first scenario, consider the following:

A researcher wishes to compare the efficacy of two stretching programs on knee range of motion in patients following ACL replacement surgery. She invites a group of 20 post–ACL replacement patients to her clinic, where she measures and records each patient's knee ROM. She then randomly divides the patients into two equally sized groups and sends them into two different rooms. In these two rooms, patients see a demonstration of the exercises in their assigned protocol, and then they practice the exercises until the researcher is confident they are performing them correctly. All patients are asked to report to the clinic three times per week for 6 weeks to perform the assigned exercises under supervision. They are also asked not to do any other exercises that might affect knee ROM during this period. At the end of the 6 weeks, all patients' knee ROMs are again measured for comparison to the original assessments.

In this second scenario, the researcher has the ability to compare knee ROM measurements taken after the experimental period to those taken before. She also has confidence that study participants are performing the stretching exercises correctly and that they are performing them the prescribed number of repetitions and times per week because the participants are directly supervised. She cannot be 100% certain that the participants did not perform any extra exercises that might affect knee ROM while outside the clinic, but at least the participants were asked not to do extra exercises. These are all ways in which the researcher was attempting to *control* the particulars of what the participants did and did not do and are considered elements of experimental control that were not present in the first scenario described. These are also the reasons why the second scenario ensures greater internal validity than the first.

---

questionnaires, or conducting interviews. No matter what the data type, researchers should collect all data within a study objectively. They should also use the same procedures. All participants should receive exactly the same instructions so that they do (and conversely, avoid) all the same things during participation in the study protocol. One of the hallmarks of good research is that if other competent researchers were to repeat the study using the same protocol with different participants from the same population, they would get the same results. In order for this to be the case, researchers must carefully control the data collection procedures as well as accurately and fully describe them when the paper is published or presented.

Step 6: Analyzing the Data with Statistical Tools

The analysis of data using statistical tools is a vitally important step in the research process. The first time you have the opportunity to examine a set of data and attempt to guess whether the data support the research hypothesis, you will fully appreciate this, because it is virtually impossible to guess

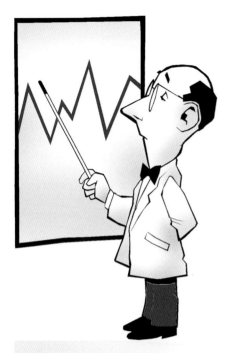

The value of statistics: 56% of the 21% who completed more than 30% of form A and 25% of form B had no opinion.

accurately. It is the statistical tests used in analyzing the data that factor in the amount of data collected, the variability in the data, and the differences in group means to determine whether differences between groups or correlations between factors are likely to exist in the population represented by the study participants. Several later chapters in the book are devoted to a conceptual overview of statistics and how to select the correct statistical test for a particular research design.

Step 7: Interpreting and Discussing the Results

The interpretation and discussion of the results of a study is usually one of the most interesting and challenging components of the scientific research process. Although there is no cookbook formula for discussing the results of a study, it is typical to talk about whether the results do or do not support the original hypotheses and to compare the findings of the study to the findings of other similar studies. Depending on the nature of the study, it may also be useful to discuss the reasons why the findings are important and to point out what practical or clinical applications may logically follow from the results.

Step 8: Deriving Conclusions from the Results

The conclusions of a study are one or more relatively concise statements that distill the results of the study into the "take-home information" that may be gleaned. It is often tempting for novice researchers to formulate grandiose conclusions that extrapolate the results of the study into much too global generalizations. Legitimate conclusions relate directly to the original hypotheses of the study. Chapter 17 will present some practical advice on appropriately deriving conclusions from the results of a study.

Cyclical Nature of the Scientific Method

As depicted in Figure 1.1, the scientific research process is often cyclical, with the results of one study providing impetus for developing logical follow-up questions that can be answered in subsequent studies. Because of this, individual researchers commonly become known for their work in a given topical area, since each new study builds on the findings of a study previously conducted in their department or lab or in another department or lab where the same topic is being studied.

The work of researchers, however, does not always follow the neat, tidy, cyclical sequence of events suggested in the simple model shown in Figure 1.1. One important step in most research work that is not typically mentioned when presenting the scientific method is the **pilot study**. A pilot study is simply a small-scale test study in which a researcher tries out a protocol on one or a few subjects to make sure that the planned procedures are workable, that the data collected can potentially address the research question, and, ultimately, that it will be a wise investment of time to conduct the full-blown study. As shown in Figure 1.2, the process of pilot testing often sends the researchers back to the drawing board to modify or refine their thinking about

Pilot Study A small scale test study undertaken to explore the workability of a research plan.

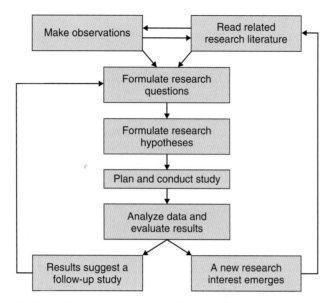

■ **FIGURE 1.1** The cyclical nature of the scientific method.

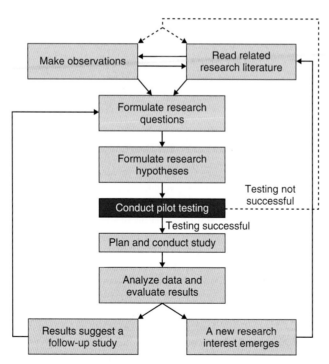

■ **FIGURE 1.2** The results of pilot testing often send the researcher "back to the drawing board!"

how best to proceed with a full-blown study in order to answer a meaningful research question. The importance of pilot testing is discussed in more detail in Chapter 4.

Developing Scientific Theories

Scientific Theory Explanation of some aspect of the natural world based on numerous research studies all confirming a given phenomenon.

A **scientific theory** is an explanation of some aspect of the natural world that is based on numerous research studies all confirming a given phenomenon. When a hypothesis has been thoroughly tested through the scientific method and is found to accurately explain a cause–effect relationship, it becomes a theory. The strength of a scientific theory is based on the extent to which it has been tested under different conditions. Theories can be improved and refined as more research is conducted. Scientists use theories to advance our scientific knowledge, as well as for applied purposes such as creating new inventions or treating diseases.

In popular culture, we often hear the word *theory* used when the speaker really means a *guess* or a *hunch*. For example, "My theory is that our professor will give us a pop quiz tomorrow if his football team loses this evening." Sometimes the word *theory* is also used when the speaker really means an *educated guess*, or a *hypothesis*. This is one example of a term (theory) having a specific and different meaning within the realm of research.

✔ Check Your Understanding

1. Why is it important to understand the findings reported in the research literature related to a topic of interest before planning a new study?
2. What are the characteristics of a good research question or problem?
3. How does the research hypothesis relate to the research question?
4. What is included in the methodology for a research study?
5. Explain the concepts of internal and external validity.
6. Why is statistical analysis of research data essential?
7. What is pilot testing and why is it important?

TYPES OF RESEARCH

Considering that research is the basic mechanism for advancing the frontier of knowledge not only in the sciences and engineering but also in the social sciences, history, philosophy, and myriad applied fields, it is not surprising that the scientific method has been modified for better utility in fields other than the basic sciences. Since the discipline of kinesiology encompasses numerous subdisciplinary specializations, it is useful to understand some of the important ways in which research approaches have become specialized for different areas of inquiry. Whereas most research in biomechanics, exercise physiology, motor control, and sports medicine follows the scientific method, research in pedagogy, sport psychology, and sport management sometimes follows different models or patterns known as **paradigms**.

Paradigms Philosophical or theoretical frameworks.

There are several recognized classification systems or taxonomies for labeling research based on different characteristics of the research, including the general purpose of the research, the nature of the independent variables, the nature of the dependent variables, and even the funding source for the research. These taxonomies are not mutually exclusive, and so any given research study could be labeled differently, based on the taxonomy being used. In this section of the chapter, we will explain the major research categories that you are likely to encounter as a beginning student of research methods.

Basic and Applied Research

The National Science Foundation[5] defines basic and applied research as follows:

> *Basic research is defined as systematic study directed toward fuller knowledge or understanding of the fundamental aspects of phenomena and of observable facts without specific applications towards processes or products in mind.*
>
> *Applied research is defined as systematic study to gain knowledge or understanding necessary to determine the means by which a recognized and specific need may be met.*

However, many people have heard the terms basic research and applied research used by the media and, accordingly, have somewhat popularized views of what these types of research entail.

We tend to think of basic research as work carried out by scientists in white lab coats in a laboratory setting, often with animal subjects. We likewise tend to think of applied research as field research carried out in settings where there is a lack of experimental control. It is important to recognize that the terms *basic research* and *applied research* do *not* denote differences in the methodological approach, but in the underlying rationale for conducting the research in the first place. Whereas **basic research** is conducted purely for the discovery of new knowledge, with little regard for whether there is an immediate application for that new knowledge, **applied research** is driven by the need to find a solution to a specific problem.

Basic Research Investigation motivated by discovery of new knowledge without regard for any immediate application.

Applied Research Investigation motivated by a desire to find a solution for an immediate problem.

From time to time, people have criticized basic research funded by federal agencies as not being a good use of taxpayer money because it seemed lacking in practical value. During the period from 1975 to 1988, for example, US Senator William Proxmire periodically announced a presentation of the Golden Fleece Award, given to projects that appeared to be significantly lacking in practical application. Table 1.1 describes some of the research projects that received the Golden Fleece Award.

In order to have received funding for research, however, the researchers had to have written a proposal for each project with a compelling rationale that convinced the people authorized to grant the funding that their projects were worthy. Although the results of basic research may not be immediately useful, they are often of great value at a later point in time. Some have criticized the research by the Nautical Aeronautics and Space Administration (NASA), the US government agency that runs the country's space program, as lacking in practicality. However, since World War II, research on spaceflight has produced countless product spin-offs that are eminently useful today in medicine, industry, and everyday living. Today, for example, hospitals are using ArterioVision software initially developed at NASA's Jet Propulsion Laboratory to examine the carotid artery for partial blockages. When plants suspended in the air aboard a spaceship grew faster than the same plants on earth, plant scientists began using aeroponic growing systems on earth, in which growing crops are suspended midair in a growing chamber in an enclosed, air-based environment where the roots are misted with a nutrient-rich spray. Other examples of products initially developed by NASA scientists include memory foam for comfortable seating, scratch-resistant lenses, and insulin pumps. Research by NASA scientists has also improved our environment, with discoveries leading to technology for superior water

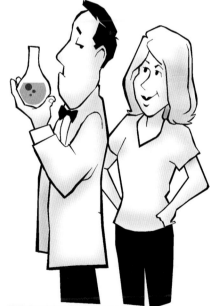

Could you take a break from research on mouse chromosomes to invent a mousetrap that works?

TABLE 1.1	Some of the Federally Funded Research Projects Given the Golden Fleece Award for Being Overly Lacking in Practical Application	
Date	**Grant Recipient**	**Research Project Description**
March 1975	National Science Foundation	For spending $84,000 to try to find out why people fall in love
October 1975	National Institute on Alcohol Abuse and Alcoholism	For spending millions of dollars to find out if inebriated fish are more aggressive than sober fish, if young rats are more likely than adult rats to drink alcohol in order to reduce anxiety, and if rats can be systematically turned into alcoholics
January 1977	Department of Agriculture	For spending nearly $46,000 to find out how long it takes to cook breakfast
February 1977	Law Enforcement Assistance Administration	For spending nearly $27,000 to determine why inmates want to escape from prison
June 1978	Federal Highway Administration	For spending $222,000 to study "Motorist Attitudes Toward Large Trucks"
December 1978	Office of Education	For spending $219,592 to develop a "curriculum package" to teach college students how to watch television
July 1981	Department of the Army	For spending $6,000 to prepare a 17-page document that tells the federal government how to buy a bottle of Worcestershire sauce

Characteristics of basic and applied research form a continuum, rather than two discrete, mutually exclusive categories.

filters, a compound called emulsified zerovalent iron that can be injected into groundwater to neutralize toxic chemicals, solar-powered appliances, improved insulation materials for residential and commercial buildings, and better fertilizer for plants.

Much of the research conducted in many fields, including kinesiology and the health sciences, has some of the characteristics that we would typically ascribe to both basic research and applied research. For example, a study to evaluate the effectiveness of two different knee braces in preventing unwanted motion at the knee (a very applied topic) might be carried out in a laboratory under very stringently controlled conditions (a basic research setting). It is therefore more appropriate to think of research along a continuum extending from the most basic to the most applied, rather than to think of basic and applied research being two discrete categories.

Translational Research
Investigation in which findings from animal studies are first tested in humans.

The term **translational research** is specific to studies in which the results of basic research studies are subsequently investigated in humans. It is common for research related to clinical applications to start with animal subjects to ensure the safety and efficacy of the research protocol before it is applied to humans. Much of the research conducted in exercise physiology is translational in that it explores whether the results of animal studies can be applied or translated to humans.

Quantitative and Qualitative Research

Quantitative Research
Investigation involving collection of numerical data.

Another dichotomy exists between **quantitative research** and **qualitative research**, based on whether the dependent variables measured are numerical or nonnumerical. Most research in kinesiology follows the quantitative approach, which is also the approach traditionally used in the natural sciences. Quantitative research designs enable description of existing conditions, analysis of relationships among different variables, and study of cause–effect relationships. Quantitative research typically begins with

Qualitative Research
Investigation involving collection of nonnumerical data.

identification of one or more research questions and related hypotheses that can be tested through collection and statistical analysis of numerical data. The methodology for the study is carefully planned in advance, and considerable effort is typically dedicated to controlling or ruling out factors other than those being studied that might influence the data. A relatively large number of observations (or data) are collected, so that the results can be viewed as indicative of the status of the population at large that the study participants represent.

Whereas research in the sciences has traditionally been quantitative, social sciences such as anthropology and sociology have long employed qualitative research techniques. This basic difference in the nature of the dependent variables also drives differences in the entire research process. Qualitative research is characterized by the collection of observations by the researchers through first hand, onsite note taking, analysis of videotapes and audiotapes, in-depth interviews, and researcher-designed questionnaires. In educational settings, an approach known as triangulation is often employed, with the opinions of students, teachers, and the researchers all compared for consistencies and differences. With qualitative research, it is generally not practical to formulate hypotheses or necessarily even a detailed methodology prior to the study, since the characteristics of the practical setting and the study participants may influence the ways in which data collections can proceed. Instead, the data are evaluated for trends or patterns that address the general questions the research is attempting to address. Within the field of kinesiology, researchers are using qualitative techniques as well as quantitative techniques in a variety of subdisciplines, but especially in pedagogy, sport history, sport psychology, and sport management. Selected studies may even employ both qualitative and quantitative approaches for assessment of different dependent variables. Use of both quantitative and qualitative approaches within the same study is termed **mixed methods**. Chapter 8 presents a comprehensive explanation of qualitative research.

Mixed Methods Investigation involving collection of both numerical and nonnumerical data.

Experimental and Nonexperimental Research

Experimental research is carried out for the expressed purpose of confirming or refuting cause–effect relationships. Experimental research questions aim at achieving *understanding* of the phenomenon being studied. Accordingly, experimental research questions often include the word *why*. The hallmark of experimental research is that the researchers are able to manipulate one or more independent variables and measure the effects of the independent variables on the dependent variables. As discussed earlier in this chapter, if the study is designed with good internal validity, any changes in the dependent variables can be attributed to the manipulation of the independent variable, and a cause–effect relationship is shown. In other words, the independent variable manipulation causes a measurable effect on the dependent variables. Special Interest Box 1.3 provides an example.

Experimental Research Investigation involving manipulation of independent variables to establish or disestablish a cause–effect relationship.

Correlation does not prove causality.

Descriptive research is nonexperimental because it does not involve any manipulation of independent variables by the researchers. Instead, the general goal of descriptive research is, as the name suggests, providing a detailed, useful description of certain characteristics of interest in a population, a group, or an individual. A descriptive study may be quantitative, qualitative, or a combination of both. Questionnaires and interviews are tools that can be used in gathering both qualitative and quantitative descriptive data, and laboratory apparatus can also be used to collect quantitative descriptive data. Numerous descriptive studies have been published that identify the characteristics of interest of selected groups of elite athletes in different sports, since lesser skilled athletes and their coaches are often interested in determining what changes might allow them to reach the elite level.

Descriptive Research Investigation conducted to provide a useful description of the characteristics of a population, group, or individual.

SPECIAL INTEREST BOX 1.3

Experimental Research

A summer camp counselor hypothesizes that having children play games of soccer will result in more improved cardiorespiratory fitness than having children do soccer drills over a 6-week period. He randomly divides a group of 50 nine-year-old campers into two groups. One group plays soccer, and the other does only soccer drills during their three times per week soccer classes. He tests both groups on the 1-mile walk/run test before and after a 6-week experimental period. A statistician compares the scores of the two groups to determine whether the counselor's hypothesis was correct.

In this study, the independent variable is the mode of exercise (soccer play vs. soccer drills). The dependent variable measured is scores on the 1-mile walk/run test. If the results of the statistical test show that the group playing soccer improved significantly more than the soccer drill group on 1-mile walk/run scores, then this suggests that playing soccer improves cardiorespiratory fitness more so than engaging in soccer drills among 9-year-old campers.

Case Study Descriptive research on a single individual.

Research designed to describe a given individual who has special characteristics or conditions, or who has responded to a clinical treatment in a special way, is termed a **case study**. The medical literature includes numerous case studies, and occasionally, case studies are reported in the literature on athletic training and adapted physical education.

Correlational Research Investigation conducted to evaluate relationships among two or more variables.

Correlational research is a form of descriptive research that can be conducted to evaluate the relationships between two or more variables. The research literature in kinesiology includes numerous examples of correlational research. For example, regular exercise has been shown to be positively correlated with VO_2max and negatively correlated with body fat, heart rate, and diastolic blood pressure.[6] Another general use of correlation in research is investigating the relationship between two different variables of interest for purposes of prediction. Since jump height is an indication of the power generating capability of the lower extremity, a measure of jump height might be used to predict sprinting ability. It is important to remember, however, that correlation is not necessarily an indicator of causality. Since growing elementary school children experience both increasing height and improving reading ability with age, we would expect there to be a positive correlation between those two variables. However, growing taller certainly does not *cause* improvement in reading ability.

Analytic Research Systematic evaluation of existing information with the goal of advancing new understanding of that information.

Analytic research is a form of descriptive, qualitative research that involves systematic evaluation of existing information with the goal of advancing new understanding of that information. Within kinesiology, the subdisciplines of sport history and sport philosophy utilize analytic research techniques. Another form of analytic research is the meta-analysis, which is a quantitative approach for analyzing a body of published literature when there are papers with results supporting opposite sides of a research question. These different types of analytic research are discussed more fully in later chapters.

✔ Check Your Understanding

1. Can a research study be both basic and applied? Explain.
2. What causes the design of a study to be described as *mixed methods*?
3. Describe the different types of nonexperimental research.

THE IMPORTANCE OF RESEARCH IN KINESIOLOGY AND THE HEALTH SCIENCES

There are two major reasons that research in kinesiology and the health sciences is important. First, as is the case in all fields, much of the research currently being conducted has implications for advancing practice in the related discipline-specific professions. These include professional endeavors in areas such as health promotion, nutrition and dietetics, health and physical education, adapted physical education, physical therapy, athletic training, and personal training. Examples of these types of research topics currently being explored include the following:

- Motor skill proficiency, physical activity, and obesity in young children
- Barriers to physical activity participation in aging populations
- Effectiveness of health coaching on high-risk mothers and their children
- Promoting walk-to-school behaviors and policies
- Efficacy of social media in promoting healthy behaviors
- Use of animal therapy to promote health among children with disabilities
- The role of fatigue in athletic injuries
- Neuropsychological effects of purposeful heading in soccer
- Biomechanical analysis of sport skills
- Motor coordination in children with autism, dyslexia, and developmental coordination disorder

Beyond advancing professional practice, however, much of the research in our fields also has broad implications for improving human health. Examples of some of these kinds of research topics currently being explored are the following:

- Diet and exercise interventions for obesity, cardiovascular disease, and cancer
- Prevention of concussions in athletes
- Psychosocial determinants of physical activity behavior
- Blood pressure regulation, diet, and exercise
- Bone health and osteoporosis
- Effects of normal aging on the nervous system
- Vascular function and dysfunction in healthy and diseased states
- Prevention and treatment of low back pain and arthritis
- Gait retraining in stroke patients
- Fall prevention in the elderly

You will recognize that many of the topics listed have received a significant amount of publicity and media coverage. Many of these topics also appear on the funding priorities lists for federal grant funding agencies such as the National Institutes of Health, the National Science Foundation, the U.S. Department of Education, and the U.S. Department of Defense. We are conducting extremely important research with major implications for public health. This is an exciting time to be working as a researcher in kinesiology and the health sciences. As a student who will be knowledgeable about research methods at the end of your course, you will be prepared to get involved and contribute to one of these cutting edge areas of research.

CHAPTER SUMMARY

- Research is a careful, systematic, and structured process for solving problems or answering questions.
- Replacing early primitive forms of reasoning, the scientific method is a series of orderly, sequential steps that provide the foundation for modern-day forms of inquiry in many fields.

- In studies employing the scientific method, independent variables are manipulated, producing differing effects on the dependent variables, which the researchers directly measure.
- The extent to which changes in the dependent variables can be attributable to the manipulation of the independent variables is termed the internal validity of the study.
- The extent to which the results of the study can be generalized to the participant population is known as the external validity of the study.
- Research can be categorized as basic or applied, quantitative or qualitative, and experimental or nonexperimental.
- Research being conducted in kinesiology and the health sciences has significant implications, not only for advancing related professional fields but for advancing our knowledge about current major human health issues.

REFERENCES

1. National Institutes of Health: http://www.nichd.nih. gov/health/clinicalresearch/references/upload/clinical_research-definitions_procedures.pdf
2. Creswell JW. *Educational Research: Planning, Conducting, and Evaluating Quantitative and Qualitative Research,* 3rd ed. Upper Saddle River, MJ: Pearson, 2008.
3. Frascatti Manual: *Proposed Standard Practice for Surveys on Research and Experimental Development,* 6th ed. Organization for Economic Cooperation and Development, 2002.
4. Kelley TL. *Scientific Method.* Columbus, OH: The Ohio University Press, 1929.
5. National Science Foundation: http://www.nsf.gov/statistics/randdef/fedgov.cfm
6. Peterson DF, Degenhardt BF, Smith CM. Correlation between prior exercise and present health and fitness status of entering medical students. *J Am Osteopath Assoc* 2003;103:361–366.

RELATED ASSIGNMENTS

1. **Select three papers from the research literature on topics of interest to you. Each paper you select must be a research paper; that is, it should contain methods or procedures, results, and discussion sections. For each paper, write a summary. You will notice that research papers usually begin with an abstract, which is another word for a short summary of a research paper. Be careful to write the abstracts using your own words and be sure that your abstracts provide more detail about the studies than the abstracts that appear at the beginning of the papers. Also, be careful to avoid using the same words that the authors used (although technical terms are okay). Since the research has already been completed, write your summaries using past tense.**

2. **Write out three researchable problem statements that are of interest to you. Each problem should meet all of the criteria for a researchable problem. The problems should identify the independent and dependent variables of interest and, if appropriate, the participant population.**

IN-CLASS GROUP EXERCISES

Directions: For each of the investigations described, identify the independent and dependent variable(s) and discuss any experimental design problems you believe could detract from internal validity.

a. A physical therapist wishes to study the effect of participation in a conditioning class on grip strength in elderly women. The grip strength of 25 participants in a conditioning class is measured and recorded at the beginning and at the end of a 16-week period.

Independent variable(s): _____

Dependent variable(s): _____

b. A researcher is interested in the effect of fatigue on running stride length in rats. A group of rats is run to exhaustion on rat treadmills. Every 2 minutes, a high-speed camera is turned on to enable measurement of rat stride length.

Independent variable(s): _____

Dependent variable(s): _____

c. The effect of participation in a running class on VO_2 max is studied. Members of a group of 40 subjects are matched as closely as possible on finish times for the mile run. The members of each matched pair are randomly assigned to groups. One group participates in a running class, and the other does not. Both groups' VO_2 maxs are tested at the end of the semester.

Independent variable(s): _____

Dependent variable(s): _____

d. A purveyor of ergogenic aids wishes to compare the effects of topically applied emu oil, ostrich oil, and snake oil on muscle strength gains. He convinces the instructors of three university weight training classes to have students rub one of these oils (one oil per class) over their triceps prior to performing bench-press exercises. At the end of the semester, he assesses maximum bench-press capability across classes.

Independent variable(s): _____

Dependent variable(s): _____

e. An elementary school teacher investigates improvement in fitness over the course of the school year by giving a group of 300 students a battery of eight fitness tests at the beginning and end of the school year.

Independent variable(s): _____

Dependent variable(s): _____

f. A clinician wishes to assess the effectiveness of two different exercises on patellar tracking in patients with chondromalacia. Patients assigned to one physical therapist do static quad sets, and patients assigned to a second physical therapist do straight-leg raises with external femoral rotation. At the end of 3 months, all patients are evaluated and scored on a 10-point scale for proper patellar tracking during knee extension.

Independent variable(s): _____

Dependent variable(s): _____

g. A hundred Labrador retrievers are randomly divided into two groups and tested for obedience. One group is then trained using milk bone rewards, while the other group is trained using verbal praise. At the end of the 6-week training period, both groups are retested for obedience.

Independent variable(s): _____

Dependent variable(s): _____

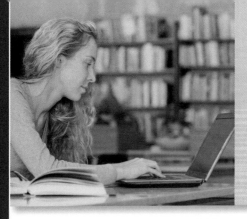

2

Research Writing Style

"The most important goal of writing is to be clear without being boring."—Aristotle, Poetics

CHAPTER OBJECTIVES

After studying this chapter, you will be able to:

1. Describe the characteristics of good research writing.
2. Explain the importance of developing a content outline before writing.
3. Demonstrate different techniques for providing transitions between ideas.
4. Utilize parallelism in composing sentences including lists.
5. Identify three common errors to avoid in research writing.
6. Compare and contrast the elements involved in different editorial styles.

■ WRITING is a critically important part of the research process. After a study is conducted, the results are of little value if they are not published in an appropriate journal where others can read about them. Just as many popular misconceptions exist about the research process, which we discussed in Chapter 1, there are plenty of erroneous notions about the nature of research writing. For example, you may be under the impression that written reports of research, by nature, must consist of long, convoluted, and jargon-laden sentences that are comprehensible only to highly educated researchers who study the same topic. If this is the case, after reading this chapter you should have a very different understanding.

You may be wondering why we chose to position this chapter on research writing so early in the book. After all, you can't begin to write a research paper describing the results of a study until you've designed the study, collected and analyzed the data, and interpreted the results. While it's true that there is a lot to learn about conducting research before you need to worry about how to write the report, there are at least two very good reasons to talk about research writing early on:

1. The initial stages of research most commonly involve writing a formal proposal that details the rationale, the specific aims, and the planned methodology for the study, as well as a proposed budget to support the related work. A sound understanding of research writing style is necessary for writing a compelling and successful proposal. In programs requiring a thesis or dissertation, graduate students are universally required to write a research proposal that must be approved by a faculty advisor and committee before being allowed to proceed with the data collection. Many undergraduates also write proposals prior to conducting research for a senior thesis or other project. Even seasoned researchers typically must have a written proposal approved by a funding agency before they have the practical ability (available funding) to conduct meaningful research.

2. Developing mastery of research writing is a process that will take time and practice. The more proposals and research reports or papers you write, the better you will become at the skill of research writing. Practicing research writing skills as you complete written assignments for this course should improve your facility with research writing.

CHARACTERISTICS OF GOOD RESEARCH WRITING

All fields of science and engineering use technical writing to clearly and concisely explain something to a particular audience. It is not supposed to be creative or engaging, like a work of fiction. Rather, it is instructive, readily comprehensible, and to the point. Good research writing shares many characteristics with good technical writing. For instance, it is grammatically correct, and follows standard rules of punctuation and spelling. It is clear, avoiding unnecessary jargon and long, complex sentences, and flowing smoothly in a logically organized progression. Also importantly, good research writing is interesting to read. The words used not only are readily comprehensible to the target audience but also communicate a meaningful concept or image.

Writing is a skill that improves with careful practice.

Another important feature of good research writing is that it tells a story. This statement may sound strange to you: after all, we've said that research writing is not like fiction. There are no imaginary characters exchanging dialogue. But in a very real way, good research writing does tell a story. It may tell a story about why a particular research topic, such as research on physical inactivity among children, is important and needed to help address a particular problem, such as the childhood obesity epidemic. It may tell a story about how a set of collected data answers an interesting question and contradicts our previous assumptions about a particular topic. For example, whereas it was once widely assumed that exercise during pregnancy was contraindicated for all women, recent research shows that 30 minutes of moderate exercise most days of the week is safe for healthy pregnant women and may have beneficial results for the offspring.[1] It may tell a story about the pros and cons of a particular argument as supported and not supported by different published studies in a body of literature. For example, there has been a long-standing debate of sorts in the literature about the benefits of stretching prior to exercise or athletic performance.[2] The bulk of recent research shows that stretching has no effect on subsequent injury incidence and furthermore, that it negatively affects muscle strength and power.

You have undoubtedly had one or more courses in English composition in which you learned the rules of grammar, punctuation, and style. So we won't review that material here. What we will address, however, are some useful strategies and tips for composing effective research proposals and reports or papers that tell interesting and meaningful stories.

Good research writing tells a compelling story.

Organization

Consider the following two paragraphs:

1. *Patients with knee pain (chondromalacia) accompanied by lateral maltracking of the patella were the object of this study. We used electromyography (EMG) to monitor activity in the vastus medialis oblique (VMO). There were 10 healthy subjects free from knee pain in the study, and these were not the aforementioned patients. The VMO is a key muscle in keeping the patella properly aligned. Eight exercises that strengthen the quadriceps muscles were studied. We had the subjects do three repetitions of each exercise. The order of the exercises was random. The results showed that static quad sets were the best (p < 0.05) at eliciting EMG in the VMO. The conclusion was that this exercise is best for these patients.*

2. *The purpose of the study was to determine which among eight different quadriceps exercises are most effective in strengthening the vastus medialis oblique muscle (VMO), a key player in preventing maltracking of the patella. Ten healthy subjects free of knee pain performed three repetitions each of these exercises, with the exercises ordered randomly, while myoelectric activity (EMG) in the VMO was monitored. The exercise eliciting the greatest (p > 0.05) amount of EMG in the VMO was the static quad set, with no other significant differences present. We concluded that this exercise is the best choice for rehabilitating patients with chondromalacia secondary to lateral maltracking of the patella.*

Composing an outline prior to writing usually saves time and results in a better end product.

The first paragraph is difficult to follow and does not seem to make much sense until you have finished reading it and then most likely have reread it at least once. The second paragraph is much more readily understandable because it is organized in a logical fashion, with the purpose of the study stated up front and events unfolding chronologically.

In good research writing, logical organization of the points you wish to convey to the reader is essential to help ensure that the reader can readily and fully understand what you wish to communicate. Why is this important? There are two compelling reasons: (1) it will save time, and (2) the end product will be much better.

One way to help ensure that what you are writing is logically organized is to start with an outline that includes the main points that you wish to convey in a well-organized fashion. No matter what the writing assignment or goal, it is invaluable to begin with at least a skeleton outline of what you would like to say. If you are writing only one short paragraph, you may be able to compose the outline in your head. If you are writing a long paragraph or more than one paragraph, it is important to have a clear written outline organizing your thoughts before you start writing. Your outline need not be formal; a simple list of points that you want to convey in the order in which you wish to present them will typically suffice. Later chapters will present some additional general guidance and specific rules for organizing each of the different sections of research proposals and papers. Special Interest Box 2.1 illustrates the advantages of outlining.

Topic Sentence Sentence, usually at the beginning of the paragraph, that states the main point of the paragraph

Another very useful thing to recall from your courses in English composition regarding organization is that each paragraph should include a topic sentence. The **topic sentence** states the main point of the paragraph. It is usually the first sentence, although it is sometimes effective to place it elsewhere. The remaining sentences in the paragraph explain and provide details about the topic of the paragraph. Many successful research writers expand their outline into a series of topic sentences, as this provides an intermediate step between the outline and composition of the text material. Special Interest Box 2.2 provides an example of a paragraph beginning with a topic sentence.

Outlining

Joe thought he had a good idea for his master's thesis research. However, when he started trying to describe his idea to his faculty advisor, his advisor asked him to put his rationale for the study in writing. The next day, Joe e-mailed the following paragraph to his advisor.

> I was a sprinter on my high school track team and we always had to stretch out before practice and before competitions. One time we were running late for a meet with another school because our bus broke down, and by the time we got there, our coach said to forget our stretching routine. It was amazing; I and several of the other guys on the team had personal best performances that day. I'm not saying it was because we didn't stretch, because maybe there was something else going on. But I would really like to try to do a study that could look at stretching versus not stretching before a sprinting performance to see if stretching makes a difference.

Joe's advisor e-mailed back the following message:

> Joe, I understand your research question and, because there is support for it in the literature, I believe we can work to refine this into a thesis topic for you. I would like you to see me tomorrow to discuss a plan and timeline. I would also like you to refine your own thinking by writing a paragraph of rationale for your thesis in research writing style. To help you get started, I'm providing the following skeleton outline for you to follow. Please provide supporting references of these statements from the research literature. This will, in turn, provide the concepts that you will expand into the introduction for your formal thesis proposal.

Outline of Rationale:

1. *Most athletes incorporate some type of stretching protocol into their workouts because stretching is generally believed to reduce injury incidence.*

2. *However, the research literature shows that stretching prior to performance results in performance decrements, especially in events requiring speed and power.*

3. *No study to date, however, has looked at both the acute and long-term effects of stretching on sprint performance.*

4. *Therefore, I propose to compare sprinting performances in two time-matched groups of sprinters, one of which will engage in a supervised stretching protocol and the other of which will serve as a control group over a period of 6 weeks during the track off-season. Sprint performance times will be recorded at the end of each of the 6 weeks.*

Topic Sentences

Research Methods is a critically important course (topic sentence). Virtually all academic disciplines require a research methods course for graduate students, and increasingly, better undergraduate programs include a research methods course as well. Certainly an understanding of research methods is essential for students planning careers in academia, but it is also extremely useful for students pursuing nonacademic careers who will need to be able to evaluate and apply research related to their professional fields. In other words, a research methods course is not just for those who wish to actually conduct research, but for all thinking professionals who want to be able to discern soundly based research findings from bogus ones.

✔ Check Your Understanding

1. What are three characteristics of good research writing?
2. Why is it often helpful to create an outline before writing?
3. What is a topic sentence?

Transitions

Transitions Clauses or sentences that provide a bridge or link between one topic and the next

Effective transitions between thoughts help the reader follow the story you are trying to tell.

Transitions are phrases or clauses that you use to help your reader follow the story you are trying to tell. In essence, they comprise bridges between different lines of thought. They therefore make your writing not only more readable but also more interesting. As you write, try to make some sort of transition between adjacent paragraphs at least.

One form of transition is a sentence that briefly summarizes what you have said and indicates what will immediately follow. Here are a few examples:

Having described the range of etiologies for low back pain, let's next focus on the related treatment options.

As discussed previously, there are good reasons to abandon the prosthetics used in the last decade for shoulder replacements and to move forward with new technology.

With this understanding of the mechanics of the normal gait cycle, let's next consider how the gait cycle is altered in children with different forms of cerebral palsy.

Another type of transition begins with a statement of a possible objection (in the mind of a reader) to what will follow and responds to it. For example:

Although stretching prior to athletic performance has long been advocated as prophylactic, the credible evidence in the research literature does not support that notion.

Some strength and conditioning specialists argue that use of free weights is the best way to improve strength during functional movements. What they fail to consider, however, is that machines offer advantages in terms of safety and proper technique.

Still another transitioning technique involves a sentence that begins by summarizing a concept just presented and then posing a question about it. The question not only provides a bridge between thoughts but stimulates added interest.

As discussed, bone responds to added mechanical stress by hypertrophying. Does this suggest that in the absence of mechanical stress, bone will atrophy?

Because the previously described intervertebral disc is avascular, it relies on a mechanical pumping action to import nutrients and export metabolic waste. What are the implications for daily living?

Finally, transitional words or clauses can be used at the beginning of a sentence to show either similarity or contrast to the preceding sentence or preceding paragraph.

In a similar study, Smith and Jones found...

In contrast, Wood and Long, in their study of stretching protocols, found...

✔ Check Your Understanding

What are three advantages of using structured transitions between different lines of thought?

Clarity

Factors such as leptin, adiponectin, and tumor necrosis factor alpha (TNF-α) feature frequently as characters in exercise physiology research.[3] This sentence is included only to illustrate that every academic discipline and every professional field has an associated body of technical terminology. Such terminology has evolved over time to facilitate accurate and explicit communication among those who work in that arena. Part of your task as a student is to master the specialized terminology associated with the academic or professional field you plan to enter. Your faculty advisor will expect that your thesis or dissertation is written using the appropriate specialized terminology for your particular field of study.

Beyond this, however, we all have considerable latitude in selecting the vocabulary we choose to use in writing. Having a large vocabulary is advantageous in that it provides more options for communicating ideas in a precise fashion. The object of any writing task, however, should not be demonstrating the extent of your vocabulary, but communicating as clearly as possible. It is important to remember that communication, whether written or oral, is a two-step process, requiring not only the sender's expression but also the receiver's comprehension. This means that the words you choose must be meaningful to your target audience in order for your message to be understood. Choice of vocabulary for an audience of Ph.D.s at a professional specialty conference should be much different than word choice for a lay audience.

Less is more! With research writing, use as few words as necessary to adequately convey what you wish to communicate.

For any target audience, however, you are most likely to achieve clarity of communication by avoiding the use of unnecessary words. If you can express the same thought using 5 words instead of 10 words, the shorter sentence is always preferable. In research writing style, words that contribute nothing to the meaning of a sentence should be omitted. Adverb and adjective modifiers are often better omitted. For example, a sentence such as "These fascinating results strongly support our hypothesis" is better stated in research writing style as simply "These results support our hypothesis."

Some words and phrases acceptable in conversation are of little practical use in research writing. Examples include "in fact," "importantly," and "hopefully." In fact, and importantly, these words usually add little or nothing to the meaning of a sentence and should be eliminated. Hopefully, this point is now clear. Special Interest Box 2.3 illustrates the importance of avoiding the use of too many words.

✔ Check Your Understanding

1. List three examples of words that are best avoided in research writing because they add no relevant meaning to a sentence.
2. What are some reasons for avoiding wordiness in research writing?

Parallelism

When you write a sentence that includes a list of phrases or clauses, state all of them in the same way. This structure, called **parallelism**, improves the clarity of the whole sentence, making it easier to read and understand. Consider the following example:

Parallelism Using parallel constructions when listing things within a sentence

> *Study participants were asked to report to the lab, then to sign informed consent forms, and then receive directions from the research assistant.*

Rewording the sentence in parallel format improves readability.

> *Study participants were asked to report to the lab, sign informed consent forms, and follow directions from the research assistant.*

Another example:

> *Conducting a research study requires understanding the related literature, the ability to collect the necessary data, the statistical analysis, and then use of research writing skills to complete the manuscript.*

SPECIAL INTEREST BOX 2.3

Avoiding Wordiness

The first assignment in Sally's Research Methods course was to write a short summary of a paper of interest from the research literature. Sally submitted the following summary:

This study was conducted in order to comparatively evaluate three different approaches to rehabilitation of ACL replacements on selected gait variables at 6, 10, and 14 weeks following a surgery conducted for replacement of the anterior cruciate ligament. There were two treatment groups, with one receiving traditional physical therapy alone (PT) and the other one receiving acupuncture in addition to traditional physical therapy (PTA). There was also a control group that received no therapy. The gait variables analyzed were measured from sagittal-view video records of patients walking at self-selected speeds, and these included stride length and the range of motion for the hip, knee, and ankle of the affected leg. The postsurgery measures were compared to those from presurgery assessments. When the statistical tests were conducted, they showed that all of the variables measured were significantly closer to presurgery values for the two treatment groups than was the case for the control group, and this was true for all three assessments. However, no significant differences between the PT and PTA groups were found for any of the assessments.

Sally's professor asked all of the students to spend a few minutes looking back at what they had written to determine if they could eliminate unnecessary words while still conveying the same information. Sally found that she was able to shorten her summary considerably, eliminating about a third of the words used in her first draft without any loss of meaning.

The purpose of this study was to compare three approaches to rehabilitation of ACL replacement patients on gait normalization at weeks 6, 10, and 14 postsurgery. Treatment groups received either traditional physical therapy alone (PT) or traditional physical therapy plus acupuncture (PTA), and a control group received no therapy. Sagittal-view video records of patients walking at self-selected speeds were analyzed for stride length and for hip, knee, and ankle ROM in the affected leg, with measures compared to those from presurgery assessments. All dependent variable measures were significantly closer to presurgery values for the two treatment groups than for the control group during all three assessments, with no significant differences between treatment groups.

Using parallel clause format, the sentence can be improved:
Conducting a research study involves understanding the related literature, collecting the necessary data, running the statistical analysis, and writing the manuscript.

✔ Check Your Understanding

What is parallelism and why is it helpful?

Research Citation Conventions

In keeping with our previous discussion on avoiding wordiness, a convention for citing the work of other researchers is to refer to the researchers by last name only. So if you wanted to discuss the similarities of your own research study to a study conducted by William J. Farquhar and Jody Greaney, you would refer to the study conducted by Farquhar and Greaney. Since Farquhar and Greaney may have published more than one study together, it is also conventional to refer to the year in which the particular study you wish to cite was published. For example, "Farquhar and Greaney (2013) investigated the role of salt sensitivity among hypertensive Afro-American men." The exact way in which you cite studies will vary with the editorial style you have selected. (Editorial styles are discussed later in this chapter.)

COMMON WRITING ERRORS TO AVOID

In addition to keeping in mind the characteristics of good research writing already discussed, it can be helpful to check your writing for some common errors. Special Interest Box 2.4 identifies a number of common errors in research writing.

If you have done much reading in the research literature, you may have seen one or more of these errors in print. Be very aware that, although the better journals employ copy editors to screen for grammatical and formatting errors, what appears in print is unfortunately not always a good example of research writing style. The next sections describe other kinds of errors in research writing style.

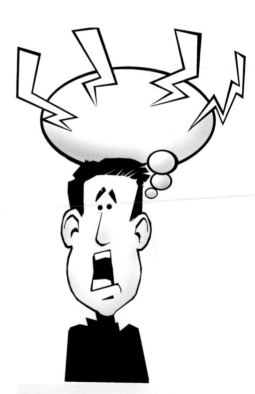

He's working on his active voice…

✔ Check Your Understanding

List some examples of sentences that are appropriate in everyday conversation, but not appropriate in research writing.

Passive Voice

Consider the following sentences:

Healing of the muscle strain was promoted by use of ultrasound treatments.

Use of the patellar tendon for the ACL graft was elected by the surgeon.

The mistake was admitted to be the fault of John.

Notice that there is a sense of vagueness associated with each of these sentences. There is no responsible party. There is no active player. There is no one home. These sentences are written in what is termed **passive voice**. With passive voice, the subject of the sentence is always acted upon.

Alternatively, we can easily rewrite these sentences so that the subject of the sentence is performing an action:

Ultrasound treatments promoted healing of the muscle strain.

The surgeon elected to use the patellar tendon for the ACL graft.

John admitted that the mistake was his fault.

Although use of passive voice is not technically an error, **active voice**—in which the subject of the sentence performs the action—is more direct and clear, and it is increasingly preferred in research writing style. Active voice

Passive Voice Sentence construction in which the subject is acted upon

Active Voice Sentence construction in which the subject performs the action

SPECIAL INTEREST BOX 2.4

Common Writing Errors

1. "Studies have shown..." (with no accompanying citation of specific studies)
In research writing style, all statements that are not considered to be common knowledge must be supported with the citation of one or more specific studies that have been published. This means that specific referencing should be provided either in or at the end of such a sentence, depending on the referencing style being used. To emphasize a study, it is also useful to mention the researchers by last names, rather than simply referring to their work as a "study" or "research" (e.g., Jones and Smith have shown that...).

2. "The study found..." or "The study concluded..."
This statement is a personification of *the study*. In actuality, it was the *researchers* who found or who concluded something.

3. "These results are significant because..."
In research writing, the word *significant* should not be used as a synonym of the word *important*. Instead, we use *significant* specifically to convey the concept of statistical significance (explained in Chapter 10).

4. "This study was similar to the one described above."
A paragraph should be able to stand alone. (The same is true of tables and figures.) In other words, if you extracted a paragraph, a figure, or a table from a paper, each should make sense without the reader having to refer back to other parts of the text. It is better to write "This study was similar to the investigation of Wood and Hall (2007)."

5. "The results showed that exercise A produced higher heart rates."
Any sentence using a comparator such as "greater," "less," "more," etc. should identify the variables at both extremes. For example, "The results showed that exercise A produced higher heart rates than were produced with exercise B."

6. "They looked at differences between men, women, and children."
The word *between* is used for comparisons of *two* groups or conditions. Whenever *three or more* entities are compared, the correct word to use is *among*. For example "There are differences in mean height among men, women, and children." And the word is *among*, not "amongst."

7. "The data was collected under three conditions."
Remember that the word *data* is plural. The correct wording is "These data were collected under three conditions." This is difficult to get used to, because the word *data* is used incorrectly by the popular media most of the time.

8. "The treatment was shown to effect the subjects."
Be careful about use of *effect* and *affect*. Both words can be correctly used as either a noun or a verb, and consequently they are often incorrectly interchanged. Here are examples of correct usage of these words.
"The treatment was shown to affect the subjects." (*Affect* is a verb meaning to influence.)
"Her affect was a little off during that conversation." (*Affect* is a noun meaning demeanor.)
"We were primarily interested in the effect of calcium on bone accrual." (*Effect* is a noun meaning a change that occurs as a result of an action.)
"Our goal was to effect change over a period of time." (*Effect* is a verb meaning to bring about.)
Affect is more commonly used as a verb, and *effect* is more commonly used as a noun.

is clearly a more powerful form of expression than passive voice. Notice that it is also more straight-forward and less wordy, which is another reason we tend to prefer active voice in research writing.

Check Your Understanding
Explain the difference between active and passive voices.

Use of Quotations

By this point in your academic career, you have no doubt been cautioned many times about avoiding **plagiarism**, or passing off someone else's ideas or words as your own. You are most likely aware that, if you wish to include a direct quotation from a published source in your own writing, you should use quotation marks around the quoted sentence or phrase, and cite the source. Failing to do so is not only unethical, but illegal when the plagia-

Plagiarism Using the thoughts or words of someone else without appropriately acknowledging the source

rized material is copyrighted, and neither ignorance nor sloppiness is a legitimate excuse. Plagiarizing from noncopyrighted documents posted on the Internet is equally dishonest, because you are still attempting to pass off the ideas and words of someone else as your own. The rule for citations is that thoughts generally regarded as "common knowledge" do not require citations, whereas all others do. If you are not sure whether something is common knowledge, it is best to cite the source. The penalty for student plagiarizing can range from a reduction in a grade on an assignment to expulsion from an academic institution. Chapter 5 is about ethics in research and includes a detailed discussion of the different forms of plagiarism.

Although using quotation marks and citing the source is the proper way to incorporate words directly from another source into your own writing, in research writing style it is almost always better *not* to quote directly from another source. Why? In keeping with avoiding wordiness, using your own words to paraphrase the content you wish to cite is typically more straightforward than is inserting a quotation. A quotation from another source also breaks the flow of your writing and is distracting to the reader. So although in research writing it is not only appropriate, but critically important, to cite ideas and content from other sources, it is better to use your own words than to directly quote the source.

Check Your Understanding
What are the reasons to avoid using direct quotations in research writing?

Failure to Proofread Carefully

Once you have completed a writing task, whether it is an assignment for a course, a research proposal, or a component of a research manuscript to be submitted to a journal for publication, it is important to keep in mind that you have not completed your writing responsibility until you have carefully proof-read the finished product and corrected all errors. Failure to *proofread*—that is, to read through the last draft (or *proof*) of your work—is an act of irresponsibility that will be noticed by everyone who reads the error-laden product. Compared to the amount of time that it takes to produce the writing, the amount of time that it takes to proofread and correct errors is minuscule.

Most word processing software now highlights misspelled words and ungrammatical constructions as you type. Certainly you should learn how to use such tools effectively. That said, relying solely on software to catch errors is a mistake. For instance, no software program will correct a misspelling that results in a viable word, such as *mead* for *mean*, or *valuable* for *variable*. Nor will software help you to spell researchers' names correctly, or avoid misplaced modifiers and many other grammatical errors. Even worse, spell checkers sometimes take a specialized term such as one you might be using

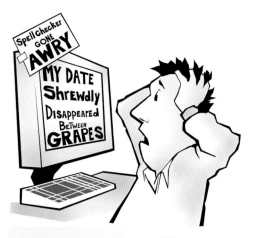

I wrote "My data showed differences between groups!"

in a research paper and convert it into a more commonly used word that has a completely different meaning. That's why it is still essential, even in the digital age, to perform a final proofreading. There is really no excuse for submitting sloppy, ungrammatical writing to another person who must be subjected to reading it. If you are not a skilled writer, it is all the more important to proofread your work. It is also important to remember that writing is a skill that improves with practice. You will not be able to get through most graduate programs without doing a fair amount of writing.

You might even consider asking trusted friends and fellow students to read your work through, give you feedback on the organization, logic, and clarity, and check for errors. The more important the body of writing that you have completed, the more important it is to have one or more other capable people read it. Of course, *you* should always carefully proofread your writing before asking someone else to read it.

✔ Check Your Understanding

Why is it important to proofread your own writing?

EDITORIAL STYLES

Editorial Style Convention that governs the formatting of the citations and reference list, as well as other aspects of a manuscript submitted to a journal for publication

Beyond the elements of research writing style discussed so far in this chapter, you should be aware of the many recognized **editorial styles** that have been adopted by published journals to establish consistency in the formatting of papers published in the journal. Editorial style governs the specific organization and formatting for elements such as

- the components of a paper and the headings for each section
- the reference list
- citation of references within the text
- figures and tables
- use of statistical symbols

Depending on the editorial style being used, an entry in a reference list can vary in many ways. Special Interest Box 2.5 illustrates differences in several commonly used editorial styles.

The ordering of references in the reference list at the end of the paper also varies according to the editorial style being used. Some list the references alphabetically, and others list references in the order in which they are cited in the text. It is important here to distinguish between a bibliography, which is any list of related sources, and a reference list, which is a specific type of bibliography that includes only those sources actually cited in the paper. Although you may have developed a habit of listing all of the sources you consulted in preparing a term paper for a class, most editorial styles require that the reference list at the end of the paper include only those sources actually cited in the paper.

You may wonder which editorial style is best or which is most commonly used. The answer is that each scientific or professional journal has adopted an editorial style and that all manuscripts published by a particular journal must be submitted in the designated style. It is therefore important to become familiar with the journals that publish work in your chosen area of interest. Table 2.1 lists many of the

SPECIAL INTEREST BOX 2.5

Common Editorial Styles

National Library of Medicine (NLM) style

Gabel L, Proudfoot NA, Obeid J, MacDonald MJ, Bray SR, Cairney J, Timmons BW. Step count targets corresponding to new physical activity guidelines for the early years. *Med Sci Sports Exerc.* 2013;45(2):314–8.

American Psychological Association (APA) style

Logan, S., Scrabis-Fletcher, K., Modlesky, C., & Getchell, N. (2011). The relationship between motor skill proficiency and body mass index in preschool children. *Res Q Exerc Sport*, 82, 442–448.

Chicago style (also known as Turabian style)

Modlesky, Christopher M., Subramanian, Stephen, and Miller, Freeman. "Underdeveloped trabecular bone microarchitecture is detected in children with cerebral palsy using high-resolution magnetic resonance imaging." *Osteoporosis International* 19 (2008): 169–176.

Harvard style

Horsak, B., Baca, A., 2013. Effects of toning shoes on lower extremity gait biomechanics. *Clin. Biomech.* 28, 344–349.

TABLE 2.1   Editorial Styles of Selected Kinesiology and Health Science-Related Research Journals

Journal Title	Editorial Style	Publisher	Content Type
Adapted Physical Activity Quarterly	American Psychological Association	Human Kinetics	Adapted Physical Education
Clinical Biomechanics	Harvard	Elsevier	Biomechanics
Human Movement Science	American Psychological Association	Elsevier	Exercise Sciences
Journal of Aging and Physical Activity	American Psychological Association	Human Kinetics	Multidisciplinary
Journal of Applied Biomechanics	American Psychological Association	Human Kinetics	Biomechanics
Journal of Applied Physiology	National Library of Medicine	American Physiological Society	Physiology
Journal of Applied Sport Psychology	American Psychological Association	Taylor & Francis	Psychology
Journal of Athletic Training	National Library of Medicine	National Athletic Trainers' Association	Athletic Training
Journal of Biomechanics	Harvard	Elsevier	Biomechanics
Journal of Electromyography and Kinesiology	National Library of Medicine	Elsevier	Exercise Sciences
Journal of Motor Behavior	American Psychological Association	Psychology Press	Motor Control

TABLE 2.1   Editorial Styles of Selected Kinesiology and Health Science-Related Research Journals (*Continued*)

Journal Title	Editorial Style	Publisher	Content Type
Journal of Sport and Exercise Psychology	American Psychological Association	Human Kinetics	Sport Psychology
Journal of Teaching in Physical Education	American Psychological Association	Human Kinetics	Physical Education Pedagogy
Medicine & Science in Sports & Exercise	National Library of Medicine	Wolters Kluwer	Exercise Sciences, Sports Medicine
Motor Control	American Psychological Association	Human Kinetics	Motor Control
Psychology of Sport and Exercise	American Psychological Association	Elsevier	Sport Psychology
Research Quarterly for Exercise and Sport	American Psychological Association	American Alliance for Health, Physical Education, Recreation & Dance	Multidisciplinary
Sociology of Sport Journal	American Psychological Association	Human Kinetics	Sport Sociology

journals that publish research related to kinesiology and the health sciences along with the editorial styles the journals require.

Because there is so much variation among editorial styles, it is useful for you (or your instructor or your major professor) to identify a particular editorial style that you will become familiar with and learn to use correctly. In preparing the manuscript for any research project, it is usually a good idea to write using the editorial style of the target journal that you hope will ultimately publish your paper. The details of the editorial style used by a particular journal appear in the instructions for authors, which are commonly listed at the end of paper copies of the journal, as well as online at the journal's Web site. Using a given editorial style consistently on your written assignments in graduate school will provide excellent practice to help you learn all the nuances of that particular style.

✔ Check Your Understanding

List three elements that vary, depending on the editorial style in use.

CHAPTER SUMMARY

- Writing is a critically important part of the research process.
- Good research writing is clear, concise, and interesting and tells a story.
- Uses of outlining and topic sentences help to develop a logical organization for what you wish to write.
- Transitions between major points help to make the writing more readable and interesting.
- Avoiding wordiness and convoluted sentence structures contributes to clarity of expression.
- Using parallel constructions when composing lists adds to clarity and readability.
- Refer to other researchers by last name only, and identify the year in which the paper you are discussing was published.
- There are a number of common writing errors to avoid.

- Active voice is generally preferred over passive voice because it tends to be more clear, concise, and readable.
- Direct quotations from others should be used sparingly, if at all.
- Always carefully proofread your own writing and correct errors before asking anyone else to read it.
- Each research journal adheres to a specific editorial style that governs the format of the reference list and the way that references are cited, among other things.

REFERENCES

1. Mudd LM, Owe KM, Mottola MF, et al. Health benefits of physical activity during pregnancy: an international perspective. *Med Sci Sports Exerc* 2013;45:268–277.
2. McHugh MP, Cosgrave CH. To stretch or not to stretch: the role of stretching in injury prevention and performance. *Scand J Med Sci Sports* 2010;20: 169–181.
3. Bell C. Pigment epithelium-derived factor: a not so sympathetic regulator of insulin resistance? *Exerc Sport Sci Rev* 2011;39:187–190.

RELATED ASSIGNMENTS

1. **Find an article in a magazine (paper or online) and make a list of the ways in which the writing is different from research writing style.**

2. **Find a research paper of interest and list the main points in the introduction section. Then take your outline of main points and rewrite the introduction in your own words.**

3. **Find three research journals of interest and identify the editorial style used by each journal (see Table 2.1). Write a paragraph explaining the advantages and disadvantages of each style.**

IN-CLASS GROUP EXERCISES

1. **Errors in Research Writing. Directions: The following sentences each contain error(s) in grammar, in construction, and/or in the use of research writing style. Working as a group, identify the error(s) for each sentence, and then rewrite the sentence using proper grammar, construction, and research writing style, without omitting any of the essential content of the original sentence. (It is acceptable to write two sentences, if necessary.)**

   a. This study hypothesized why many struggle to quit smoking.
   b. It is suggested that this may be a limitation of the Theory of Planned Behavior.
   c. This insightful statistical analysis makes it intuitively clear that the critical differences were between the relatively harder surfaces and the relatively softer surfaces.
   d. Hopefully, the results are in agreement with those of Hall.
   e. In summary, although there are some good points in the content, the general disorganization and lack of presentation of study limitations depressingly impact the strength of the discussion.
   f. Smith and Jones' research paper on asymmetrical sweating patterns (or lack thereof) among children and adolescents with cerebral palsy is for the most part a compelling and well thought out body of work, although it is not without its flaws.
   g. The very topic of this paper would grab the interest of anyone who has suffered a knee injury, as well as medical care providers.

2. **Composing Topic Sentences. Directions: Working within your group, write what might be the topic sentence of an introduction to a paper given each of the following purpose/problem statements:**

   a. The purpose of this study was to compare the effectiveness of two different static stretching protocols on hamstring flexibility.

   b. The purpose of this study was to evaluate the relationship between regular exercise participation and high blood pressure.

   c. The purpose of this study was to describe the biomechanical factors that distinguish normal gait from gait in Parkinson's patients.

   d. The purpose of this study was to determine what factors are associated with compliance to a weight loss diet program.

   e. The purpose of this study was to examine the effects of three treatment protocols on perceived pain in ACL reconstruction patients 3 hours postsurgery.

3. **Have each member of your group write what might be the first sentence of an introduction to a paper on a topic of personal interest. Once everyone has completed this, trade papers with the person seated next to you and make suggestions for improving your neighbor's sentence.**

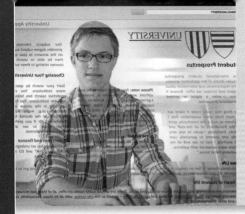

3

Reviewing and Critiquing the Literature

"If I have seen farther than others, it is because I stood on the shoulders of giants."—Isaac Newton

CHAPTER OUTLINE

CHAPTER OBJECTIVES

After studying this chapter, you will be able to:

1. Explain the different purposes that literature reviews can serve.
2. Describe strategies for searching the published literature.
3. Critique the quality of papers in the published literature.
4. Write a literature review on a topic represented in the published literature in your area of interest.

■ You may have wondered if there are available sources for learning about the current state of research on a given topic. A **literature review** is a body of writing that provides an overview of the state of current research on a topic of interest. Depending on the purpose of the review and the nature of the topic, it may be comprehensive and lengthy or it may be focused on one aspect of the topic and short. Reviews of literature commonly are incorporated in the introduction to a research paper as part of the rationale for the

Literature Review Writing that presents a view of a topic based on summary and commentary on previously published research papers related to that topic.

Published literature review papers are valuable because they enable the reader to become familiar with a topic without having to identify, collect, and read multiple papers on that topic.

Original Research Paper Writing that includes introduction, methods, results, and discussion of findings for a research study conducted by the authors.

Abstract Concise summary of a paper that appears before the beginning of the paper.

Introduction Beginning section of a paper that introduces the topic and explains the rationale for the paper.

Methods Section Section of an original research paper that presents a detailed description of all procedures used in the study.

Results Section Section of an original research paper that objectively presents the findings of the study.

Discussion Section Section of an original research paper in which the authors provide interpretations related to the findings of the study.

Conclusions Concise list of one or more generalizations that may be directly drawn from the findings of the study and that either confirm or fail to confirm the original hypotheses for the study.

study. It is important that the researchers show how the results of the study will build on what is already known and also how the results are expected to expand the knowledge base. For the same reason, literature reviews are also commonly used as part of the introductory portion of a thesis or dissertation. Entire papers consisting of literature reviews on topics of interest are also published in research journals.

Literature review papers are different from **original research papers**. An original research paper typically describes a single research study. Organizationally, most original research papers are very similar and include the following ordered components (see Chapter 17 for more details):

- An **abstract** that presents a concise summary of the work at the very beginning of the paper
- An **introduction section** describing the rationale for and purpose of the study, with the rationale typically involving some short review of closely related literature
- A **methods section** explaining what the researchers did
- A **results section** presenting the outcomes of the study
- A **discussion section** interpreting the results of the study
- Sometimes, there is a subtitled **conclusions** section at the very end of the paper. In the absence of this, conclusions of the study are discussed within the discussion section.

Literature reviews, in contrast, discuss a number of related original research papers. Although a literature review paper usually starts with an introduction, there are no methods or results sections, and the entire paper is a discussion of a particular topic area, based on specific references to published research papers.

Literature reviews published in journals typically provide a perspective on an exciting topic area that is receiving current attention in the research literature. A published literature review is quite valuable for interested readers, since it presents the essential elements of a number of published works on the chosen topic all in one paper. Many journals that primarily publish original research papers also occasionally publish literature reviews. A few journals, such as *Exercise and Sport Sciences Reviews* and *Sports Medicine*, publish only literature reviews. Reading a literature review from such journals enables you to quickly become familiar with the primary issues related to a particular area of research.

The goals of published literature reviews vary. Some are written to inform readers about one or more important recent discoveries in the field. Sometimes a literature review is written to foster appreciation for the historical development of a line of research. Other literature reviews present opposing viewpoints on a subject, both with support from the literature. The author of a literature review may take a neutral perspective in summarizing the findings reported, or the author may choose to construct the review in such a way as to support a particular perspective on the subject.

A few examples of recently published review literature reviews include the following:

1. Gunter KB, Almstedt HC, Janz KF. Physical activity in childhood may be the key to optimizing lifespan skeletal health. *Exerc Sport Sci Rev* 2012;40:13–21.
2. Gorman MW, Feigl EO. Control of coronary blood flow during exercise. *Exerc Sport Sci Rev* 2012;40:37–42.
3. Opar DA, Williams MD, Shield AJ. Hamstring strain injuries: factors that lead to injury and re-injury. *Sports Med* 2012;42:209–226.

Notice that, although a number of papers have recently been published on these topics, the topics are not so broad that it would take an entire book to adequately address them.

As mentioned, a literature review is also a required component of most theses and dissertations. In these works, a good literature review sets the stage for the thesis/dissertation proposal by explaining what is already known of direct relevance to the topic and explaining where one or more gaps exist in the knowledge base that the thesis/dissertation will address. It is important to remember that you must support this explanation based on citation of published papers from the research literature, however, and not based on your own logic or opinion.

For students preparing to undertake a research project, the literature review has a somewhat different set of purposes from those of literature reviews published in journals. The first step in identifying the specific question you design your research to answer is acquiring a solid, thorough understanding of the related, published literature. Such understanding is necessary to make it clear what important questions related to your topic remain unanswered (i.e., knowledge gap), as well as to ensure that your proposed study has not already been done. Sometimes the literature review can also help demonstrate that the approach, procedure, or instrumentation that you plan to use is valid, since other published researchers have also used it. And finally, the written literature review helps to demonstrate that your own knowledge of the literature related to the topic you're proposing to study is sufficient.

Literature review papers are based primarily on original research papers.

Check Your Understanding

1. Explain how literature reviews differ from original research papers.
2. List three different approaches that authors may take in writing literature reviews for publication.
3. What are three reasons for students to write a literature review?

STRATEGIES FOR LITERATURE SEARCHES

If you're like most students, you've probably developed the habit of consulting a broad range of sources, including books, journals, online sources, apps, and sometimes the popular news media, when preparing a term paper or oral presentation. Although all of these sources, as well as professional conference proceedings, can be helpful in furthering your understanding of a topic area, the literature review paper is primarily based on original papers from research journals. There are two important reasons why this is the case.

1. Published original research papers have been thoroughly vetted through a peer review system, so that studies with poor designs or erroneous conclusions tend not to be published. This means that you can have much more confidence in the content of a published research paper than in material from most other sources that typically has not been subjected to stringent review.

2. And after all, what you are summarizing is what we know about *research* on a given topic, not what you may piece together from various, undocumented sources. As mentioned, although other kinds of sources can help you develop a general understanding of your topic, it is research-based information about your topic that goes into a literature review.

Find out what electronic databases and search engines are available to you through your campus library.

Discussion of a published review paper in your own literature review is also appropriate, so long as you clearly identify the paper as a review. It is also important if mentioning opinions stated by the authors of review papers to clearly identify them as such and to not treat these as the same as the results of original research papers. Fortunately, there are a number of convenient resources available to assist you in locating both original research papers and review papers related to your topic.

Online Search Engines

The first step in performing a literature search is to identify an appropriate online search engine that you can utilize to quickly search the published literature on your topic of interest. Here are some online search engines commonly used:

- For life sciences, exercise science, and biomedical topics, the best starting place is usually PubMed,[1] which is a free, online service provided by the U.S. National Library of Medicine. PubMed supplies links to abstracts and, in some cases, to full-text articles and related resources for over 21 million citations from the biomedical literature dating back to the 1950s.
- The National Center for Biotechnology Information (NCBI)[2] provides free, online access to biomedical and biological research publications and data, including PubMed, and enables researchers to set up automatic searches on a monthly or weekly basis.
- For topics related to physical education, a good starting place is the Education Resources Information Center (ERIC).[3] Like PubMed, ERIC is a free, online service that provides links to bibliographic records of journal articles and other education-related materials with links in some cases to full-text articles. ERIC is sponsored by the U.S. Department of Education, Institute of Education Sciences, with access provided to more than 1.2 million sources.
- A more generic, free, online search engine is Google Scholar,[4] which indexes full-text papers from peer-reviewed, online journals across a broad spectrum of disciplines.

There are also a growing number of apps downloadable from iTunes that can assist with quick identification of a research paper on a topic of interest. A few to mention are COREMobile, PubChase, and Questia. However, these tend to be not as well developed as the previously mentioned online search engines that provide multiple delimiters to refine searches.

Several publishing companies also offer paid subscriptions for online literature search engines to individuals and institutions. It is worthwhile finding out if your institution's library has a subscription that will enable you access to one of these. Some examples include the following:

- ScienceDirect,[5] provided by Elsevier, provides access to over 8 million articles from the physical sciences and engineering, life sciences, health sciences, social sciences, and humanities.

Sparky always searches online first.

- Ovid,[6] a product owned by publishing conglomerate Wolters Kluwer, enables searches of hundreds of databases, more than 1,200 journals, and books from dozens of publishers, all related to the health sciences or health care.
- The Web of Science,[7] published by Thomson Scientific, enables access to five databases, including Science Citation Index,[8] Social Sciences Citation Index,[9] Arts & Humanities Citation Index,[10] Index Chemicus,[11] and Current Chemical Reactions.[12] These databases link to over 8,000 journals in the areas of science, technology, social sciences, arts, and humanities. The three citation databases include references that have been cited by other articles, which can be useful if you want to find an earlier paper cited in a paper you are reading.
- For topics related to education and physical education, there are the Physical Education Index,[13] a subscription-based, online service provided by Cambridge Scientific Abstracts, and the Wilson Education Index,[14] a subscription-based, online service provided by EBSCO Publishing.
- SPORTDiscus,[15] provided by EBSCO Publishing, is a comprehensive source of full text for sports and sports medicine journals, providing full text for more than 530 journals.

✔ Check Your Understanding

Which search engines are most likely to be useful for finding papers related to your own research interests? Why?

Delimiting the Search

Once you have found an appropriate online literature search engine and familiarized yourself with its features, you will need to determine the best ways to *delimit* (limit the scope of) your search. If your search topic is too broad, the service will return a list of thousands of related citations.

There are two common ways to limit your search. First, identify your topic as specifically and narrowly as possible. For example, if you are interested in existing exercise programs that target childhood obesity, do not search for "obesity" or even "childhood obesity." Search for "childhood obesity" and "exercise programs." Second, limit the number of years through which you want the engine to search. For many topics, papers published more than 10 years ago contain outdated information that may be of little use or interest. However, if there are related older papers that are considered to be seminal, that is, they were important enough to have spawned a new line of research on a particular topic, it would be important for you to acknowledge them. The relevance of older papers varies by topic area. For example, some topics still of current interest were thoroughly explored 10 or more years ago, and so there are not many recent papers on the topic. If in doubt, consult your faculty advisor as to the importance of older papers on your topic. Special Interest Box 3.1 illustrates the importance of delimiting a search.

Using reference management software to organize and manage reference citations can save you a lot of time!

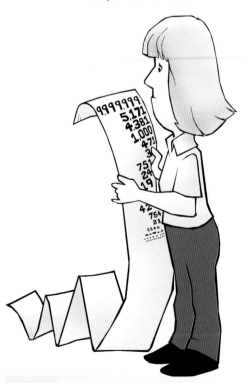

Delimit or die!

SPECIAL INTEREST BOX 3.1

Delimiting a Literature Search

Conducting a literature search on PubMed on the topic of "knee + injury" for the years 2002 to 2012 generates a list of 12,656 citations, which is likely to be a few more than you probably hope to write about in your literature review. If we search more specifically over that time interval for "'anterior cruciate ligament' + injury," we turn up only 3,953 citations, which is still a somewhat unmanageable number. Placing the following *delimiters* (limiting terms) on the search in a sequential fashion dramatically reduces the number of citations generated.

Delimiter	Number of Citations
English language only	3,640
Term appears in title or abstract	2,010
Term appears in title	527

At this point, it is usually wise to look through the titles of those 527 papers to develop an understanding of the range of topics included. If we were to further modify the search, using all of the delimiters listed above but with the key terms "anterior cruciate ligament + athlete," the search returns only 41 citations. Online literature searches are fast, so you can refine your search using different key terms with different delimiters without wasting a lot of time.

✔ Check Your Understanding

1. What key terms best describe your own research topic or interest?
2. What delimiters are likely to be useful with a search on your own topic?

Reference Management Software

Reference Management Software software that enables storing, organizing, and formatting reference lists.

Another handy tool related to literature searches is **reference management software** (also known as *citation management software* or *personal bibliographic management software*). This software enables you to store and organize lists of references, and so gives you the ability to generate a specific reference list for a paper or chapter you are writing and is compatible with most word processing software. The more sophisticated packages will also format the reference list in one of hundreds of choices of journal editorial styles. Anyone who has undertaken the tedious task of converting a reference list from one editorial style to another can readily appreciate the saving of time and angst that this feature provides.

Some of the commercially available reference management packages are Biblioscape,[16] Bookends,[17] EndNote,[18] Papers,[19] ProCite,[20] Reference Manager,[21] RefWorks,[22] and Sente.[23] A number of free versions of reference management software can also be downloaded from the Web. Wikipedia, the well-known online encyclopedia, has a table that compares reference management software features across software packages, providing descriptive information about cost, operating system support, import and export file formats, citation styles, word processor integration, and database connectivity. To locate it, Google "comparison of reference management software" + Wikipedia.

EVALUATING PUBLISHED RESEARCH REPORTS

In selecting papers to consider for inclusion in your literature review, you should first make sure that each paper is either an original research paper or a review paper related to your chosen topic.

As previously described, an original research paper is one that includes an abstract, introduction, methods section, results section, and discussion section, with a summary or conclusions sometimes also placed under a subheading at the end. A **research journal** is a journal that primarily publishes either original research papers or research review papers. However, there are also other types of articles sometimes found in research journals, such as follows:

Research Journal A publication that includes original research papers and/or research review papers.

- Editorial position statements, in which the journal editor in chief writes what is usually a short piece designed to help orient readers to either a descriptive overview of the papers published in that particular issue or a new direction or format that the journal is adopting
- Letters to the editor, which usually consist of commentary on a previously published paper in the journal. If the commentary is critical, the journal editor invites the authors of the paper being criticized the opportunity to write a response that appears following the letter of criticism.
- Rapid communications, which represent research that may not yet have been peer reviewed at the same level of rigor of an original article, but have the potential for impact in the field

Although editorial position statements and letters to the editor are often quite interesting to read and may be thought provoking, the opinions expressed in these types of articles should not be confused with the data-based results of original research papers. It is not appropriate to include these types of communications in a literature review for a thesis or dissertation.

Another important distinction is between research journals and **professional journals**. The *Journal of Physical Education, Recreation and Dance* and *Strategies: A Journal for Physical and Sport Educators* are examples of professional journals that publish papers related to practical aspects of these professions. Some of the papers published in these journals offer advice or suggestions from the authors on a professionally related topic and in support of their views cite previously published research papers. Such papers may be described as being **research based**. It is not usually appropriate to cite research-based papers in a literature review. If in doubt about whether a paper is an original research paper, as compared to being research based, remember that original research papers have the structured format that includes a description of methods and results from a specific study.

Professional Journal A publication that includes articles of practical interest to professionals in a particular field.

Research Based Term describing papers that cite original research papers to support the authors' contentions.

Be cautious about accepting the validity of research that is only published online.

Once you have identified the original research and possibly research review papers related to your topic, the next step is screening these papers for quality. The quality of published research papers varies widely. Of the papers that you identify through online searching, not all of them will be necessarily of sufficiently high quality to merit citation in your literature review. So how do you evaluate the quality of a given paper? A first step is to evaluate the quality of the journal in which it is published.

✓ Check Your Understanding

1. What are the differences between an original research paper and a research-based paper?
2. What are the differences between a research journal and a professional journal?

The Journal Peer Review Process

Peer Review Process through which research manuscripts submitted to journals are reviewed by knowledgeable researchers and typically revised by the authors in accordance with reviewer suggestions prior to the publication.

Most reputable journals use what is called a **peer review** process, in which research manuscripts submitted to the editor to be considered for publication are sent out for review. Typically, the journal engages three researchers who are known to be knowledgeable about the topic area addressed in the paper. These reviewers usually respond in writing with their opinions regarding the suitability of the work for publication and a list of suggestions for revising and improving the paper. Reviewer recommendations may include incorporation of substantive changes related to content, modification of the statistical methods, or improvement of writing clarity, although it is not the job of the reviewer to correct grammatical errors. The editor then sends the paper back to the authors, along with the reviewer comments and suggestions, as well as a letter that typically indicates that the paper is accepted for publication, accepted for pending revision in accordance with the reviewer suggestions, or not acceptable for publication in its current form. It is not unusual for a paper to be reviewed and revised more than once before it is accepted for publication.

As you can imagine, papers almost always improve significantly after the authors incorporate suggestions from knowledgeable reviewers. For this reason, peer-reviewed journals are deemed superior in quality to journals that do not employ a peer review process. How can you tell if a journal is peer reviewed? This is usually stated somewhere in the instructions for authors that appear at the back of the journal or on the journal's Web site.

 Check Your Understanding

What is the peer review process?

Other Indicators of Journal Quality

Acceptance Rate Ratio of number papers accepted for publication in a journal to number of papers submitted to the journal.

Another indication of journal quality is the journal's **acceptance rate**, or the percentage of submitted papers that are eventually accepted for publication as compared to those that are rejected. A high-quality journal may accept only 15% to 20% of the papers submitted to it. Journals do not usually disclose their acceptance rates in writing because, for one thing, the acceptance rate tends to vary throughout the calendar year. It may also be dramatically different for domestic as compared to foreign submissions, and for certain types or categories of papers compared to others.

Journal Impact Factor A number that reflects the average number of times that papers published in a journal within the past two years have been cited in subsequent published papers.

Journal impact factor is another tool available for evaluating journal quality. This quantitative measure is published annually in *Journal Citation Reports*[24] for all journals indexed by the Thomson Institute for Scientific Information. Journal impact factor can be thought of as the average number of citations in a year, based on those papers in a journal that were published during the 2 preceding years. For example, if

A = the number of times papers published in a journal in 2009–2010 were cited in indexed journals during 2011 and

B = the number of all papers published in the journal in 2009–2010, then

A/B = the 2011 impact factor.

The more important or interesting the results of studies published in a given journal, the more likely these papers are to be cited by others, and the higher the journal impact factor. Journal impact factors vary somewhat from year to year, but tend to remain consistently high for prestigious journals.

A confounding factor—and a reason that use of the journal impact factor has been criticized—is that more narrowly focused journals publishing papers from highly specialized fields tend to have their papers cited less frequently than more general journals. This is explained simply by the fact that there are fewer researchers working in highly specialized fields than in general fields. For example, we would expect that papers published in the *Journal of the American Medical Association (JAMA)* would be cited more frequently than papers published in the *Journal of Biomechanics*, because there are more people working in medical research in general than in biomechanics research. The 2011 impact factors for journals in kinesiology and the health sciences are listed in Table 3.1.

A cautionary note regarding research papers appearing online is in order. Many print journals have adopted an online presence that enables electronic publication of accepted research papers in advance of the printed issues of the journal. In such cases, the papers appearing online have been subjected to the rigor of the peer review process normally employed by the journal. However, an increasing number of online-only journals exist that do not have a coexisting printed version. As with print journals, it is important to evaluate the quality of an online journal and to remember that in the absence of a peer review process the quality of the papers is not likely to be high. There is also an abundance of what may appear to be "research-based" online papers on virtually any topic. These may be useful in leading you to reputable published sources, but keep in mind that there is no vetting process for information posted on the Web.

Organize your literature review around a theme or perspective. Never simply present summaries of papers in chronological order!

TABLE 3.1	2011 Impact Factors for Selected Journals Related to Kinesiology and the Health Sciences
Impact Factor	**Journal Title**
3.1	Acta Physiologica Scandinavica
1.2	Adapted Physical Activity Quarterly
4.7	American Journal of Physiology: Endocrine and Metabolism
3.9	American Journal of Physiology: Heart and Circulation
3.8	American Journal of Sports Medicine
1.5	Applied Ergonomics
2.2	Applied Physiology, Nutrition, and Metabolism
1.1	Applied Psychological Measurement
2.8	Applied Psychology: An International Review
2.4	Behavior Research Methods
3.5	British Journal of Sports Medicine
2.0	Clinical Biomechanics
2.1	Clinical Journal of Sports Medicine
2.4	Clinics in Sports Medicine
1.1	Current Sports Medicine Reports
1.4	Ergonomics
2.2	European Journal of Applied Physiology
2.4	Exercise and Immunology Reviews
3.8	Exercise and Sport Sciences Reviews

TABLE 3.1 **2011 Impact Factors for Selected Journals Related to Kinesiology and the Health Sciences** *(Continued)*

Impact Factor	Journal Title
2.3	Gait & Posture
2.2	High Altitude Medicine & Biology
2.0	Human Movement Science
5.8	International Journal of Epidemiology
2.2	International Journal of Sport Nutrition and Exercise Metabolism
1.0	International Journal of Sport Psychology
2.4	International Journal of Sports Medicine
1.2	International Journal of Sports Physiology and Performance
1.1	International Journal of Sports Science and Coaching
1.8	Journal of Aging and Physical Activity
1.1	Journal of Applied Behavior Analysis
1.7	Journal of Applied Behavioral Science
1.1	Journal of Applied Biomechanics
4.2	Journal of Applied Physiology
4.0	Journal of Applied Psychology
1.3	Journal of Applied Sport Psychology
2.0	Journal of Athletic Training
2.5	Journal of Biomechanics
2.4	Journal of Electromyography and Kinesiology
3.0	Journal of Epidemiology and Community Health
2.7	Journal of the International Society of Sports Nutrition
1.5	Journal of Leisure Research
1.7	Journal of Motor Behavior
2.0	Journal of Occupational and Environmental Medicine
2.5	Journal of Orthopaedic and Sports Physical Therapy
5.1	Journal of Physiology
2.5	Journal of Science and Medicine in Sport
2.8	Journal of Sport and Exercise Psychology
1.9	Journal of Sports Sciences
1.8	Journal of Strength and Conditioning Research
4.1	Medicine and Science in Sports and Exercise
1.2	Motor Control
1.1	Pediatric Exercise Science
1.1	Physical Therapy in Sport
2.2	Psychology of Sport and Exercise
1.2	Research Quarterly for Exercise and Sport
2.8	Scandinavian Journal of Medicine and Science in Sports
5.1	Sports Medicine

As a novice researcher and a student of research methods, you will need to rely on your faculty advisor for guidance as to which journals are considered to be of high quality related to your topical area of interest. As you learn more about research design and research writing, you will develop the ability to read the research literature more critically and you will begin to personally appreciate which journals are publishing high-quality work that is of most relevance and interest to you.

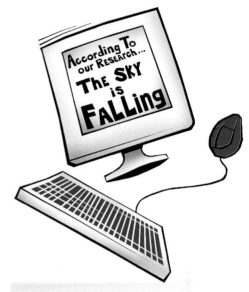

✔ Check Your Understanding

What are some indicators of the quality of a research journal?

Critiquing a Research Paper

In addition to techniques for evaluating the quality of a journal, you need strategies for evaluating the papers they publish. As a novice researcher and research writer, you might feel daunted by the thought of having to discern the strengths and weaknesses of published papers. However, you can begin by asking a few simple questions.

Maybe we can't believe everything that appears on the Web.

First, read the paper through to follow the story, which we mentioned in Chapter 2 as an element that every good research paper should have. Initial questions to ask and answer include the following:

- Was I able to follow the story?
- Was the story interesting?
- Was it logically developed?
- Did the writing flow smoothly?
- Did the paper seem well organized?
- Was it clear to me why the study was conducted in the first place?
- Do the results seem important or useful?

In Chapter 17, we will discuss in detail what appropriately goes into the various components of a research paper. In the meantime, here are some questions to consider as you begin to critique the published papers that you may wish to include in your review of literature (Special Interest Box 3.2).

✔ Check Your Understanding

1. List five general questions that might be asked in determining the quality of an original research paper.
2. List two general questions that might be asked about each subsection of an original research paper.

Use titled subsections within the body of the review to identify for readers the main idea of the subsection.

WRITING THE LITERATURE REVIEW

Whether for a thesis, the introduction to a research paper, or an entire literature review paper, a good literature review organizes and synthesizes the important information relevant to the topic of the review. A common

Remember that a summary includes no new information!

SPECIAL INTEREST BOX 3.2

Critiquing a Research Paper One Section at a Time

Questions about the Introduction:

Do the first several sentences capture the reader's attention?

Is a compelling rationale for the study presented?

Is it clear how the present study fits within the body of existing literature?

Is the purpose of the study clearly and concisely stated?

Questions about the Methods section:

Are the participants' characteristics clearly identified?

Is the apparatus (or instruments) described in sufficient detail that another researcher could repeat the study?

Is the experimental protocol clearly spelled out?

Are the statistical procedures explained?

Questions about the Results section:

Is the description of the results complete, concise, and well organized?

Are tables and graphs appropriately used to supplement the text without being redundant?

Are tables and graphs clearly labeled and do they contain enough information to "stand alone?"

Are interpretive comments saved for the Discussion section?

Questions about the Discussion and Conclusions sections:

Are the results related back to the hypothesis?

Are the results explained within the context of the results of similar studies?

Are limitations of the study that confine the applicability of the results mentioned?

Are any unexplained factors or loose ends addressed?

Are the conclusions appropriate given the results and delimitations of the study?

General questions:

Is the reader left with the feeling of "So what?"

Is it clear that this study was worth conducting?

Was the study interesting?

Was the paper well written?

Did the study uncover new information?

Do the results of this study form the basis for new research questions?

error in student literature review sections for theses is stringing together a series of disjointed paragraphs, with each paragraph describing an individual research paper. Instead, a good literature review is organized by subtopics that flow in a logically organized fashion. Related research studies under each subtopic are mentioned and cited, but are not usually presented in the form of what might be the abstract for the paper. If you are a novice researcher faced with the task of constructing a literature review for a thesis or other research project, do not use another student's thesis as a model for your literature review. Instead, in consultation with your major professor, find a published literature review on a topic similar to yours to use as a model.

Every literature review is written for a particular purpose, and so it may be useful to actually write out the purpose of your literature review before you begin to write it. As a student, the general purpose of your literature review is likely to explain the following:

- Why your topic is of interest or importance
- What related research has been published on your topic
- Which important question remains unanswered

(Answering this important, unanswered question will then be the purpose of your study.)

Beyond this, however, you may have other purposes in mind, such as

- Documenting that little to no research has been done in a new, emerging area
- Demonstrating that there is controversy or disagreement surrounding a particular practice
- Explaining why a study using new, state-of-the-art instrumentation or methodology is needed to reevaluate an existing belief

A clear understanding of the story that you wish to tell through the literature should serve as your guide for organizing the literature review and determining which published papers to cite in it.

To assist you in selecting a theme and organizational superstructure for your literature review, it is worth searching the literature to determine if there are any published literature reviews related to your topic or a similar topic. Reading a published review may help you organize your own thoughts. Search engines such as PubMed give you the ability to search for review papers only. If you are able to find a good review paper related to your own topic, scrutinize the paper's reference list to determine if there are any related published papers that you somehow missed in your own searching. Finally, it's a good idea to check with your faculty advisor and with other professors who may be knowledgeable about your topic to make sure that you are on the right track before you write the review.

Once you have a clear understanding of what you want to accomplish with the literature review, the next step is to prepare an outline. Virtually all literature reviews start with an introduction and end with a summary. In between the introduction and summary is the body of the review, which is usually organized into several titled subsections. The skeleton outline you will begin with, then, will look something like this:

Introduction
Body
    Subsection A
    Subsection B
    Subsection C
Summary

But how do you develop this skeleton into a working outline for your paper? Let's explore each section separately.

✔ Check Your Understanding

What are the two first steps in preparing to write a literature review?

Developing the Outline for the Introduction

In developing the outline for your introduction, keep in mind the following purposes of the introduction. The first is to capture the reader's interest. This means that the first sentence, and possibly the entire first paragraph, should clearly describe why the topical area is of interest and/or importance.

The second purpose of the introduction is to identify for the reader the major subtopics included in the body of the review and explain why they are relevant. Depending on how many subtopics you address, this explanation may require one or several paragraphs.

Sometimes it is helpful as well to explain to the reader what potentially related subtopics will *not* be included and why. For example, "This review will include sections on the incidence of low back pain, the causes of low back pain, and the anatomical structures involved in low back pain. It will not address treatment protocols...."

✔ Check Your Understanding

What should be accomplished in the introduction to the literature review?

Determining Numbers and Titles of Subsections

To determine how many subsections you will need in the body of your paper, and what you should call them, think carefully about two things: the purposes of the review and the available relevant papers that you have selected from the literature. These considerations should drive your choice of an organizational "superstructure" for the body of your paper. Assign each subsection its own descriptive subtitle. For instance, your subsections could discuss the following:

- Different methodological approaches to a problem area
- Different subtopics within the larger area of your particular interest
- Areas of agreement and areas of controversy in the related literature

As you construct the outline for the body of your paper, jot down the titles of the papers you intend to discuss beneath the subsection heading(s) where you plan to discuss them. If you find that you have one paper that does not logically seem to fit anywhere, you may decide to exclude that paper from the review. Similarly, if you find that you have too few papers to reference in one subsection, you may need to go back and search further for appropriate papers on that one subtopic. It is better to err on the side of being overly inclusive than to leave out one or more papers of potential importance.

Also under each subsection title in your outline, jot down all of the main points you wish to make there. A subsection that rambles on and meanders with no clear story or direction is not only ineffective but frustrating to read! So be sure that the points you plan to make beneath each subtitle support the topic the subtitle promises. For instance, if the subsection title refers to the etiology of low back pain, each paragraph beneath it should contribute to an understanding of that subject. It is much better to organize each subsection around the ideas you wish to convey than to doggedly march through one paper after another in sequential fashion with no logical thread for the reader to follow. Stringing together a series of paragraphs, with each paragraph summarizing a single study, is not an effective way to accomplish the purpose of a literature review. Again, each subsection should tell a story about what is known based on the published research literature on that topic.

Keep in mind, too, that your job is not simply to summarize what was done in each of the papers you are reviewing, but also to interpret the findings within the context of the theme or perspective that you have chosen. If you do, you'll naturally find yourself including more detail about the key investigations under review and less detail about studies that are peripheral to your interpretation. In describing the studies you have chosen to include, keep in mind that you should write in past tense, since the studies have already been done.

Finally, let's return to an important point made in Chapter 2. It is rarely appropriate to include direct quotations of text from a paper you are reviewing. Careful paraphrasing that avoids plagiarism is almost always preferred.

✔ Check Your Understanding

What literature body subtitles might be appropriate for your own research topic or interest?

Developing the Summary

The summary is usually confined to one paragraph. When planning this section, it is instructive to think about what the word *summary* means! This is the section where you highlight the main points that you have already detailed in the subsections of the paper. It is not intended to be the place where you introduce new information or share your plans for your own study. It is intended to reinforce the take-home messages from the literature review.

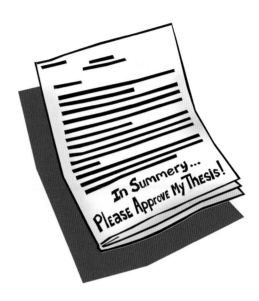

Depending on the goal of the literature review and the preference of your faculty advisor, the final section may be entitled something like "Summary and Conclusions" or "Summary and Recommendations," rather than simply "Summary." If this is the case, then *after* presenting a summary highlighting your main points from the body of the review, you will construct a short additional paragraph that relates the gap you have identified in the literature to the proposed plans for your own study.

✔ Check Your Understanding

In what ways are a summary and conclusions similar and different?

CHAPTER SUMMARY

- A literature review presents a view of a topic of interest based on summary and review of previously published research papers related to that topic.
- The purpose of a published literature review is to summarize a body of literature from a particular perspective.
- For students, there are the additional purposes of demonstrating comprehensive knowledge of a topical area and highlighting a gap in the literature, which can potentially be filled by the thesis or dissertation project.
- There are a variety of online search engines and other tools available for identifying published papers related to a topic.
- Once related papers have been identified, it is important to screen for quality, since published papers are not necessarily free from flaws.
- There are a number of general questions (discussed in the chapter) that can be asked in critiquing any research paper.
- The first steps in writing a literature review are determining the perspective or underlying themes that will unify the review and then developing an outline.
- The general organization of most literature reviews consists of an introduction; the body of the review, which is usually divided into subsections; and then a summary and conclusions at the end.

REFERENCES

1. PubMed.gov: http://www.ncbi.nlm.nih.gov/pubmed/
2. National Center for Biotechnology Information (NCBI): https://www.ncbi.nlm.nih.gov/
3. Educational Resources Information Center (ERIC): http://www.eric.ed.gov/
4. Google Scholar: http://scholar.google.com/
5. ScienceDirect: http://www.sciencedirect.com/
6. Ovid: www.ovid.com
7. Web of Science: http://thomsonreuters.com/web-of-science/
8. Science Citation Index: http://thomsonreuters.com/science-citation-index-expanded/
9. Social Sciences Citation Index: http://thomsonreuters.com/social-sciences-citation-index/
10. Arts & Humanities Citation Index: http://www.thomsonscientific.com/cgi-bin/jrnlst/jloptions.cgi?PC = H
11. Index Chemicus: http://thomsonreuters.com/index-chemicus/
12. Current Chemical Reactions:http://ip-science.thomsonreuters.com/cgi-bin/jrnlst/jloptions.cgi?PC = CR
13. Physical Education Index: http://www.csa.com/factsheets/pei-set-c.php
14. Wilson Education Index: http://www.ebscohost.com/academic/education-full-text
15. SPORTDiscus: http://www.ebscohost.com/biomedical-libraries/sportdiscus-with-full-text
16. Biblioscape: http://www.biblioscape.com/
17. Bookends: http://www.sonnysoftware.com/
18. EndNote: http://www.endnote.com
19. Papers: http://www.papersapp.com/papers/
20. ProCite: http://www.www.prosites.com
21. Reference Manager: http://www.refman.com/
22. RefWorks: http://www.refworks.com/
23. Sente: http://www.thirdstreetsoftware.com/site/SenteForMac.html
24. Journal Citation Reports: http://thomsonreuters.com/journal-citation-reports/

RELATED ASSIGNMENTS

1. **Using either online access or a visit to your school library, identify the available search engines and, using each one in turn, perform a search on a topic of interest to you. Prepare a list of the search engines and provide the citation for one paper you identified through each engine. Perform a second search with all of the available search engines, this time using the same key terms for all searches. Compare and contrast the results.**

2. **Critiquing a Published Paper. Select a research paper from the published literature on a topic of interest to you. The paper you select must be a research paper; that is, it should contain Methods or Procedures, Results, and Discussion sections. Do not select a paper that is a review paper or a position paper. Using the criteria for critiquing a paper discussed in the chapter, write a critique of the paper you have selected. Your critique should not include a summary of the paper. Write with the assumption that the reader has read the paper itself. Target length for the critique is approximately two to three pages (typed in a 12-point font, double-spaced, with 1.5-inch margins on all sides). The heading should include the complete citation for the paper, for example:**

   A Critique of: Blair SN, Ellsworth NM, Haskell WL, et al. Comparison of nutrient intake in middle-aged men and women runners and controls. *Med Sci Sports Exerc* 1981;12:310–315.

   Your critique should be written in formal, scientific writing style. Finally, submit a photocopy of the paper along with your critique.

3. **Searching the Literature. Prepare a bibliography of 20 citations of papers from the research literature on a topic of interest to you. Use the editorial style of a journal that you would like to publish your own work in. Restrict your bibliography to the more current papers that appear to be most directly relevant to your topic.**

4. **Write a short literature review paper based on six to eight important and directly related research studies that have been published relating to your area of interest. The papers included in the review must be research papers (describing a research study, with methods and results reported) and should not be review papers. Papers from conference proceedings, unpublished sources, and the Web are not acceptable. When summarizing the papers you**

are reviewing, write in past tense since the research has already been completed. Use the organizational structure discussed in the chapter and include a reference list at the end in the format of a journal you would like to publish in. The paper should be typed, double-spaced, with 1.5-inch margins.

IN-CLASS GROUP EXERCISES

1. Within your group, identify three topics appropriate for literature reviews. For each topic, then decide what approach (chronological review, opposing viewpoints, or position based) would be most interesting for each topic. Then, identify three main subtopics to be covered in the review. Report the results of your discussion to the class.

2. Within your group of two to three students, prepare for one side of a point–counterpoint debate on a topic assigned by your instructor. The arguments you prepare should be based both on the results of original research papers related to the topic and on your own logic. Following an adequate preparation period, class time may be used for oral debates, or the groups can write research-based position papers.

3. After all group members have read an assigned original research paper, work as a group to critique the paper, using the criteria identified in the chapter. Discuss the paper as though you were serving as reviewers for a journal. Would your advice to the journal editor be to (a) accept the paper as is, (b) recommend that the paper be revised, or (c) reject the paper?

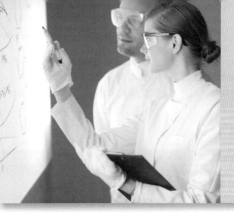

4

Developing a Research Proposal

"Research is to see what everybody else has seen, and to think what nobody else has thought."
—*Albert Szent-Gyorgyi, 1937 Nobel Prize for Medicine*

CHAPTER OBJECTIVES

After studying this chapter, you will be able to:

1. Explain the importance of a sound research question or problem.
2. Describe the purpose and organization of each of the components of a typical research proposal in detail.
3. With the assistance of a faculty advisor, write a convincing research proposal.
4. Describe the different purposes and associated target audiences for research proposals.

■ BEFORE a research study is conducted, the researchers write a proposal that must be approved by a person or group of authority in order for the study to proceed. A good research proposal clearly identifies what the researcher wishes to investigate, presents a compelling rationale as to why the proposed study should be conducted, explains how it will be conducted, and sometimes projects what the results are likely to be and why they will be important. Some proposals also include a budget for the projected costs associated with conducting the study along with an explanation as to why these costs are necessary. In the absence of a good proposal, a study is not likely to be approved by a faculty advisor or to be funded by a granting agency. Accordingly, writing a sound research proposal is a critically important part of the research process.

Once approved or accepted, the research proposal serves two main purposes. First, it provides the action plan, including exactly what the researcher plans to do at every sequential step along the way in conducting the study. Second, it serves as a contractual agreement between the researcher and those who approve the proposal. Once a proposal has been approved, any nontrivial changes to what has been approved must be agreeable to both the researcher and those who approved the original proposal.

✓ Check Your Understanding

1. List three characteristics of a strong research proposal.
2. What are the two major purposes of an approved research proposal?

TOPIC SELECTION

For students, the first, and often daunting, step in developing a research proposal is determining the general topic area to research. Whereas established researchers are typically working on a line of related studies within an area of research in which they have strong interest and have developed expertise, this is not the case for most beginning students of research. Accordingly, selection of a sound research topic is quite important and can be a somewhat time-consuming task.

There are many approaches for selecting a topic area for a thesis, dissertation, or other research project. If you are a graduate student, you are likely to have a strong interest in the kind of research your advisor is doing and you may be participating as an assistant with your advisor's research. If this is the case, your advisor may assign you a topic for your master's thesis or may provide strong guidance in discussing some different topic possibilities. At the Ph.D. level, students are expected to function more autonomously and be capable of developing researchable questions independently, although there still may be an understanding that the work will be generally in line with the kind of research the advisor or major professor is doing.

Whether you are an undergraduate or graduate student, if you are expected to suggest a topic on your own, you are well advised to talk extensively with your advisor and possibly other professors about different possibilities, depending on your own interests. Your participation in these discussions will be much more profitable if you have already done some reading in the research literature on one or more topics that seem interesting to you. If you are able to attend a professional conference where research is being presented in your general area of interest, this can also serve to stimulate your thinking. Researchers presenting papers at conferences often suggest topics for follow-up studies to answer new questions that have

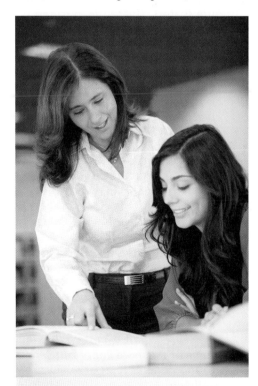

Faculty advisors are a valuable source of helpful information and advice for beginning researchers.

emerged during their own work. The most unlikely scenario, however, in the absence of reading the research literature and talking with your advisor and others, is that you simply will wake up one morning with a good topic in mind. Even when a thesis topic is assigned, your advisor will expect you to become highly familiar with the research literature related to your topic and to become competent in collecting the kind of data that your project will require. Special Interest Box 4.1 illustrates how the process of selecting a topic area for a research project might be initiated.

SPECIAL INTEREST BOX 4.1

Exploring a Topic Area for a Thesis

Jean had taken figure skating lessons for several years as a young girl, and she had been following figure skating competitions and prominent skaters avidly. She was quite interested when she read an article describing how both 1996 U.S. Figure Skating champion Rudy Galindo and 1998 Olympic gold medal winner Tara Lipinski had both had double hip replacements, Galindo at the age of 32 and Lipinski at the age of 18. The article went on to describe how the incidence of overuse injuries among figure skaters is increasing, with most involving the lower extremity and lower back. Thinking back to her own training as a figure skater, Jean knew that her hips were sometimes sore after practice, especially when she had been practicing jumps. A quick search using PubMed for "figure skating + injuries" revealed several papers in the medical literature documenting a high incidence of lower extremity injuries among figure skaters. This led Jean to send the following e-mail message to her advisor, Dr. Strictly:

Hello, Dr. Strictly,

As you know, I've been thinking about a topic for my thesis, and I think I have an idea that might work. You know I've always been interested in figure skating, and it occurs to me that figure skaters seem to have a lot of overuse-type hip injuries. I'm wondering if there are a safe number of jumps that figure skaters can execute during practice, with performing more than that safe number of jumps leading to hip injury. I was wondering if we could somehow estimate the forces acting at the hip during landings from some of the different jumps and then based on published force values in the literature for bone fracture, figure out what the safe number of jumps is. I'll try to catch you in your office for a follow-up discussion.
Thanks for your time,
Jean

Dr. Strictly responded:

Whether there is a "safe" number of jumps that a skater can perform during a given practice session is an interesting question, and if we could answer that question, the information would certainly be valuable. However, the answer is likely to depend on the age, weight, and bone status of the skater, as well as landing kinematics and kinetics, the shock absorbing characteristics of the skates, and the time intervals between jumps, just to name a few variables of influence. In other words, it is a complicated problem. However, I think we might do some pilot testing to see if it might be possible to focus on some of the more important variables and come up with a researchable question related to this general topic area. Fortunately, we do have the motion analysis equipment and software available in our lab to enable estimating forces on the hips during landing using inverse dynamics. Please see me tomorrow during my office hours if you are free.
Dr. Strictly

✓ Check Your Understanding

List several strategies for identifying a topic area for a research study.

The Research Question

Once you have identified a general area of research interest, the next step is developing the research question. As discussed in Chapter 1, the research question is the focal point, or driving force for the study. It is also sometimes referred to as the problem statement, since it is, in fact, usually presented in the form of a statement rather than a question. For example, if we were interested in studying the effect of salt consumption on hypertension among African American men, we could pose the general research question, "How much salt intake is required to significantly increase blood pressure in African American men?" Refining this into a more specific, researchable question, we might pose "Is blood pressure significantly elevated in African American men aged 20 to 40 years following 6 weeks of a 3% sodium diet?"

In a research proposal or paper, however, it is more common to present a specific problem statement than a research question. As described in Chapter 1, the problem statement contains the major independent and dependent variables of interest and also, if important, identifies the population being studied. Our problem statement might be "The purpose of the proposed study is to compare three levels of chronic salt consumption on blood pressure in African American men aged 20 to 40 years." Here *The research problem statement clearly identifies the independent and dependent variables being studied.*

the independent variable, or variable being manipulated by the researcher (defined in Chapter 1), is salt consumption; the dependent variable, or variable being measured, is blood pressure; and the population being studied is obviously African American men aged 20 to 40 years. Another problem statement related to the same general research question might be, "The purpose of the study is to investigate the acute effect of an injection of 3% saline solution on blood pressure in African American men with a predetermined sensitivity to salt." Alternatively, we might wish to investigate whether there is a correlation between blood pressure and salt intake, in which case we might write, "The purpose of the study is to investigate the relationship between blood pressure and salt intake among..." Note that all problem statements clearly identify both independent and dependent variables being studied.

As you can surmise from the example in Special Interest Box 4.1, the development of a good research question is often quite a process. Not only it must be of interest and importance to some population it must also be delineated specifically enough that it can be answered, at least potentially, through the collection and analysis of data. This typically requires some preliminary experimentation to determine which of the dependent variables that can be measured are likely to yield the best information relative to an independent variable of interest. It is also, of course, important that the necessary equipment and expertise be available for studying the problem of interest. Special Interest Box 4.2 presents a list of criteria typically associated with a good research question.

We cannot overemphasize that **a good problem statement is the heart of a strong research proposal**. In the absence of meeting the criteria listed, most proposals are doomed to failure. Accordingly, you should plan on spending considerable time and effort developing and refining the problem

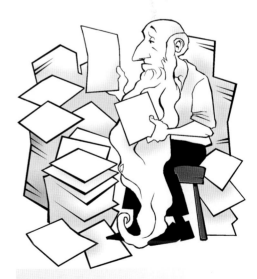

His master's thesis is a 50-year, longitudinal study.

SPECIAL INTEREST BOX 4.2

Criteria for Identifying a Good Research Problem

A good research problem should be

- **Important**: clearly important or of potential value or use either generally or to some group for a particular reason

- **Interesting**: of interest either generally or to some group for a particular reason. If this is going to be your thesis topic, it had better also be pretty interesting to you, because you are going to be spending lots of time working on it!

- **Novel**: one that has not specifically been answered in the research literature

- **Researchable**: one that can be addressed through the research process, that is, through the collection and analysis of data

- **Practical**: one for which the necessary equipment, expertise, access to participants, and time for completing the study are all available

- **Clearly stated**: written in a straightforward, readily comprehensible manner using appropriate research writing

- **Timely**: one that addresses a current problem or issue

- And for proposals submitted to funding agencies, **in line with the priorities of the funding agency**: one that clearly falls within the criteria stated in the request for proposals

---

The single most important element of a strong research proposal is a sound problem statement (research question) or specific aims.

statement for your research project. **Make sure that your advisor has approved not only the idea but also the exact wording of your problem statement before you proceed with writing the rest of your research proposal.** Note that you should arrive at a well-worded problem statement first, before writing any of the remainder of your research proposal.

 ## Check Your Understanding

What are the characteristics of a good problem statement?

The Research Hypothesis

Research Hypothesis
Statement expressing the researcher's expectation for the outcome of a study (effect of the independent variable[s] on the dependent variable[s]).

The next step in developing a research proposal is the identification of one or more hypotheses associated with the problem statement or research question. As described in Chapter 1, a **research hypothesis** is the researcher's own expectation as to the outcome of the study. This expectation should be based on understanding of the research problem and analysis of what is known about the topic based on the related literature. Specifically, you should be able to explain the rationale for your research hypothesis based on the results of previously published research and/or results from pilot studies. The research hypothesis typically follows directly after the problem statement. Here are some examples of hypothetical problem statements followed by research hypotheses:

- The purpose of the study is to evaluate the relationship between the number of hours spent studying and performance on a research methods exam. Our hypothesis is that there will be a direct, positive correlation between study time and exam performance.
- The purpose of the study is to compare the effects of isotonic and plyometric resistance training on peak torque and power in the knee extensors following a 6-week training intervention. We hypothesize that both forms of training will result in significant improvements in these variables. We further hypothesize that isokinetic training will produce significantly better results than isotonic training.
- The purpose of the study is to characterize attitudes of K-6 classroom student teachers before and after a 3-day workshop on physical education activities for classroom teachers. We hypothesize that the student teachers will have a significantly more positive attitude toward physical education activities following the workshop.

Notice that in all cases the hypotheses can be confirmed (accepted) or not confirmed (rejected) based on the results of the study. This must be the case for all legitimate research hypotheses. Special Interest Box 4.3 presents some problem statements and hypotheses taken from papers published in research journals.

SPECIAL INTEREST BOX 4.3

Research Problem Statements and Hypotheses

Problem Statement
Given the mixed findings of the previous literature, the primary purpose of the current study was to test the effects of acute aerobic exercise on long-term memory.

Hypothesis
We hypothesized that participants engaging in acute exercise would perform better on the recall task than those not performing any exercise.
(From Labban JD, Etnier, JL. Effects of acute exercise on long-term memory. *Res Q Exerc Sport* 2011;82:712–721.)

Problem Statement
The purpose of this study was to conduct a functional analysis to examine how teachers' use of task adaptations differs in teaching stronger versus weaker instruction units.

Hypothesis
We hypothesized that quality and appropriateness of adaptations would vary relative to the content expertise (stronger vs. weaker instruction units).
(From Ayvazo S, Ward P. Pedagogical content knowledge of experienced teachers in physical education: functional analysis of adaptations. *Res Q Exerc Sport* 2011;82:765–684.)

Problem Statement
Is there a relationship between BMI and MABC-2 percentile in preschoolers?

Hypothesis
We hypothesized there would be a negative relationship, which would suggest that as BMI increased, motor proficiency would decrease.
(From Logan SW, Scrabis-Fletcher K, Modlesky C, et al. The relationship between motor skill proficiency and body mass index in preschool children. *Res Q Exerc Sport* 2011;82:449–457.)

✔ **Check Your Understanding**

Using your own words, define *research hypothesis*.

Specific Aims and Related Hypotheses

Much of a well-written research proposal can be used with only minor modifications in the thesis/dissertation or manuscript submitted to a journal for publication after the study has been completed.

Specific Aims Two or more related specific research problems proposed for investigation in a study.

Although it is perfectly acceptable to have one strong research question or problem statement for an undergraduate or master's thesis, researchers often conduct projects to investigate two or more related questions termed **specific aims**. Each specific aim has one or more research hypotheses associated with it. If we were interested in studying the effects of stretching protocols on ankle function, for example, we might investigate the following related specific aims and associated hypotheses:

Specific Aim I: To determine the effects of 30-, 60-, and 120-second static stretches on ankle range of motion after 0, 10, and 20 minutes

Hypothesis I: Ankle range of motion will increase with increased stretch duration.

Specific Aim II: To determine the effects of 30-, 60-, and 120-second static stretches on plantar flexor peak torque after 0, 10, and 20 minutes

Hypothesis II: Plantar flexor peak torque will decrease with increased stretch duration.

If we wanted to investigate ways to promote the development of throwing ability among girls aged 5 to 7 years, we might propose the following specific aims and related hypotheses:

Specific Aim I: To evaluate the effects of daily expert instruction over a 2-week period on throwing accuracy to a target

Hypothesis I: Throwing accuracy will improve following instruction.

Specific Aim II: To measure the effects of 15 minutes of daily throwing practice over a 2-week period on maximum throwing distance

Hypothesis II: Maximum throwing distance will improve with practice.

✔ **Check Your Understanding**

1. What is the difference between a research question and a research problem?
2. How is a specific aim similar to and different from a research problem?

DEVELOPING THE RATIONALE FOR THE STUDY

Composing an outline prior to writing the different sections of a proposal usually saves time and results in a much better end product.

Once the wording has been agreed upon for the research problem/aims, the next step in the development of a research proposal is writing the rationale for the proposed study. The rationale is presented in the introduction to a thesis as well as in the introduction to a research paper. A well-crafted proposal introduction can be used as written for the introduction to a thesis and/or as the introduction section for the research manuscript that is submitted to a journal for publication after the study has been concluded.

A good rationale for a proposal begins by introducing the topic of the study and making it clear why it is of interest or importance. Next, through references to what is known in the closely related research literature, a logical rationale is developed that leads the reader down a path to the conclusion that ends with a clear understanding as to why the proposed study should be conducted. The problem statement or specific aims, followed by one or more hypotheses, then actually conclude the introductory section.

There are two important points to keep in mind when writing the rationale for a proposal. First, as discussed in Chapter 2 and in keeping with good research writing style, it is invaluable to begin with a basic outline of the sequential points you wish to make in leading the reader to understand why the proposed study should be conducted. Second, whereas it is typically useful to cite studies of direct relevance in making your points, this is *not* the place for a full-blown review of related literature. You do not want the reader to be distracted or misled by including a meandering citation of too many studies that have only tangential relevance to the logical rationale you hope to compose. A good proposal rationale is relatively concise.

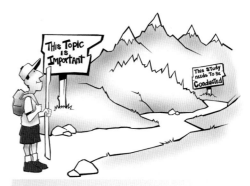

A well-written introduction leads the reader down a path, convincing them that this is an important study that needs to be done.

If we were to compose a hypothetical rationale for our two specific aims related to three stretching durations for the ankle plantar flexors, for example, we might start with the following basic outline:

1. Reasons why stretching protocols are thought to be useful
2. Reasons why stretching protocols may not be useful
3. Reasons to investigate effects of different stretching durations
4. Reasons to monitor effects of stretching on range of motion and strength

A short rationale for this proposed study might then read as follows:

Stretching regimens are commonly performed prior to athletic and fitness-related activities due to a long-standing belief that increased range of motion at a joint will reduce the likelihood of injury. Research, however, has not supported this notion, and some studies have even documented a temporary decrement in stretched muscle's ability to produce force. Because stretching protocols are of different durations, the length of the poststretching period of effect on either range of motion or strength may vary. Pilot testing in our lab indicates that stretch durations of 30, 60, and 120 seconds are sufficiently different to elicit different immediate effects on both range of motion at the ankle and plantar flexor strength. Because the effects of these different durations of stretch on range of motion and strength after 10 or 20 minutes have not been previously reported, yet could have a practical effect on performance, we therefore propose the following specific aims for our study.

Notice that the rationale statement is concise, but that it adequately conveys the rationale for the specific aims. It begins with a brief explanation as to why this problem is of interest and importance. Next, it explains what gap in the existing knowledge base the results of the proposed study could potentially fill. These are key elements that should appear in all specific aim rationales. If this were the rationale for a real study, it would be somewhat longer, primarily because a few specific examples of studies showing a decrement in muscle force generating capacity would be described.

One line of rationale that students are advised against using is trying to make the case that a problem is important solely because "it has never been studied before." No one has ever studied "how to extract one's own appendix" and for good reason! The rationale statement, specific aims, and related hypotheses for a real research proposal appear in Special Interest Box 4.4.

SPECIAL INTEREST BOX 4.4

Specific Aims from a Research Proposal

Note: *This section on specific aims is provided courtesy of Dr. Bill Farquhar at the University of Delaware from a proposal that was funded by the NIH National Heart, Lung, and Blood Institute through the R15 mechanism.*

Hypertension is a major health problem in the United States; recent statistics suggest that 65 million Americans have hypertension, and the total hypertension prevalence rate in the United States is 31.3% (Fields, 2004). These data are estimated from the years 1999 to 2000 and represent a 30% increase from the 1988 to 1994 data (reviewed in the aptly titled manuscript *The Burden of Adult Hypertension in the United States 1999 to 2000: A Rising Tide*) (Fields, 2004). While many studies support the general link between sodium intake and blood pressure, the mechanisms underlying this relationship remain unclear. Certain segments of the population appear to be more "salt sensitive" than others. For example, African American adults have a high degree of salt sensitivity, as do older adults (Weinberger, 1996). Salt sensitivity occurs in both normotensive and hypertensive adults.

Recent data in experimental animals suggest that modest increases in plasma sodium concentration activate centrally located osmoreceptors that trigger sympathoexcitation (Brooks, 2005; O'Donaughy, 2006). This sympathoexcitation may be one of the mechanisms underlying salt sensitivity of blood pressure. Furthermore, inappropriately high angiotensin II levels (i.e., failure to suppress this hormone in the presence of a volume load) may facilitate this sympathetic activation, leading to further elevations in blood pressure. These hypotheses have not been tested in humans.

In the context of studying the mechanisms underlying salt sensitivity of blood pressure, it is important to highlight the clinical relevance of this problem. Influential studies by Weinberger et al. have reported that not only sodium sensitivity is associated with increased mortality in hypertensive and normotensive adults (Weinberger, 2002) but sodium sensitivity may also *predict* future hypertension in normotensive adults (Sullivan, 1991). Understanding sodium sensitivity may provide tremendous insight into the pathophysiology of hypertension, *but sodium sensitivity alone is gaining renewed attention because of its association with the development of cardiovascular and renal diseases* (Bigazzi, 1996; Chiolero, 2001; de la Sierra, 1996; Weinberger, 2001).

Using the gold standard technique of salt sensitivity classification (2-week controlled sodium diet coupled with ambulatory blood pressure monitoring), we will classify a cohort of middle-aged adults as either salt sensitive or salt resistant and subsequently examine neural and hormonal differences in their responses to a sodium- and volume-loading protocol. These studies will translate recent experimental findings in various animal models to humans and provide insight into the mechanisms underlying salt sensitivity of blood pressure.

Specific Aim I
Purpose: To examine the osmotic regulation of sympathetic nervous system activity in salt-sensitive and salt-resistant individuals
Hypothesis: Increases in plasma osmolality will lead to *greater increases* in muscle sympathetic nerve activity and circulating norepinephrine in salt-sensitive compared to salt-resistant individuals.

Specific Aim II
Purpose: To examine the volume regulation of circulating angiotensin II and aldosterone in salt-sensitive and salt-resistant individuals
Hypothesis: An acute volume load will cause angiotensin II and aldosterone concentration to *decline less* in salt-sensitive compared to salt-resistant individuals.

Check Your Understanding

What should be the first step in writing the rationale for a study?

PLANNING THE METHODOLOGY FOR THE STUDY

A methods section is a key component of both the research proposal, written before the study is conducted, and the research paper manuscript, written after the study is conducted. In the case of theses and dissertations, this means that if the proposal includes a careful, detailed, and comprehensive description of the methods and nothing occurs during execution of the data collection to necessitate a modification of the proposed methods, when you write up the thesis/dissertation, all you may need to change within the methods section is the verb tense. The methods section for a research proposal, of course, is written in future tense, since the study is being proposed, and the methods section for the thesis/dissertation/manuscript is written in past tense because the data have already been collected and analyzed.

The Methods section of a proposal, thesis/dissertation, or manuscript for publication should be written in sufficient detail that another competent researcher could follow it to replicate the study.

   Once you have a clear, sound, and detailed understanding of exactly what you wish to propose, the methods section is typically the quickest and easiest section of the proposal to write. Getting to that point of clear, sound, and detailed understanding, however, is typically a process. What level of detail is required for the methods section of a research proposal? The general answer to this question is that upon reading your methods section, any other competent researcher familiar with your topic area should be able to precisely replicate your study methods. This means that every step along the proposed path of action for your study must be reported in sufficient detail. Methods sections are commonly organized into three main sections describing the participants, the research protocol, and the statistical analyses.

Check Your Understanding

1. What general information should be included in the methods section of a proposal?
2. How much detail is required in the methods section of a proposal?

Describing the Participants

The number of participants (also referred to as subjects) must be specified, and all important relevant participant characteristics must be reported. Descriptive data for participants normally include the means and standard deviations of participant ages, heights, and weights or body masses, as well as the gender breakdown. Any other participant characteristics of particular relevance to the study should also be reported in this section. For example, if the study involves physical training, the training status of the participants (sedentary, recreationally active, trained, or elite) should also be documented in as a detailed fashion as possible. If the study involves an intervention of any kind, the preintervention means and standard deviations of the dependent variables should be presented along with the description of participants. The procedures by which participants were selected for inclusion or exclusion should also be clearly delineated. As will be discussed in Chapters 6 to 9, the research design used for the study will determine the ways in which the study participants are selected and, if appropriate, placed into groups. Most commonly, a statement assuring that all participants signed informed consent documents is also required. Informed consent forms explain what the study is about and specify what each participant will be expected to do. The concept of informed consent is explained in detail in Chapter 5. Special Interest Box 4.5 includes a sample hypothetical description of participants for a methods section.

SPECIAL INTEREST BOX 4.5

Hypothetical Participants Component of a Methods Section

Forty postmenopausal women (62 ± 5 year; 155 ± 6 cm; 80 ± 11 kg) volunteered for this study by responding to posted solicitation notices in the community and were randomly divided into equally sized training (TRN) and control (CON) groups. All participants were sedentary, although apparently healthy and free from diagnosed musculoskeletal diseases or injury within the past 6 months. Prospective participants who reported walking or other mild to moderate exercise as much as once per week were excluded. All participants signed institutionally approved statements of informed consent prior to participation in the study.

✔ Check Your Understanding

List all of the characteristics of study participants that should be described in a proposal methods section.

Describing the Protocol

The protocol section is where all study-related procedures are described. This includes everything that participants are required or expected to do, as well as who will collect the data, and how, when, and where data will be collected. If your problem statement for a thesis proposal includes any term that is at all ambiguous or for which the definition may be context specific, you will need to provide what is known as an **operational definition** for that term. For example, a "static stretch" of the plantar flexors might be operationally defined as "a maximal passive stretch performed by a trained physical therapist" or, alternatively, as "a voluntary active stretch performed by the participant to the point of discomfort." In order for your protocol to be completely and accurately described, operationally defining such terms is imperative. Operational definitions are usually only required for terms that appear within the problem statement or that are used in describing key elements of the protocol. It is not necessary or appropriate to provide a special definition for every term you use in describing the study protocol.

Operational Definition
Explanation of a term specifically within the context of a proposed study.

In crafting the protocol description, it is also important to convey that standardized procedures will be used and that every participant will be treated identically and without bias. As you will no doubt recall from reading Chapter 1, this is essential for convincing the reader that the proposed study is designed to have strong internal validity. If the directions given to participants are very complicated at all, it is best to state that a set of standardized written instructions will be read to each participant so it is clear that each participant was told the same things. Generally speaking, and particularly for novice researchers, it is better to err on the side of including too much detail in this section, rather than too little.

A secondary purpose for the protocol part of the methods section is often to convince the readers that you, the researcher, are sufficiently knowledgeable and skilled to competently carry out the proposed study. This translates to accurately and appropriately describing your proposed protocol in detail and, where appropriate, citing any specialized techniques you will be using that have been previously reported in the literature. This will require not only that you have a sound understanding of the protocol you are proposing but also that you are conversant with any specialized or technical terminology best used to describe your protocol to other knowledgeable researchers.

The protocol must also describe in detail all **apparatus** and/or **instruments** that will be used for data collection. Although you may have the impression that these two terms are interchangeable, within the realm of research, they have very different and specific meanings.

Apparatus is the term used to refer to any piece of laboratory equipment, such as a treadmill, force plate, isokinetic strength testing machine, or even a handheld goniometer. In describing apparatus, you should normally include the manufacturer name and model number. Depending on the level of detail required for your proposal format, you may also need to identify the address of the manufacturer.

Instrument, on the other hand, is the term we use specifically to refer to questionnaires, whether they will be completed with pencil and paper, on a computer, or through interview format. If you will be using one of the numerous published, standardized questionnaires, your description of the instrument should include the questionnaire name and the published reliability figure for the questionnaire. For example, there are various published reliability figures for the Minnesota Multiphasic Personality Inventory (MMPI), based on the population and purpose for which it is being used. There should be a citation of the original publication in which the instrument was introduced in your reference list.

Depending on how complicated the study protocol is, this part of the methods section may be divided into several subsections. This is particularly likely to be the case if several different dependent variables are being measured using different laboratory apparatus and/or instruments.

> **Apparatus** Laboratory equipment used in a research investigation.

> **Instruments** Questionnaire used in a research investigation.

Assumptions, Limitations, and Delimitations

Some proposal formats require statements disclosing the researcher's knowledge of **assumptions**, **limitations**, and/or **delimitations** associated with the proposed study protocol. There are commonly assumptions associated with most studies involving human participants, with most of these having to do with assuming that the participants will do what they are asked to do and will respond honestly to any questions. For example, participants are often asked to verify that they meet the entrance criteria for a study, to prepare for a data collection in some way before reporting to a lab, or to carry out instructions on their own away from direct supervision as part of their participation. In each case, the researcher should be aware that there is an assumption being made that the participants are cooperating in good faith. The stronger the internal validity of a study (as described in Chapter 1), the fewer such assumptions must be made. For example, a study that requires participants to report to a lab setting for supervised exercise or other intervention has much better internal validity than a study in which participants are sent home and asked to exercise or perform the intervention on their own.

> **Assumptions** Things a researcher must trust that are true in the absence of actual verification.

> **Limitations** Problems associated with a research protocol.

> **Delimitations** Boundary conditions intentionally selected by a researcher in designing a study.

Most study proposals also have limitations associated with them. In this context, a limitation is an unavoidable drawback that constitutes a weakness in the study. The better designed the study, the fewer the limitations that will typically emerge, and for this reason, of course, careful planning is important. Having a sample size that is too small for the statistical tests to work properly, for example, would be a serious limitation. Researchers should identify how many participants are likely to be needed and plan accordingly before wasting time on a data collection that will not yield

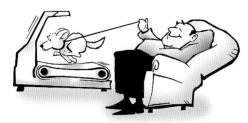

A home exercise intervention gone awry!

any information of use. Sometimes, however, limitations crop up through no fault of the researcher. Participants may choose or need to drop out of a study prior to completing it for extraneous and unanticipated reasons. Equipment may malfunction, with the resulting data being unusable. On the whole, however, at the proposal level, the number of limitations can be minimized through careful planning.

Although the word *delimitation* sounds a lot like the word limitation, it is a completely different concept. Delimitations can be thought of as boundary conditions that are deliberately chosen or set by the researcher. Typically, delimitations set constraints on the external validity or generalizability of the results of a study, as discussed in Chapter 1. For example, if we were proposing to collect data on participants with special characteristics, we could generalize our results only to the population at large with those same characteristics. Accordingly, the results of a study of elite cyclists, children aged 4 to 6 years, or individuals with hip replacements would be delimited to those same specific populations. Choices that researchers must make in limitations and delimitations influencing internal and external validity will be discussed in more detail in Chapter 6. Special Interest Box 4.6 includes a hypothetical protocol component of the methods section of a proposal.

✔ Check Your Understanding

Give an example of an assumption, limitation, and delimitation for a research study.

The Importance of Pilot Testing

Pilot Testing Preliminary, small-scale experiments conducted during the planning of a study.

Pilot testing is an important step for a well-designed study.

The term **pilot testing** refers to preliminary experimentation carried out during the planning stages for a study and before the "real" data collection commences. There are numerous potential reasons to conduct pilot testing. As alluded to by Dr. Strictly, it is sometimes necessary to do pilot testing to determine which dependent variables are important to measure and/or practical to measure. Other reasons to do pilot testing include learning how to operate the apparatus you will be using for collection of data, determining

---

SPECIAL INTEREST BOX 4.6

Hypothetical Protocol Component of a Methods Section

Participants in both training (TRN) and control (CON) groups were placed on a controlled diet for the 6-month duration of the intervention. A registered dietitian packed daily food rations including all minimum recommended vitamin and mineral content for postmenopausal women and with caloric content calculated to maintain body weight for each participant. These were available for participant pickup between 6:00 and 7:00 AM each day. All participants reported to the lab once each week for body weight assessment.

The TRN group participated in a supervised walking program 5 days per week. Between 3:00 and 5:00 PM each day (M–F), each participant walked on an indoor track at individually preferred walking speed for a distance of 3.22 km (2 mile). To promote adherence, participants were encouraged to walk in pairs or small groups and to converse while walking. One participant was dropped from participation due to an illness causing her to miss more than the agreed upon allowable absences of 10% of days walking.

Within 1-week, pre- and postintervention measures of bone mineral density (BMD) were made at the lumbar (L3), total hip, tibial plateau, and distal radius sites. All measures were taken by a certified technician using DEXA at a university research facility.

how long it will take to test each participant, determining whether the data you plan to collect are likely to enable you to address the problem you wish to study, and determining generally whether the data collection will proceed as you envision. If your study involves the development of an instrument, pilot testing is crucial to make sure that the questionnaire items are clear and understandable to the target audience and that they yield optimal information. Pilot testing of a few participants can also give you a preliminary estimate of the variability you can expect within the data set, which is necessary for calculating the number of participants you will need to test, or your **sample size**, based on the level of statistical power required for your study (discussed in detail in Chapter 10).

Sample Size The number of participants involved in a study.

The title of a proposal should accurately convey the essence of the proposed study without being a repeat of the problem statement.

Reporting of supporting pilot data within a research proposal dramatically strengthens the proposal, because it shows not only that you are capable of doing what you propose but also that the preliminary data tend to support your research hypothesis. Indeed, there are some types of research proposals that require the reporting of supporting pilot data, and without it the proposal will not even be considered. There are clearly numerous good reasons to incorporate pilot testing into any research plan.

✔ Check Your Understanding

What is *pilot testing* and why is it important?

Describing the Statistical Analysis

The final section of the methods is generally a description of all statistical analyses planned for the study. You may be surprised to learn that you will need to know exactly how you will be analyzing your data before they are even collected. This is absolutely essential, because it is important that all data you collect can be analyzed using conventionally accepted tests, with the results supporting or not supporting your research hypotheses. For a large, complicated study, it may be necessary to break the statistical analysis section down into subsections, although one paragraph is usually sufficient. Chapters 10 to 13 explain what you will need to know about commonly used statistical tests.

PROPOSAL TITLE AND ABSTRACT

You may wonder why this section on the proposal title and abstract is near the end of this chapter when the title and abstract are the first things the reader of a proposal sees. The answer is that in developing a research proposal, these are usually the last things written. If you start writing a proposal by writing the title, there is a strong likelihood that you will be revising the title multiple times as your thoughts on your research problem become more focused and refined.

A good proposal title captures the reader's attention and accurately, but concisely conveys the essence of the proposed research problem. Many poor thesis titles are basically a restatement of the research problem and hence are too long and unwieldy. An example of such a title might be "The effects of 24 hours of sleep deprivation on pre- and postintervention reaction time, choice reaction time, and MABC-2 scores." A much better title would be "Effects of sleep deprivation on measures of motor proficiency."

A proposal abstract may or may not be required, depending on formatting requirements and proposal length. The longer the proposal, the more likely it is that an abstract will be required (and useful). The proposal abstract is typically a one paragraph summary that includes a brief rationale, the statement of the problem, and an overview of the proposed procedures.

✔ Check Your Understanding

What are the characteristics of a good proposal title?

THE TARGET AUDIENCE FOR A RESEARCH PROPOSAL

Research proposals are written in different lengths and formats, depending on the target audience. There are several common target audiences for research proposals. When a study involving human participants will be conducted at a college or university, at a hospital or clinic, or at a research institute, one important target audience that *must* approve all research proposals is the **Institutional Review Board** (IRB). Studies involving animal subjects must similarly be approved by an animal protection review committee. As mandated by federal law, IRB approval of a research proposal must occur prior to collection of data. Consequently, when planning a timeline for a research project, it is important to find out how often the IRB at your institution reviews proposals, when they are scheduled to meet, and how much lead time they require for review of proposals prior to their meetings. It is also important to find out what proposal format is required by the IRB at your institution. For example, some institutions have a proposal form that investigators must complete, some simply have a required proposal format that must be followed, and some are more open ended in terms of proposal format and length. It is typically helpful to get a copy of a proposal that has been successfully reviewed by your institution's IRB and to use it as a model for your own proposal to the IRB. It is also useful to learn what review procedures are used by your institution's IRB. Some require that the lead investigator for a proposed study do a brief oral presentation of the proposal at the IRB meeting or be in attendance to respond to questions, while others may send written questions for the investigator to respond to. IRB requirements are described in more detail in Chapter 5.

Institutional Review Board Official body that must approve all proposed research studies involving human participants and conducted at a college/university, hospital, or other research facility.

Another common target audience for research proposals is a funding source for the proposed research, which may be a college or university, a professional organization, a state or federal agency, or a foundation. Once again, it is critically important to find out the length and format for proposals required by the funding source, since a proposal that is not submitted in the preferred format is likely to be returned or discarded without even being read. It is also very important to make sure that the topic area for your proposal is in line with the stated interests of the funding source. Having a proposal that has been previously funded by the source to which you are applying to use as a model is invaluable. It is also crucial to know the funding source's deadline for proposal submission. Some funding sources entertain proposals once a year, while others may review proposals more than once per year or on a rolling basis. Many institutions offer some financial support to assist with theses/dissertations, sometimes on a competitive basis. Speak with your faculty advisor to find out if there is a reasonable opportunity for you to write a proposal to fund your research. Successfully acquiring funding is something you can list on your resume, beyond the fact that it will reduce the financial burden of your project on your academic department.

As a student proposing a thesis or dissertation topic, you will also be required to develop a written research proposal that must be approved by your advisor and your thesis/dissertation committee. Your college or university is likely to have format guidelines for thesis/dissertation proposals, and it is a good idea to become acquainted with those before you start writing. Beyond the institutional requirements, your advisor may also have a preferred format for proposals, so it is clearly a good idea to check in with your advisor on that topic. Your advisor is likely to have available one or more model proposals that you can access. At many institutions, there is also an oral component to the thesis/dissertation proposal process, which we will discuss in Chapter 17.

CHAPTER SUMMARY

- A good research proposal presents a compelling rationale and detailed plan of action for conducting a study based on a strong research problem that is important, interesting, novel, researchable, and practical.
- Proposals begin with an introduction that logically leads the reader down a path of understanding where the proposed research problem fits within the context of what is known, based on the related research literature, as well as why the projected results of the proposed study are of potential importance.
- The introductory section ends with a clear statement of the research problem, or the specific aims, and related research hypotheses.
- The proposed methods section includes a description of the study participants, the study protocol, and the planned statistical analysis.
- Strong proposals typically include pilot data that demonstrate the viability of the research hypotheses and help document the investigator's competence for conducting the study.
- Research proposals vary in length and format, depending on the target audience, which may be a thesis/dissertation committee, an IRB, or a potential funding source.

RELATED ASSIGNMENTS

1. **Meet with your faculty advisor to discuss your ideas for a research proposal. Following the meeting, please complete the following:**
   a. State your research problem or specific aims and associated research hypotheses.
   b. What independent and dependent variable(s) do you plan to focus on in your study?
   c. Write a paragraph explaining the rationale for this study.
2. **Write a research proposal that includes the following titled subsections in the order listed:**

   Title Page (to include your proposal title, your name, and the submission date)

   ABSTRACT

   SPECIFIC AIMS

   BACKGROUND AND SIGNIFICANCE

   RESEARCH DESIGN AND METHODS

       Participants
       General Procedures
       Statistical Analysis
       Limitations
   LITERATURE CITED

IN-CLASS GROUP EXERCISES

1. **Working in a small group, write a researchable problem statement for each of the following general research questions:**

   a. What motivates people to regularly work out at health clubs?
   b. What are the most common barriers to successful student teaching in health and physical education?
   c. Which exercises are most effective in addressing maltracking of the patella?
   d. Is there a relationship between dehydration and prerace hydration level prior to a marathon?
   e. Are there important differences between treadmill running and overground running?

2. **For each of the problem statements your group has written, write two different research hypotheses.**

3. **For each of the problem statements your group has written, write a brief outline for a rationale for a hypothetical study.**

5

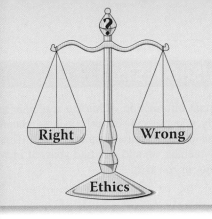

Right | Wrong

Ethics

Understanding Research Ethics

"Always do right—this will gratify some and astonish the rest."—Mark Twain

CHAPTER OBJECTIVES

After studying this chapter, you will be able to:

1. Explain what constitutes plagiarism and how to avoid it.
2. Describe the appropriate range of measures for dealing with data outliers.
3. Properly handle and store research data in accordance with federal regulations.
4. Construct documents of informed consent and assent that comply with federal regulations.
5. Engage in an informed way in discussion of appropriate authorship on research manuscripts.
6. Make ethically informed decisions on other topics often confronting students.

■ THE field of ethics, also known as moral philosophy, is a major branch of philosophy, and there are philosophers who specialize in fields such as medical and research ethics. Accordingly, it would be a vast overgeneralization to suggest that ethics is as simplistic as being about right versus wrong. In this chapter, the focus is on a range of ethical issues that students may encounter as part of the research process, as well as in navigating the path through school and career decisions. Being informed about these issues is the first step in enabling smart, as well as ethical, decision making.

ACADEMIC DISHONESTY

Any misrepresentation or nonreporting of important information within the academic setting can be characterized as academic dishonesty. Interestingly, many specific ethical concerns related to academic dishonesty are pertinent issues not just for students but for faculty members as well. This underscores the advisability of seeking advice from a faculty member should you find yourself in what you perceive to be an ethical dilemma related to academics or research.

Plagiarism

Plagiarism Presenting words, drawings, or ideas of someone else as though they were your own.

Plagiarism is the dishonest act of presenting intellectual property, including a piece of writing, a drawing, or an idea, that originated with someone else as if it had originated with you. In the United States, the copyright law protects most published writings, making plagiarism not only unethical but illegal. Unfortunately, the ready availability of writings on a multitude of topics on the Internet has made opportunities for plagiarism more plentiful and inviting. At the same time, penalties to students for commission of plagiarism on an assignment such as a term paper can range from a reduction in the grade on the paper to dismissal from the institution, depending on the circumstances. Plagiarism in a published research paper can ruin the career of an academician, leading to termination of employment and permanent stigma. Yet within the realm of research, we are continually referring to and trying to build upon knowledge that has originated through the published work of other investigators. It is therefore critically important that students develop a clear understanding of the difference between plagiarism and properly citing the work of others.

As with most legal and ethical issues, ignorance of what constitutes plagiarism and commission of plagiarism through laziness or sloppiness are not deemed valid excuses for committing it. This translates to two important points for students. First, it is necessary to carefully keep track of which references are associated with which ideas and concepts if you are taking notes or otherwise storing information to be used later. Second, you must be careful with selection of wording in your own writing, such that you do not present something advocated by the authors of a published paper as your own thought. For example, a paper recently published in *Medicine and Science in Sports and Exercise* by Yang et al.[1] ends with the statement, "Individuals should be encouraged to participate in regular physical activity as early as possible to prevent the risk of developing metabolic syndrome and related adult-onset diabetes and cardiovascular diseases." If you wanted to express this same concept in your own writing, it would be necessary to cite Yang et al.

Paraphrasing Restating in your own words.

It is important to read a source before citing it, rather than trusting that it has been accurately represented when cited by someone else.

As discussed in Chapter 2, however, it is usually best to avoid direct quotations, lest your own paper end up awkwardly reading as a disjointed series of statements made by others. **Paraphrasing** is the act of restating someone else's words in your own words. It requires changing both the keywords used and the sentence structure, without changing the content. Referring back to the quotation from the paper by Yang et al.,[1] an appropriate paraphrase might be "According to Yang et al., the risk of cardiovascular health deficits later in life can be minimized by early participation in regular exercise."[1] Note that it is still necessary to cite the source, even though you are paraphrasing the words used in the original source. Here is another example. Valiante and Morris published a paper on the sources of self-efficacy among male professional golfers in which they reported "enactive mastery experiences were the most powerful source of self-efficacy."[2] Appropriate paraphrasing of this finding might be written as "Valiante and Morris determined that the primary source of feelings of self-efficacy among male professional golfers was previous experience of masterful play."[2] Notice that in both of these examples, the content of the sentence is reworded, although it is okay to reuse a technical term such as *self-efficacy*. Notice also that the authors of the study being referenced are both mentioned by name and cited. If you are not already proficient at paraphrasing and citing sources, these will be important skills for you to develop as early as possible as a college or university student. Many universities have writing centers where students can go for assistance with learning how to develop skill in paraphrasing and otherwise avoid plagiarism.

The topic of paraphrasing brings up another cautionary note for students. When researchers paraphrase the findings of other researchers in a published paper, they occasionally misrepresent the original findings or do not present the original findings in their entirety. This underscores the importance of reading the entire original source—not just the abstract—if you intend to cite it. You will appear to be sloppy and possibly even foolish if you perpetuate a misinterpretation of a published source. Always remember that the publication of a paper does not guarantee that all statements made by the authors are correct or true.

You may wonder under what circumstances it is *not* necessary to cite a published paper for something you want to write about. The general rule is that anything regarded as "common knowledge" does not need to be cited. For example, today we regard the notion that smoking cigarettes is unhealthy to be common knowledge. Historically, of course, this was not always the case. However, after hundreds of studies showing links between cigarette smoking and multiple forms of cancer and other negative health consequences, we now regard this as common knowledge. If you are not sure whether you can properly label something as "common knowledge," it is always safest to find a citation for it.

✔ Check Your Understanding

1. Using your own words, define *plagiarism*.
2. Why is paraphrasing preferable to always quoting directly from the source?
3. Under what circumstances is it *not* necessary to cite the research literature in your own writing?

Data Management

At many universities, there is an expectation that faculty members will engage in an active program of research or scholarship that results in publication of papers contributing to the knowledge base in peer-reviewed journals. Unfortunately, some professors have succumbed to the temptation to falsify or fabricate data to enhance their publication records. In November of 2005, Luk Van Parijs, a faculty member described as "a rising star" in the Department of Biology at the Massachusetts Institute of Technology (MIT), was dismissed from the university in disgrace following his admission that he had fabricated and falsified data in grant applications, submitted manuscripts, and one published paper.[3] Not only is falsifying data dishonest but the consequences of being discovered make it a risk not worth taking—not for a faculty member and not for a student. This is not an ethical, honest, or *smart* thing to contemplate, and in many cases, discovery of such an act at the graduate student level would result in nonconferral of your degree.

Another related ethical question regarding data management has to do with appropriate handling of outliers. An **outlier** is a measurement or observation that is way out of line with the rest of the data set. Outliers can result from a transient malfunction of data collection apparatus, a "bug" in software, or from collection of data on a participant who has characteristics that are markedly different in some way from the other participants. It is

> **Outlier** A datum that is sufficiently different from the rest of the data set to arouse suspicion as to its validity.

important to look over your data set as you are collecting it so that you are alerted to any outliers, particularly if they may indicate a calibration issue or other problem with the apparatus you are using. If there were a hardware or software problem during data collection for a particular participant, it would unquestionably be appropriate to discard the faulty data, make sure everything is working properly, and ask the participant to be retested. Similarly, if a participant was not feeling well or was unable to meet the inclusion criteria for the study on a particular day, it would be appropriate to discard the faulty data and ask the participant to be retested. An example of inappropriate data management, however, would be scanning the data set for values that simply do not support your research hypothesis, labeling those values "outliers," and discarding them. It is useful to keep in mind that sometimes it is the results that you did not expect that turn out to be the most interesting and also publishable.

You should also be aware that, increasingly, there are federal regulations governing the storage and management of data collected on human participants, particularly when the data are health related. The Health Insurance Portability and Accountability Act (HIPAA), signed into law in 1996, regulates the ways in which **protected health information** (PHI) can be stored and utilized. PHI is any information related to the past, present, or future health of an individual. Many studies in kinesiology and the health sciences rely on such information either for screening purposes or as a primary data source. Researchers may access PHI legally following a participant sign off on an authorization form that includes the required HIPAA authorization language. Alternatively, researchers can use PHI that has been deidentified in blinded studies such that the researcher is not aware of which information is associated with a particular participant while collecting data. Use of personal nonpublic information (PNPI), such as social security numbers, is also federally regulated. Such information should not be used for participant identification. Beyond HIPAA and PNPI issues, most institutions require that the original data set be stored in a secure location for a minimum of 3 years following completion of the work/publication.

Protected Health Information Information pertaining to past, current, or future health of an individual; regarded as confidential and protected by federal law.

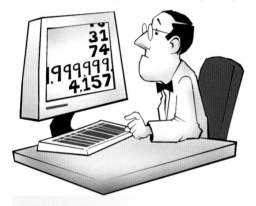

Too bad this data outlier isn't a deposit in my checking account!

✔ Check Your Understanding

1. Should all outliers be discarded? Explain why or why not.
2. Define and briefly explain HIPAA, PHI, and PNPI.

PROTECTION OF PARTICIPANTS

As mentioned in Chapter 4, in the United States, every college or university, hospital, and research institute at which investigators engage in research on human participants must have an institutional review board (IRB) that is responsible for reviewing all research proposals involving human participants. The Code of Federal Regulations administered by the U.S. Department of Health and Human Services[4] mandates the role of the IRB. This code, referred to as 45CFR46,[4] also requires training for the protection of human participants in research for all researchers (faculty, students, staff) who will be directly interacting with research participants or who will have access to identifiable private information. Before you will be allowed to be involved in research including human subjects, you will need to have completed such a training session. Most universities offer these online as well as in live formats.

It is wise to decide who will be included as co-authors on a paper early in the research process.

The criteria established in the United States for IRB approval of research proposals include the following (as adapted from Title 45 Public Welfare, Part 46 Protection of Human Participants, from the Code of Federal Regulations[4]):

1. Risks to participants are minimized by using procedures that are consistent with sound research design and that do not unnecessarily expose participants to risk.

2. Risks to participants are reasonable in relation to anticipated benefits, if any, to participants, and the importance of the knowledge that may reasonably be expected to result.

3. Selection of participants is equitable. In making this assessment, the IRB should take into account the purposes of the research and the setting in which the research will be conducted and should be particularly cognizant of the special problems of research involving vulnerable populations, such as children, prisoners, pregnant women, mentally disabled persons, or economically or educationally disadvantaged persons.

4. Informed consent will be sought from each prospective participant or the participant's legally authorized representative.

5. Informed consent will be appropriately documented.

6. The research plan makes adequate provision for monitoring the data collected to ensure the safety of participants.

7. There are adequate provisions to protect the privacy of participants and to maintain the confidentiality of data.

Items 1 and 2 refer to the risks and benefits to the participants in a study. There are two separate, though related, concepts here. The first is that the researchers should plan in every way practically possible to minimize any risks to participants participating in a study. This translates to ensuring that data collection conditions are as safe as possible and that the likelihood of injury to participants is minimal. This requires knowledge on the part of the investigators about any special concerns or needs associated with special populations such as children, the elderly, or those with medically diagnosed conditions. In the case of training interventions, it also requires knowledge of sound exercise durations and loading increments. You do not want to plan a training protocol that will result in so many injuries that you lose many of your participants.

The second concept is known as the **risk/benefit ratio**. Simply stated, any known or potential risks incurred by participants by virtue of participation in a study should not outweigh any benefits for the participants. A single serious risk is not likely to be outweighed by any number of perceived benefits. Benefits to participants may include monetary compensation or gifts, particularly in studies where participants must be tested for a lengthy period or on several different occasions, or must travel a distance to come in to be tested. College student participants, alternatively, may be willing to participate in a study without compensation because they are interested in the project or wish to learn more about the research process. The risk/benefit ratio is an important consideration when an IRB deliberates whether to approve a proposed research investigation. Known or potential risks to participants are taken very seriously, and if such risks cannot be well managed, a proposed study is not likely to be approved.

> **Risk/Benefit Ratio** Weighted analysis of the risks associated with participation in a research study in relation to the benefits of participation.

Item 3 is designed to ensure that the participant population has been selected because it is the most appropriate population for participation, given the research problem being studied. There have been unfortunate cases in the past where researchers used prisoners for medical experiments, not because they were especially appropriate as participants but because they had no ability to object to the treatments. Suffice it to say, this egregiously unethical behavior on the part of researchers is part of the reason that today we have federal and international standards for protection of human participants in research.

✔ Check Your Understanding

1. Explain the risk/benefit ratio.
2. Why is the selection of a particular population type for a study an ethical issue?

Informed Consent

Items 4 and 5 refer to the concept of **informed consent**. Generally speaking, informed consent means that each participant is fully apprised about what they will be expected to do if participating in a study and, being fully informed, gives his or her consent to participate. As adapted from the U.S. Code of Federal Regulations,[4] the elements of informed consent stipulate that the following information shall be provided to each participant:

1. A statement that the study involves research, an explanation of the purposes of the research and the expected duration of the participant's participation, a description of the procedures to be followed, and an identification of any procedures that are experimental
2. A description of any reasonably foreseeable risks or discomforts to the participant
3. A description of any benefits to the participant or to others that may reasonably be expected from the research
4. A statement describing the procedures by which confidentiality of records identifying the participant will be maintained
5. For research involving more than minimal risk, an explanation as to whether any compensation and an explanation as to whether any medical treatments are available if injury occurs and, if so, what they consist of or where further information may be obtained
6. An explanation of whom to contact for answers to pertinent questions about the research and research participants' rights and whom to contact in the event of a research-related injury to the participant
7. A statement that participation is voluntary, refusal to participate will involve no penalty or loss of benefits to which the participant is otherwise entitled, and the participant may discontinue participation at any time without penalty or loss of benefits to which the participant is otherwise entitled
8. Anticipated circumstances under which the participant's participation may be terminated by the investigator without regard to the participant's consent
9. The approximate number of participants involved in the study

Although all of these elements of informed consent must appear in the form to be signed by participants prior to a study, the wording of each element is specific to what participants will actually be doing in the study. Moreover, the language used in informed consent forms must be lay language that will be readily understandable by the participants (as a rule of thumb, write at an 8th grade level). Copying the technical language directly from the methods section of the research proposal is therefore not appropriate for describing the research on an informed consent form. Although the informed consent form is signed by the participant and the investigator, it is not a legal document, and the formatting requirements vary from institution to institution. Special Interest Box 5.1 shows an informed consent form used in a Ph.D. dissertation study at the University of Delaware.

✔ Check Your Understanding

1. List at least five elements of informed consent.
2. Who can make the decision to terminate a participant's participation in a study?

Protection of Minor Participants

When the participants in a study will be children under the age of 18 years, an informed consent form must be developed for signature by each participant's parent or legal guardian. Additionally, a separate

SPECIAL INTEREST BOX 5.1

Sample Informed Consent Form

(Provided courtesy of University of Delaware Ph.D. student Kat Arbour.)

INFORMED CONSENT FORM

"How Jump Type, Repetitive Jumping, and Muscular Strength Affect Tibial Shock
in Takeoff and Landing Legs of Competitive Skaters"

Kat Arbour, MS, MPT, CSCS, Michelle Provost-Craig, PhD and Todd Royer, PhD
Department of Health, Nutrition, and Exercise Sciences, University of Delaware

1. PURPOSE/DESCRIPTION OF THE RESEARCH

The purpose of this research is to measure the relationship between jumping impact of takeoff and landings, leg muscle strength, and your ability to jump when exerting yourself, similar to when you are doing your program. The first step is to measure on-ice jump impact in five (5) participants between the ages of 10 and 25 in a separate pilot study. You will be one of these 5 participants. After this portion is completed, you may volunteer to participate in the full study. If you agree to do so, you will be one of approximately 30 participants between the ages of 10 and 25 who are participating in this study. To participate, you need to be a figure skater able to consistently land jumps through double axel and at least one triple jump. You are not eligible for the study if you have been injured in the last 6 months or cannot land a double axel and at least one triple jump on most days. You will be asked to fill out a Skating and Training History Questionnaire including some questions about your height, width, and weight.

The pilot study will consist of one meeting on the ice and is described below in "Day 1 Data Collection." The full study will consist of three total meetings. Two will take place on the ice, the first lasting up to 1 hour and the second up to 30 minutes. The fee for ice time will be covered for you. The first on-ice session will measure the impact of the various jumps you are able to land consistently. The second on-ice session, on a separate day, will measure 10 jump impacts while working at a high intensity similar to a run through of your program. The goal is to complete a jumping pass every 30 seconds and stroke to a preset tempo in between jumps, for about 5 minutes. The final meeting will be in the Human Performance Lab behind the Fred Rust Arena to measure the strength in your legs and will take less than 45 minutes.

Equipment will be taped directly to the skin on your shins, which will need to be clean-shaven. You should wear skating pants or footless tights for the on-ice testing and comfortable clothing for the off-ice testing session. Your participation is entirely voluntary. If you decide at any point that you do not wish to continue, you may withdraw from the study without penalty.

Day 1 Data Collection: Measuring On-Ice Jump Impact (Approximately 1 Hour)

A small measuring device (19 × 13 × 11 mm) weighing about one-third on an ounce (10 g) will be taped to each of your shins, and a wire will connect each device to a small 13-oz computer that will be worn on your lower back. The shin will be shaved prior to the attachment of the measuring device. For this reason, you will need to wear skating pants or footless tights for your on-ice sessions to cover the wires connecting the measuring device on your shins to the small computer on your back. The measuring device records the fast motion in the legs (acceleration) associated with jump takeoffs and landings.

You will be asked to warm up and get used to the equipment for up to 15 minutes, and then, when you feel comfortable, you will start jumping. The order of the jumps will be

(Continued)

chosen at random by pulling numbers out of a bag. Each number will correspond to a different jump type and revolution, such as single toe-loop or triple salchow. If you miss a jump you can usually land, you will have up to five attempts to land it. In addition, jumps will be videotaped to aid analysis of the acceleration data. If at any time during the testing you feel that you need to rest, you may do so until you feel ready to continue.

Day 2 Data Collection: The Effect of Jump Repetition on Jump Impact

The equipment setup is exactly the same as is in the first meeting, as described above. In addition, you will also wear a heart rate monitor to record heart rate during the testing. You will need to wear skating pants or footless tights for your on-ice sessions to cover the wires connecting the measuring device on your shins to the small computer on your back. Once you get used to the equipment again, then testing can begin. The test setup and warm-up will take about 20 minutes, and the on-ice test will take 5 minutes.

You will be asked to complete stroking at a preset tempo and a double axel jumping pass every 30 seconds for 10 jumps while working at an intensity similar to a run through. You will be asked how hard you feel you are working, on a scale of 1 to 10, after every other jump. You will be encouraged to continue the test at a high exercise intensity. However, if you need to stop due to pain, injury, illness, or for any reason, you should do so. If you do stop, it will not be possible for you to resume the testing, and you will not participate in any further study activities.

Day 3 Data Collection: Isokinetic Strength Testing and 30-Second Jump Test (45 Minutes)

You will come to the Human Performance Lab to measure the strength in your legs. Lower body strength is measured on a Biodex machine that is similar to standard equipment in any gym and is connected to a computer. You will be seat-belted into the chair and asked to bend or straighten your knee with your greatest effort for three repetitions, and then the test is repeated on the opposite leg. You can stop the test at any time for any reason. Throughout the test, you will be holding the kill switch that will shut down the equipment immediately if you press the button. After strength testing, you will complete the 30-second jump test. The goal of the test is to jump as high as possible as many times as able in 30 seconds.

2. CONDITIONS OF PARTICIPANT PARTICIPATION

The results from your tests will be kept confidential. All data will be stored either as password-protected computer files or as paper documents that will be kept in a locked cabinet. The videocassettes will also be kept in a locked file cabinet. All data and videos will be kept indefinitely. Your own results and the group averages will be returned to you. It will not be shared with your coach. All published results will be reported as group data; participants will not be individually identified in any resulting publication. Should an injury occur during testing procedures, you will receive first aid. You will be responsible for the cost of any further medical treatment if required. You may withdraw from the study at any time without penalty.

3. RISKS AND BENEFITS

There is a chance that you could be injured while completing the jumps or during stroking. Minor skin irritation from the tape adhesive may occur as the result of sensitivity to the adhesive. The strength testing may cause immediate or delayed onset muscle soreness.

There are several benefits to participating in the study. For the pilot study, your jumps will be ranked from lowest to highest impact, allowing you to know how much more or less impact one jump delivers compared to your other jumps. If you participate in the full study, after it is completed, you will receive the group averages for each of the different jumps, muscle strength testing, and muscular endurance testing. In addition, you will receive the results of your own jump impacts, muscle strength test, and muscular endurance test. You will also learn how your jump impact changes as you tire while doing a mock program.

4. FINANCIAL CONSIDERATIONS

You will not be compensated for your time or participation.

5. CONTACTS

If you have any questions about the research study, you may contact Kat Arbour (302) 456-2000 (Primary Researcher) or Dr. Shelley Provost-Craig (302) 789-1000 or Dr. Todd Royer (302) 234-5678, Associate Professors, Department of Health, Nutrition, and Exercise Sciences. If you have questions regarding the rights of individuals who agree to participate in this research, you may call the chair of the University of Delaware Human Participants Review Board (302) 456-3000.

6. PARTICIPANT'S ASSURANCES

I have read the above informed consent document. The nature, demands, risks, and benefits have been explained to me. I knowingly assume the risks involved. I understand that my participation is completely voluntary and that I may withdraw my consent and discontinue my participation at any time without penalty or loss of benefit to myself. A copy of this consent form has been given to me.

7. CONSENT SIGNATURES

I have read and understand the procedures and the instructions outlined in the attached informed consent form, which describes the current study. Questions concerning these procedures have been answered to my satisfaction. I understand that I am free to withdraw from the study at anytime and that I can decline to answer any question or questions during the evaluation process without penalty or prejudice to me.

I understand that if I am injured in any way while participating in this study, immediate onsite first aid will be provided. In addition, if I require additional medical treatment, then I will be solely responsible for the costs incurred. Neither the investigator nor the University of Delaware will be responsible for additional medical costs incurred by me due to participation in this research study.

_____

Signature of Participant   Date

I certify that I have explained to the above individual the nature and purpose, the potential benefits, and possible risks associated with participation in this research study; have answered any questions that have been raised; and have witnessed the above signature. I have provided the participant with a copy of this informed consent document.

_____

Signature of Investigator   Date

_____ Yes, my contact information may be kept on file so that I can be contacted for future research studies.

_____ No, my contact information may not be kept on file. Please do not contact me for future research studies.

Participant's initials/Date _____   Investigator's initials/Date _____

Assent Form Document explaining the requirements, risks, and benefits of participation in a research study in language appropriate for child participants.

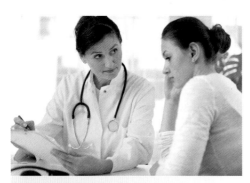

Researchers should carefully explain informed consent forms and offer to answer any questions.

form, called an **assent form**, must be developed for signature by each child participant. Whereas the informed consent form should be written using appropriate lay language for adults, depending on the age range of the child participants, the language on the assent form may need to be simplified further. When researching young children who have limited or no ability to read, researchers may need to read the assent form to them. Young children may not be able to sign the form, either, so a check box may be substituted. Special Interest Box 5.2 includes an assent form for child participants in a study, and Special Interest Box 5.3 shows the corresponding required informed consent form for the parent or guardian of a child participant.

✔ Check Your Understanding

1. Should the protocol section of a research proposal be used on the informed consent form to describe to a potential participant what he or she will be expected to do? Explain why or why not.

2. What is the difference between *informed consent* and *informed assent*?

Protection of Animal Subjects

Just as federal and institutional policies exist for protection of human participants, so do standards for the protection and humane treatment of animals used as research subjects. The Guide for the Care and Use of Laboratory Animals,[5] published by the National Academy of Sciences, advocates the following:

1. Design and performance of procedures on the basis of relevance to human or animal health, advancement of knowledge, or the good of society
2. Use of appropriate species, quality, and number of animals
3. Avoidance or minimization of discomfort, distress, and pain in concert with sound science
4. Use of appropriate sedation, analgesia, or anesthesia
5. Establishment of experimental end points
6. Provision of appropriate animal husbandry directed and performed by qualified persons
7. Conduct of experimentation on living animals only by or under the close supervision of qualified and experienced persons

Many universities have an Animal Subjects Protection Committee assigned the responsibility of reviewing all research proposals within the institution that involve animal subjects.

✔ Check Your Understanding

Using your own words, list at least three standards for appropriate use and care of animals used in research studies.

SPECIAL INTEREST BOX 5.2

Sample Assent Form

(Provided courtesy of University of Delaware Ph.D. student Kat Arbour.)

"How Jump Type, Repetitive Jumping, and Muscular Strength Affect Tibial Shock in Takeoff and Landing Legs of Competitive Skaters"

Kat Arbour, MS, MPT, CSCS, Michelle Provost-Craig, PhD and Todd Royer, PhD

Department of Health, Nutrition, and Exercise Sciences, University of Delaware

1. PURPOSE/DESCRIPTION OF THE RESEARCH

Kat Arbour is going to measure how hard my skates hit the ice on the takeoffs and landings of various jumps.

I will be asked questions about how often I skate and train. After this, measuring devices will be taped to my shins, and a small computer pack will be worn in a backpack. Next, I will get my skates on stroke around the ice to get used to wearing the equipment. When I feel comfortable, I will continue my warm-up with some single jumps. After about 15 minutes, I will start to practice the various jumps that I can land consistently. My jumps will be video-taped during the testing session.

On a separate day, I will wear the same equipment and complete the on-ice warm-up. This time, I will attempt a jump every 30 seconds for 5 minutes, similar to a program run through.

Finally, on the third day, I will complete an off-ice leg strength test and a jump test.

2. CONDITIONS OF PARTICIPANT PARTICIPATION

I am volunteering for the study. I can quit the study whenever I want to.

3. RISKS AND BENEFITS

I understand that I will be asked to skate with my best effort, but if I get too tired while skating during the first day of testing, I should stop to take a break and rest. I also understand that if I stop on the second day of testing during the 5-minute task, it will not be possible to restart the test.

4. CONTACTS

If I have any questions about the research study, I may contact Kat Arbour (302) 456-2000 (Primary Researcher) or Dr. Shelley Provost-Craig (302) 789-1000 or Dr. Todd Royer (302) 234-5678, Associate Professors, Department of Health, Nutrition, and Exercise Sciences. If I have questions regarding the rights of individuals who agree to participate in this research, I may call the chair of the University of Delaware Human Participants Review Board (302) 456-3000 and Review Board (302) 831-2136.

5. PARTICIPANT'S ASSURANCES

I understand the activities I will do in this study. I may ask questions at any time. I may quit the study at any time. A copy of this assent form has been given to me.

6. ASSENT SIGNATURES

Participant Signature: _____   Date: _____

I certify that I have explained to the above individual the nature and purpose, the potential benefits, and possible risks associated with participation in this research study; have answered any questions that have been raised; and have witnessed the above signature. I have provided the participant with a copy of this informed consent document.

Signature of Investigator: _____   Date: _____

SPECIAL INTEREST BOX 5.3

Sample Informed Consent Form for a Parent or Guardian

(Provided courtesy of University of Delaware Ph.D. student Kat Arbour.)

PARENT/LEGAL GUARDIAN INFORMED CONSENT FORM

"How Jump Type, Repetitive Jumping, and Muscular Strength Affect Tibial Shock in Takeoff and Landing Legs of Competitive Skaters"

Kat Arbour, MS, MPT, CSCS, Michelle Provost-Craig, PhD and Todd Royer, PhD
Department of Health, Nutrition, and Exercise Sciences, University of Delaware

As the parent or legal guardian, please read the following material to make sure that you are informed of the nature of this research study and how your child or the child you are responsible for will participate. For the remainder of this document, if you are the legal guardian, the child that you are responsible for will simply be referred to as your child. Signing this form will indicate that you understand what the study entails and that you have decided to allow your child to participate in this study at the Fred Rust Ice Arena and at the University's Human Performance Lab.

The University of Delaware is conducting research examining the relationships that exist between jump impact on takeoff and landings; jumping ability with physical exertion, similar to when your child is doing his or her program; and leg muscle strength. The current study described in this consent form will provide new knowledge about which jumps place the most stress on the skater and will assist skaters and coaches in identifying what may be a safe number of jumps to perform daily, during a growth spurt or while recovering from an injury.

1. PURPOSE/DESCRIPTION OF THE RESEARCH

The purpose of this research is to measure the relationship between jumping impact of takeoff and landings, leg muscle strength, and jumping ability with physical exertion, similar to when your child is doing his or her program. The first step is to measure on-ice jump impact in five (5) participants between the ages of 10 and 25. Your child will be one of these five participants. After this portion is completed, your child may volunteer to participate in the full study. If you agree to do so, your child will be one of approximately 30 participants between the ages of 10 and 25 who are participating in this study. To participate, your child needs to be a figure skater able to consistently land jumps through double axel and is working on at least one triple jump. Your child is not eligible for the study if he or she has been injured in the last 6 months or cannot land a double axel and at least one triple jump on most days. Your child will be asked to fill out a Skating and Training History Questionnaire including some questions about your child's height, width, and weight; you may assist with this.

The pilot study will consist of one meeting on the ice and is described below in "Day 1 Data Collection." The full study will consist of three total meetings. Two will take place on the ice, the first lasting up to 1 hour and the second up to 30 minutes. The fee for ice time will be covered through the research project. The first on-ice session will measure the impact of the various jumps your child is able to land consistently. The second on-ice session, on a separate day, will measure ten jump impacts while working at a high intensity similar to a program run through. The goal is to complete a jumping pass every 30 seconds and stroke to a preset tempo in between jumps for about 5 minutes. The final meeting will be in the Human Performance Lab behind the Fred Rust Arena to measure lower body strength and power and will take less than 45 minutes.

Equipment will be taped directly to the skin on the shins, which will need to be clean-shaven. Have your child wear skating pants or footless tights for the on-ice testing and comfortable clothing for the off-ice testing session. Your child's participation is entirely voluntary. If you or your child decides at any point to not continue, you may withdraw from the study without penalty.

Day 1 Data Collection: Measuring On-Ice Jump Impact (Approximately 1 Hour)

A small measuring device (19 × 13 × 11 mm) weighing about one-third on an ounce (10 g) will be taped to each shin, and a wire taped to the leg will connect each device to a small 13-oz computer that will be worn on the lower back. The shin will be shaved prior to the attachment of the tibial accelerometer. For this reason, your child will need to wear skating pants or footless tights for the on-ice sessions to cover the wires connecting the measuring device taped to the shins to the small computer on the back. The measuring device records the fast motion in the legs (acceleration) associated with jump takeoffs and landings.

Your child will be asked to warm up and get used to the equipment for up to 15 minutes, and then, when your child feel comfortable, he or she will start jumping. The order of the jumps will be chosen at random by pulling numbers out of a bag. Each number will correspond to a different jump type and revolution, such as single toe-loop or triple salchow. Skaters are given up to five attempts to land a jump before moving on to the next jump. In addition, jumps will be videotaped to aid analysis of the acceleration data. If at any time during the testing your child feels the need to rest, he or she may do so until he or she feels ready to continue.

Day 2 Data Collection: The Effect of Jump Repetition on Jump Impact

The equipment setup is exactly the same as in the first meeting, as described above. In addition, the skater will also wear a heart rate monitor to record heart rate during the testing. Your child will need to wear skating pants or footless tights for the on-ice sessions to cover the wires connecting the measuring device on the shins to the small computer on the back. Once the skater gets used to the equipment again, then testing can begin. The test setup and warm-up will take about 20 minutes, and the on-ice test will take 5 minutes.

Your child will be asked to complete stroking and a double axel jumping pass every 30 seconds for 10 jumps while working at an intensity similar to a run through. Your child will be encouraged to continue the test at a high exercise intensity. However, if the skater needs to stop due to pain, injury, illness, or for any reason, the skater should do so. If the skater stops, it will not be possible to resume the testing, and your child will not participate in any further study activities.

Day 3 Data Collection: Isokinetic Strength Testing and 30-Second Jump Test (45 Minutes)

Your child will come to the Human Performance Lab to measure lower body strength. Lower body strength is measured on a Biodex machine that is similar to standard equipment in any gym and connected to a computer. Your child will be seat-belted into the chair and asked to bend or straighten one knee for three repetitions, and then the test is repeated on the opposite leg. Your child can stop the test at any time for any reason. Throughout the test, your child will be holding the kill switch that will shut down the equipment immediately by simply pressing the button on the kill switch. After strength testing, your child will complete the 30-second jump test. The goal of the test is to jump as high as possible as many times as able in 30 seconds.

(*Continued*)

SPECIAL INTEREST BOX 5.3 *(Continued)*

2. CONDITIONS OF PARTICIPANT PARTICIPATION

The results from your child's tests will be kept confidential. All data will be stored either as password-protected computer files or as paper documents that will be kept in a locked cabinet. The videocassettes will also be kept in a locked file cabinet. All data and videos will be kept indefinitely. Your child's results and the group averages will be returned to you and your child. It will not be shared with the skater's coach. All published results will be reported as group data; participants will not be individually identified in any resulting publication.

Should an injury occur during testing procedures, your child will receive first aid. You will be responsible for the cost of any further medical treatment if required. You may withdraw from the study at any time without penalty.

3. RISKS AND BENEFITS

There is a chance that your child could be injured while completing the jumps or stroking. Minor skin irritation from the tape adhesive may occur as the result of sensitivity to the adhesive. The strength testing may cause immediate or delayed onset muscle soreness.

There are several benefits to participating in the study. For the pilot study, your child's jumps will be ranked from lowest to highest impact, so that it can be determined how much more or less impact one jump delivers compared to the other jumps. If your child participates in the full study, after it is completed, you and your child will receive the group averages for each of the different jumps, muscle strength testing, and muscular endurance testing. In addition, you and your child will receive the results of his or her own jump impacts, muscle strength test, and muscular endurance test. Your child will also learn how jump impact changes as he or she tires while doing a mock program.

4. FINANCIAL CONSIDERATIONS

You or your child will not be compensated for the time or participation.

5. Contacts

If you have any questions about the research study, you may contact Kat Arbour (302) 456-2000 (Primary Researcher) or Dr. Shelley Provost-Craig (302) 789-1000 or Dr. Todd Royer (302) 234-5678, Associate Professors, Department of Health, Nutrition, and Exercise Sciences. If you have questions regarding the rights of individuals who agree to participate in this research, you may call the chair of the University of Delaware Human Participants Review Board (302) 456-3000.

6. PARTICIPANT'S ASSURANCES

I have read the above informed consent document. The nature, demands, risks, and benefits have been explained to me. I knowingly assume the risks involved. I understand that my child's participation is completely voluntary, and that my child or I may withdraw consent and discontinue participation at any time without penalty or loss of benefit to my child or myself. A copy of this consent form has been given to me.

7. CONSENT SIGNATURES

I have read and understand the procedures and the instructions outlined in the attached informed consent form, which describes the current study. Questions concerning these procedures have been answered to my satisfaction. I understand that my child is free to withdraw from the study at anytime and that my child can decline to answer any question or questions during the evaluation process without penalty or prejudice to my child or me.

SPECIAL INTEREST BOX 5.3 (*Continued*)

I understand that if my child is injured in any way while participating in this study, immediate onsite first aid will be provided. In addition, if my child requires additional medical treatment, then I will be solely responsible for the costs incurred. Neither the investigator nor the University of Delaware will be responsible for additional medical costs incurred by me due to participation in this research study.

Signature of Parent/Guardian (if participant under 18)   Date

I certify that I have explained to the above individual the nature and purpose, the potential benefits, and possible risks associated with participation in this research study; have answered any questions that have been raised; and have witnessed the above signature. I have provided the participant with a copy of this informed consent document.

Signature of Investigator   Date

ETHICAL CONSIDERATIONS WITH OTHER ISSUES

Students must make a number of decisions in navigating through educational programs and subsequent careers, and it is useful to have an understanding of the ethical implications associated with some of these types of decisions. Some of the issues you may encounter in working with a faculty advisor at the undergraduate or graduate levels may be similar to issues you will encounter after starting a career in your field of interest. Similarly, there may be ethical issues associated with choosing a graduate program or a job.

Authorship

As a student, you have probably not given much thought to the authorship of published research papers, including the order of the authors listed on a given paper, and not to mention who gets named as an "author" on the paper in the first place. However, since the ultimate goal for all quality research, including theses and especially dissertations, is publication in an appropriate scientific or professional journal, this may become of personal interest to you. In many established labs or other working research environments, there are understandings regarding who will be listed as authors and in what order they will be listed on papers. In the absence of this, however, communication regarding authorship and ordering of authorship is important, and the ideal time for this understanding to take place is during the planning stages of a project and, in all cases, before the research group submits a manuscript to a journal. Why is this an issue? Within academia, more credit is ascribed to first, or senior, authors on research papers than to coauthors. Typically, the first listed author had the underlying idea for the study and who was most instrumental in getting the study conducted. Paradoxically, some fields and some labs list the senior author last. The only way to ascertain the senior author is by being familiar with the field or lab in question. Similarly, being listed as one of three or four coauthors on a paper carries more weight than being listed as one of 20 authors on a paper.

There are widely different philosophies regarding inclusivity of authors. The fact that papers have been published with 20 or more authors suggests that everyone who had anything to do with those projects was listed as a coauthor. More commonly, however, coauthors are those who were

Selection of a faculty advisor is one of the single most important decisions to be made by graduate students.

involved with planning the study, interpretation of the results, and the actual writing of the paper. Those serving as technicians to assist with data collection or as statistical consultants are not necessarily sufficiently involved to warrant authorship.

If you are interested in publishing your thesis in a scholarly journal (which, if at all possible, you should be—see Chapter 17), you should engage your advisor in a conversation about authorship, including who should be listed as coauthors on the paper and in what order. Many professors have standing policies that they will be first authors on theses, especially if they have provided the research problem, the overall direction, and the funding for the project. At other institutions, the expectation is that the student will be the first author on the master's thesis and that the faculty advisor will be listed as a coauthor. Whether members of your thesis committee are also listed as coauthors is a matter of how much each person may have contributed to the work, as well as the authorship philosophy of your advisor. On doctoral dissertations, the expectation is definitely that the student will have taken a leadership role with the project(s) and will be the lead author on the resulting publications.

✔ Check Your Understanding

Who all should be included as coauthors on a research paper?

Multiple Submissions

Another set of ethical issues related to authorship has to do with multiple submissions of the same work. If you want to get your thesis project published, it might seem like a good idea to send your manuscript out to several different journals at once and learn which one might accept it first. However, this is not only a bad idea but also a practice that would be viewed as unethical.

As described in Chapter 3, when a research manuscript is sent to a professional journal to be considered for publication, the manuscript usually goes out to three reviewers who have expertise specifically related to the paper topic. In this peer review process, the reviewers serve on a voluntary basis but devote a fair amount of time and work to the manuscript review. For this reason, it is not appropriate to send a manuscript for consideration to a second journal unless the first journal unequivocally rejects it. Once a paper has been accepted for publication in a journal, under no circumstances is it appropriate to try to publish the same work in a different journal, even if the manuscript is rewritten with a different emphasis. A study in which several dependent variables are measured on the same participants is almost always best presented as a single publication (and/or conference presentation), rather than as two or more papers. A similar but different situation exists when a large, multifaceted study is undertaken that generates more data than can logically be packaged into a single paper. This is often the case for Ph.D. dissertations that encompass two to four related but separate studies. In such cases, the authors should clearly reference the related publications to clarify what linkages do and do not exist across the data sets.

✔ Check Your Understanding

1. Why is it unethical to submit a research manuscript to more than one journal at the same time?
2. When you have published one paper based on a given data set, why is it unethical to publish a second paper from the same data set with a different emphasis in a different journal?

Interacting with Your Faculty Advisor

The importance of one of your earliest decisions, selecting an appropriate graduate program and faculty advisor, cannot be understated. This is important at the master's level and crucial at the doctoral level. Keep in mind that many graduate programs will not accept a student unless a specific faculty member has agreed to advise them.

How can you identify the best professor to work with? Talk with faculty at your undergraduate institution, and ask whom they might recommend, given your interests and the geographical range within which you are willing to consider a graduate program. Internet resources (described in detail in Chapter 3) make it relatively quick and easy to search databases of published literature to find out which professors affiliated with which institutions are publishing work related to your interests. You can also go to university Web sites and usually learn who the faculty members are in a given department and what their research interests are. Attending professional conferences is also a very good way to meet faculty members and graduate students doing work in a given area of interest.

You should have a good understanding of your potential faculty advisor's research interests and make certain that you have compatible interests. An in-person interview with a potential faculty advisor is well worth the time and any expense involved. Indeed, many professors require the in-person interview before agreeing to accept a student. Prior to an interview, you should carefully review the graduate program course requirements on the university Web site. Going into the interview, be prepared to ask a number of questions that will make it clear what your life will be like if you are working with that professor. Here are some examples:

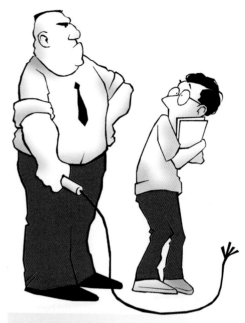

I should have been more careful in choosing an advisor...

- Aside from the graduate program requirements, does the professor have expectations for other courses you should take?
- What hours will you be expected to spend in the lab or the field?
- To what degree you will be supervised or expected to work independently?
- Will you be working with other faculty members or other graduate students on a routine basis?
- How can you expect to be spending your time during a typical day?
- How many other students is the professor supervising?

If you are being offered a graduate assistantship, there are additional questions to ask:
- What responsibilities are you expected to fulfill with the assistantship?
- For what period and under what conditions will your funding support continue?
- By what criteria your work will be judged?

Do your best to find out as much as you can about the culture of the department you will be a part of. Talking with current or recently graduated students who have worked with the same professor is an invaluable source of information. Finally, you should also keep in mind that the interview with a potential faculty advisor is a two-way street. You want to be well prepared and appropriately dressed for an interview with a potential advisor, or the professor may not wish to accept you as a graduate student.

So what if you find yourself in a situation where you realize that you have made a mistake or your interests or situation change and you are not pleased with the way things are going between you and your faculty advisor? You have a number of options. First, it is important not to make a hasty decision. If your interests are in line with the work you are doing but there seem to be personality issues, plan to have a courteous, objective conversation on a professional level with your advisor to express your concerns and seek resolution. It may also be a good idea to seek the advice of the department head, but only after you have spoken personally with your advisor. Alternatively, if you decide that you are not getting the education and experience that you wanted, you should make every effort to complete the work associated with any contract that you have signed, but give notice that you will not be continuing. If you think you want to switch and work with a different major professor either at the same institution or at a different one, you should be every bit as careful and cautious in your selection process as was previously described.

✔ Check Your Understanding

1. Why is it important to make a careful choice regarding a faculty member to work with as a graduate student?
2. What questions would you ask a prospective faculty advisor during an interview?

Interviewing for a Job

At some point, you are likely to be seeking employment. Once again, you may be faced with decisions for which there are ethical implications. You may find yourself in a situation where you have applied for several positions and you are invited to interview for more than one of these. Be sure to talk with your advisor and others about how to best prepare for professional interviews. In all cases, you should be going into an interview knowing what to expect in terms of the interview format and being well prepared to answer questions about yourself and your professional goals. If you are interviewing for a faculty position, you should be prepared to give an oral presentation explaining your research interests.

Suppose you find yourself in a situation where you have interviewed for three positions. You decide that you are definitely not interested in position A, you think position B has potential and would be acceptable, but the one you really hope to get is position C. Recognizing that employers A, B, and C have doubtlessly interviewed other candidates, you should realize that the courteous, professional (and ethical) thing to do is to consider sending a polite letter to employer A and withdrawing from the search process. Employer A will appreciate this because if they were seriously considering you for the position following the interview, they will now quickly be able to move on to consider their other candidates. Suppose you then receive a phone call with a job offer from employer B. The courteous, professional (and ethical) thing to do is to explain to employer B that you have also interviewed elsewhere (you need not specify where) and that whereas you are pleased to have B's offer, you would like some time to find out if you may also have an offer from "elsewhere" to consider. Employer B is likely to give you a period of time, which may be relatively short or not depending on their circumstances, within which to make a decision on their offer. Your next step is to politely check in with employer C, indicate that you have received a job offer from "elsewhere," and ask if C can provide an update on their search process. Employer C will be pleased to either let you know that (a) you are not being recommended for their position or (b) indicate that they remain interested in hiring you but have not yet completed their search process. All things considered, it is not a good idea to accept a job you really do not want if you have other prospects.

✔ Check Your Understanding

What things would you do to prepare for a job interview?

CHAPTER SUMMARY

- Plagiarism, or presenting the writing or ideas of someone else as though they were your own, is one example of unethical behavior.
- Other examples include willing falsification of data and intentional mishandling of outliers or data that are out of line with the rest of the data set.

- Federal regulations govern the handling and storage of data, protection of human participants, and protection of animal subjects, and it is imperative that students develop a good understanding of the regulations relevant to their own research interests.
- There are also ethical issues related to authorship on research papers, including who should be included as an author and in what order authors should be listed.
- Other decisions with potential ethical implications for graduate students include selecting a faculty advisor and selecting a job offer.

REFERENCES

1. Yang X, Telama R, Hirvensalo M, et al. The longitudinal effects of physical activity history on metabolic syndrome. *Med Sci Sports Exerc* 2008;40:1424–1430.
2. Valiante G, Morris DB. The sources and maintenance of professional golfers' self-efficacy beliefs. *Sport Psychol* 2013;27:130–142.
3. Couzin J. Scientific misconduct. *Science* 2005;310:5749.
4. U.S. Department of Health and Human Services, Code of Federal Regulations: http://www.hhs.gov/ohrp/human-subjects/guidance/45cfr46.html
5. National Research Council. *The Guide for the Care and Use of Laboratory Animals.* Washington, DC: National Academy of Sciences, 1996.

RELATED ASSIGNMENTS

1. Write a one-page paper explaining, in detail, what constitutes plagiarism and describing how to avoid it. Be sure to include treatment of Internet, as well as published sources.

2. Write a paragraph explaining the concept of an "outlier" and describing appropriate and inappropriate ways to handle outliers.

3. Write a paragraph explaining what federal law requires with regard to appropriate handling and storage of research data.

4. Construct a document of informed consent for participation in a hypothetical (or real) research study that meets the format specifications for your institution.

5. Write a paragraph explaining your personal philosophy with regard to inclusion and ordering of authors on a research paper.

IN-CLASS GROUP EXERCISES

1. Working in a small group, write a paraphrase for each of the following statements that might have been taken from the research literature, remembering that you must change not only the wording but the sentence structure:

   a. Numerous investigators have documented specific differences in both kinematic and kinetic variables for treadmill running compared to overground running.
   b. These results demonstrate that when severe or repeated ankle sprains are not properly treated, functional ankle instability can result.
   c. Adherence to conventional exercise regimes is typically improved when psychosocial variables are known to influence the experience in a positive way.
   d. Instructional strategies for elementary physical education can only be optimized when the instructor has been sensitized to the culture of the student mix.
   e. A sound understanding of functional anatomy lies at the heart of the athletic training and physical therapy curricula.

2. **Within your group, discuss what you believe should happen in each of the following situations:**

   a. A student confides in her friend that she has downloaded the paper she is turning in for a writing assignment from the Internet. What should the friend do?

   b. A graduate student is ready to collect data on his last participant for a research project. He hopes to analyze the data and write an abstract for a conference presentation that must be submitted the following day. When the participant arrives, she is pale and announces that she has the flu.

   c. The situation is the same as in (b) above, but the participant does not show up.

   d. A student has coded computer software that generates biomechanical gait analysis data for a project comparing elite and subelite sprinters. After completing the data collection, analyzing the data, and writing a complete manuscript, he discovers that there was an error in his software.

   e. A graduate student completes her master's thesis project after working on it, with little input from her advisor, for approximately 18 months. Her advisor lists his name as first author on the manuscript being submitted to a journal for publication, because he provided the research question and the funding for the project.

   f. A student enters a prestigious graduate program working with a faculty advisor who is internationally known for her research. After the first year, the student realizes that although she enjoys the research work, she cannot stand the faculty advisor.

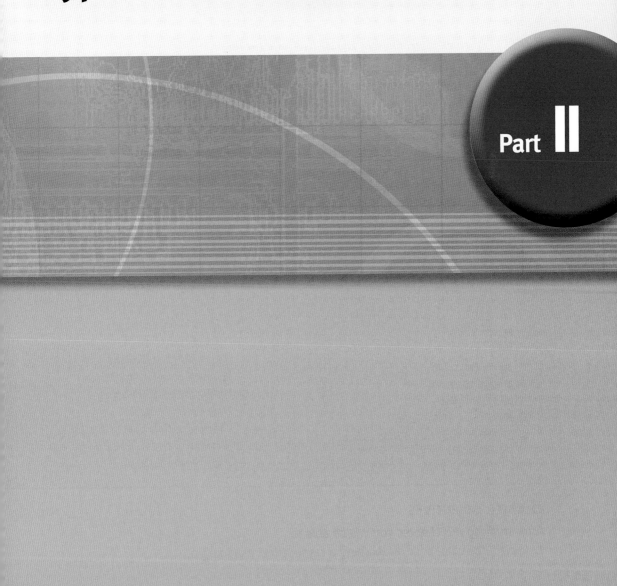

Understanding Different Types of Research

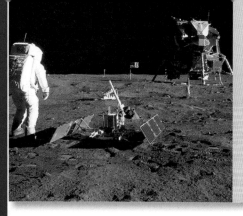

Part II

Experimental Research

"Research is creating new knowledge."—*Neil Armstrong*

CHAPTER OBJECTIVES

After studying this chapter, you will be able to:

1. Explain the criteria for establishing a cause–effect relationship.
2. Discuss the role of experimental control in designing research studies.
3. Describe the general categories of threats to internal and external validity.

4. Characterize the differences among preexperimental, true experimental, and quasi-experimental designs.

5. List the steps in the experimental research process.

■ THIS chapter discusses the many considerations that researchers must pay attention to in designing experimental research studies. Experimental research asks the "why?" question. In scientific contexts, it is also referred to as **mechanistic research**, because the general goal is to discover the underlying mechanisms or processes that explain how something works. Whereas descriptive research studies have documented a relationship between tobacco smoking and lung cancer, experimental studies have taken the next step to document the mechanisms through which smoking *causes* lung cancer. In other words, the purpose of experimental research is exploring **cause–effect relationships**. This can translate to documenting that a cause–effect relationship does exist, showing that one does not exist, or finding inconclusive results that suggest more research on the topic is needed.

A number of conditions must be met in order to demonstrate a cause–effect relationship.

Mechanistic Research
Research aimed at discovering or explaining underlying mechanisms of causation

Cause–Effect Relationship
Defined association between two variables in which one variable precedes and leads to the other in a predictable fashion

THE ELEMENTS OF EXPERIMENTAL RESEARCH

Suppose a researcher wants to investigate the effects of sleep deprivation on reaction time, movement time, and fine motor ability. In such a study, the potential causal factor is sleep deprivation, and the effects of sleep deprivation are measured on reaction time, movement time, and fine motor ability. As introduced in Chapter 1, we term the "cause" factor the **independent variable** and the "effect" variables the **dependent variables**. Another way to think about this is that the independent variable is the variable of interest, or what is driving the reason for the study. The dependent variables are those things being measured that are expected to change in some way due to the influence of the independent variable.

The independent variable is also what the researchers manipulate. In a simple study of sleep deprivation, there might be one group of participants, known as the **experimental group**, who are tested on the dependent variables (reaction time, movement time, and manual dexterity) before and after a prescribed period of sleep deprivation. In this case, the researchers make the decision as to the most appropriate period of sleep deprivation, or they manipulate the amount of sleep deprivation that occurs prior to posttesting. The exact amount or dosage of sleep deprivation that the participants will undergo in the course of the study is referred to as the **experimental treatment**.

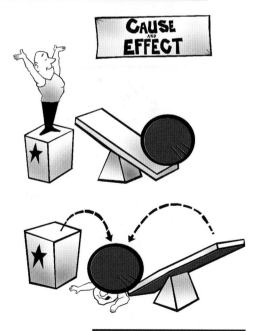

Independent Variable Factor of interest that researchers manipulate to determine measured effects on other factors

Dependent Variables Factors that are measured to evaluate the effects of the independent factors being manipulated in a study

Experimental Group Participants in a study receiving a specific dosage of the independent variable

Experimental Treatment The particular dosage of the independent variable that participants in an experimental group receive

Cause–Effect Relationships

You can probably think of many examples where there is a relationship between two factors, but no cause–effect relationship. As elementary school–aged children grow, we would normally expect there to be concomitant increases in height, weight, running speed, reading ability, etc. If we were to do a study looking for relationships between weight and running speed or height and reading ability among elementary school–aged children, we would most certainly find strong positive correlations. However, no one would suggest that these represent cause–effect relationships. Clearly, other variables serve as the cause for these changes. Height and weight in children typically increase as a function of growth. Running speed potential increases with maturation of the neuromuscular system. Reading ability increases by virtue of reading instruction and practice.

What does it take to conclusively demonstrate a cause–effect relationship between two variables? For a cause–effect relationship to exist, there must first be a well-documented relationship between the cause and the effect. As noted, however, a relationship alone does not show a cause followed by an effect. There is also no statistical analysis that can prove a cause–effect relationship. In order for a cause–effect to exist, all of the following must be true:

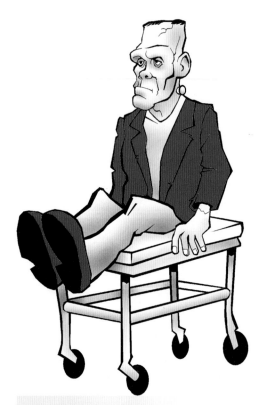

- There is a strong correlation between the cause and the effect.
- The cause precedes the effect.
- The cause always produces the effect (in the absence of some other simultaneously acting factor intervening).
- There is not a viable alternative explanation for the effect.

Cause–effect relationships can only be shown through well-controlled experiments with sound, logical interpretation of the results. This chapter discusses the factors that must be considered and, when possible, controlled in designing strong experimental research.

✔ Check Your Understanding

1. Using the terms highlighted in bold, explain the purpose of experimental research.
2. What is a cause–effect relationship, and what conditions are necessary in order to document one?

Experimental Control

Considering our study of sleep deprivation, it may occur to you that there are a number of things that the researchers should take into account in order for the results to be meaningful. For example, it would be important to make sure that all of the participants were tested under the same conditions. We would not want for some of the participants to have been exhausted before beginning the study, while others were

Experimental control gone awry!

well rested. It would be important for none of the participants to be taking medication for colds or allergies that might make them more drowsy than usual. These types of considerations are what we refer to as **extraneous variables**, because they can affect the measures of the dependent variables but are not part of the study. Taking steps to ensure that extraneous variables such as these are not an issue is referred to as **experimental control**. Appropriate experimental control, eliminating as many as possible sources of data contamination, is necessary in order for us to have confidence in the results of a study.

In another scenario for the sleep deprivation study, the researchers might have two groups of participants, one that is sleep deprived and one that is not sleep deprived, with both groups getting pre- and posttests of the dependent variables. In such a case, the non–sleep-deprived group is considered to be the **control group**, providing a set of comparison data that will help to more definitively show the effects of sleep deprivation on the experimental group of sleep-deprived participants. The inclusion of a control group is typically invaluable in an experimental research study.

In some instances, variables may exist that can potentially affect the outcome of the study, but for various reasons, the researchers cannot eliminate them. If some of the participants were very experienced at taking the tests of the dependent variable, for example, this would tend to improve their performances but would not likely be known to the researchers. In our example, some participants may have faster reaction times than others. Such factors, which may influence the results but are not eliminated, are known as **confounding variables**.

Extraneous Variables Factors other than the independent variables that can exert an effect on the measures of the dependent variables

Experimental Control The ability to eliminate all influences other than the independent variable that can affect the dependent variables

Control Group Participants who are measured for the dependent variables but do not receive an experimental treatment

Confounding Variables Uncontrolled factors other than the independent variables that influence the measures of the dependent variables

✓ Check Your Understanding

1. Explain what is meant by "experimental control."
2. Describe a research study for which it would be important to have a control group.
3. For the study you describe in #2 above, can you identify potential extraneous and confounding variables?

INTERNAL AND EXTERNAL VALIDITY

Good research studies produce results that accurately reflect the effects of the independent variables on the dependent variables in the population being studied. When these conditions are met, the results of the study can be said to have strong **validity**. In order for the results of a study to be valid, the researchers must carefully plan for two major elements—internal validity and external validity.

Validity The ability of a research study to faithfully reflect the true state of the variables being studied in the population of interest

Internal Validity

Internal validity is the extent to which any changes measured in the dependent variables can be directly attributed to manipulation of the independent variables. In order to have "good" internal validity when planning the research design, researchers attempt to control all extraneous factors that

Internal Validity The ability to conclude that only the independent variables affected any differences in measures of the dependent variables across groups or across tests on the same group

SPECIAL INTEREST BOX 6.1

Considerations Affecting Internal Validity

Consider the following example:

A researcher wishes to compare the efficacy of two stretching programs on knee range of motion in patients following ACL replacement surgery. She invites a group of 20 post–ACL replacement patients to her clinic to view a demonstration of both stretching programs. She then asks each patient to choose either program A or program B and gives each patient a prepared list of the exercises in the program selected. She then instructs the patients to perform the stretching exercises three times per week and to return in 6 weeks for an assessment of knee range of motion.

What is wrong with this research design? (You will need to make quite a list!) Here are a few suggestions:

- What if patients who were not very motivated tended to choose program A because they perceived it to be easier?
- What if the patients who tended to choose the more difficult or time-consuming program were less likely to faithfully perform the exercises at home than those who chose the other program?
- What if the patients in both groups did not really understand the exercise protocols and were exercising with widely different versions of the programs?

All of these factors could affect the outcome of the research, detracting from our ability to determine cause–effect relationships. To better appreciate how poor the internal validity is for this first scenario, consider this second scenario:

A researcher wishes to compare the efficacy of two stretching programs on knee range of motion in patients following ACL replacement surgery. She invites a group of 20 post–ACL replacement patients to her clinic, where she measures and records each patient's knee ROM. She then randomly divides the patients into two equally sized groups and sends them into two different rooms. In these two rooms, patients see a demonstration of the exercises in their assigned protocol, and then they practice the exercises until the researcher is confident they are performing them correctly. All patients are asked to report to the clinic three times per week for 6 weeks to perform the assigned exercises under supervision. They are also asked not to do any other exercises that might affect knee ROM during this period. At the end of the 6 weeks, all patients' knee ROMs are again measured for comparison to the original assessments.

In this second scenario, the researcher has the ability to compare knee ROM measurements taken after the experimental period to those taken before. She also has confidence that study participants are performing the stretching exercises correctly and that they are performing the prescribed number of repetitions and times per week because she directly supervises the participants. She cannot be 100% certain that the participants did not perform any extra exercises that might affect knee ROM while outside the clinic, but at least the participants were asked not to do extra exercises. These are all elements of experimental control that were not present in the first scenario described, and these are all reasons why the second scenario ensures greater internal validity than the first.

might affect the dependent variables. Special Interest Box 6.1 illustrates the importance of controlling for internal validity.

In the scenarios described in Special Interest Box 6.1, the research hypothesis is most likely that one of the stretching protocols will result in greater knee ROM than the other. When there is a reason-able possibility that the dependent variables could have been affected by a factor other than the independent variable, a **plausible rival hypothesis** can be constructed. With the first scenario, for example, a plausible rival hypothesis might be that the participants in one group did not perform the exercises correctly because the exercises were too complicated or were not well explained, negating the ability to really compare the effects of the two protocols. Another plausible rival hypothesis might be that the patients who were not very motivated to participate all chose the exercise that appeared to be easier, but then, since they were not really motivated in the first place, they did not faithfully perform the stretching exercises. In a well-designed study, the researchers have carefully planned such that any change in the dependent variables can *only* be attributed to the treatment dose of the independent variable and there are no plausible rival hypotheses.

Plausible Rival Hypothesis Proposal that something other than the independent variable affected measures of the dependent variables

✔ Check Your Understanding

1. Using your own words, define internal validity.
2. Explain the concept of the plausible rival hypothesis.

External Validity

The second important underlying consideration in designing research methodology is **external validity**. External valid-ity is simply the extent to which the results of a study can be generalized beyond the participants. One consideration is always the extent to which the participants represent the general **population**. We tend to think of a population as being a very large group. However, in research, we have the luxury of defining a population of interest. If we wish to study elite wheelchair basketball players, we would select only elite wheelchair basketball players as participants in our study, and the results of the study could then be general-ized to our specified population, which, in this case, consists only of elite wheelchair basketball players. We refer to the group of partici-pants selected as being representative of a given population as the **sample**. Participants involved in a research study are considered to be a representa-tive sample of the larger population.

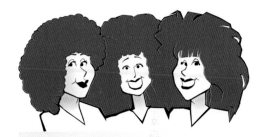

"Sample of the BIG hair population."

Suppose we have conducted a study comparing two different leg strength training protocols over a period of 6 weeks among college-age males. The results show the two protocols to both increase knee extension torque as mea-sured on a dynamometer, with no difference in the efficacy of the two proto-cols. Does this mean that these leg strengthening techniques will work equally well for everyone? The answer is "no." We cannot say, based on the results of this study, that the techniques will work for people who are older than college age or younger than college age. We also cannot say that the techniques will work for college-age females. We can only generalize the findings to college-age males with the same characteristics as those who participated in the study.

External Validity Ability to generalize the results of a study to the sample population in a real world setting

External validity is diminished when the researchers try to simulate "real world" conditions in a controlled laboratory environment.

Population Defined, large group to which the results of a study conducted on a sample of that group may be generalized

Sample Group of participants in a study selected as being representative of a defined population

Inclusion Criteria List of characteristics that individuals must possess in order to qualify as participants in a study

Exclusion Criteria List of characteristics that individuals cannot possess in order to qualify as participants in a study

This example highlights the importance of choosing appropriate **inclusion criteria** and **exclusion criteria** when selecting participants for a given study. Inclusion criteria are a list of characteristics that individuals must have, and exclusion criteria are a list of characteristics that individuals must not have in order to qualify for participation in a study. Inclusion criteria often include things such as age range, gender, and training status (sedentary or regularly exercising). Exclusion criteria may include having had a recent injury, being a tobacco smoker, or being obese. The longer the list of inclusion and exclusion criteria, the more narrowly defined the population to which the results of the study can be generalized.

Good external validity is based in part on making sure that the study participants are accurately representative of the population to which you want to be able to generalize the results. The larger the population of interest, the more difficult it can become to make sure that your sample is truly representative. Think about the range of heights, weights, health habits, training statuses, etc. among American men aged 22 years. In order to have perfect external validity for this population, the composition of your sample would need not only to reflect the diversity of characteristics in that population but also to reflect all characteristics in the same proportions in which they occur in the population. So, for example, if 27% of the population is overweight, 27% of the sample should be overweight if body weight status has any influence on any of the dependent variables being collected.

One way that researchers can have confidence that their sample is truly representative of the population is to randomly select participants from the population. If the population of interest were all students at a certain university, then a sufficiently large random sample of all students at that university would help to ensure strong external validity. Obviously, the larger the population, the more difficult it becomes to utilize true random selection of participants.

The other major component of external validity is the extent to which the testing conditions in the study are representative of "real-world" conditions. In a study where the testing conditions closely mimic real-world conditions, the study is said to have good **ecological validity**. If you want to study the ways in which children interact on a playground, you will need to figure out a way to unobtrusively observe children out on a real playground. A study in which researchers bring children into a laboratory environment and ask them to pretend they are on a playground would have very poor external validity, because it is very unlikely that the children would behave as if they were actually on a playground or as if they were not being observed. Similarly, researchers wishing to document the movement characteristics of world class track and field performances at an international competition are going to have to actually be present at such a competition with cameras. Asking elite athletes to perform in a noncompetitive environment is not likely to yield a truly maximum effort.

Ecological Validity The extent to which the testing conditions in a study are like the conditions in the environment being studied

There are certainly advantages, however, to testing or observing participants in a controlled laboratory environment. If you are recording participant movements with a camera, for example, you can make certain that you have optimum lighting and viewing perspectives in a lab. Alternatively, when filming at an event such as the Ironman Triathlon, you cannot guarantee that a car will not pass in front of the camera just as a participant is running by, as one of these authors well knows!

✔ Check Your Understanding

1. Using your own words, define external validity.
2. When designing a research study, what is the population?

CONTROLLING THREATS TO VALIDITY

Researchers achieve good internal validity by carefully planning to control all factors in the data collection environment and achieve good external validity by collecting data in the field, where there is little ability to control things. These two concepts are clearly at odds. Therefore, when planning a study, the researchers must make decisions regarding the study design with sensitivity to the implications for internal and external validity. No study design will optimize both. Intelligent decision making in designing a study hinges in part on understanding the factors that can threaten the integrity of internal and external validity.

Threats to Internal Validity

Campbell and Stanley[1] have described eight general threats to internal validity, and Rosenthal[2] has identified an additional one. These are described in this section of the chapter and summarized in Table 6.1.

HISTORY

When an experimental treatment extends over a period of time, there is a possibility that something going on simultaneously other than the treatment will affect the dependent variables being measured. For example, if the treatment involves an exercise protocol and some of the participants are getting additional exercise through participation in an organized sport, this could influence the results and would constitute a history threat to the internal validity of the study. For this reason, exercise intervention studies should include sport participation among the exclusion criteria to ensure that this does not happen unbeknownst to the researchers.

MATURATION

A similar threat to internal validity, termed maturation, refers to things naturally occurring with the passage of time that can influence data. This most commonly refers to the fact that over an extended experimental period, the participants age and develop over time. This is particularly an issue for studies involving children; since as children grow, they are becoming bigger and stronger and acquiring more advanced skills. For these reasons, we would expect elementary school children to perform better

TABLE 6.1 Threats to Internal Validity	
Threat	**Description**
History	Events or processes other than the planned experimental treatment
Maturation	Effects related to the passage of time, such as aging
Testing	Beneficial practice effects for repetitions of the same test
Instrumentation	Effects of reliability problems with equipment or observers
Statistical regression	Extreme scores tend to regress toward the mean upon retest
Selection bias	Comparison groups are not equal at the beginning of the study
Experimental mortality	Loss of participants from a study
Selection–maturation interaction	Maturation affects groups within the study differently
Expectancy	Rater expectations influence data

on fitness tests at the end of a school year than at the beginning of that school year irrespective of the quality of physical education that they may have received during the year. Maturation can also be an issue in studies involving elderly individuals who may experience declining height, strength, and reaction time as a function of aging. Other factors that can constitute maturation threats with the passing of time are changes in daylight over the course of a day, changes in the weather over the course of a year, or increasing participant fatigue over an extended data collection period.

TESTING

Testing constitutes a threat to internal validity in studies involving one or more repetitions of the same test because of the potential practice effect. That is, taking the test the first time essentially served as practice on the test, and so performance on a repetition of the same test is likely to be better. This is especially common for tests of physical skills.

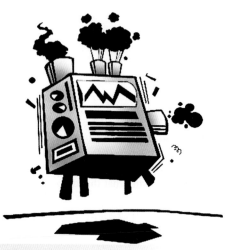

"D' ya think instrumentation was a problem?"

INSTRUMENTATION

The instrumentation threat includes all potential sources of data error resulting from the data collection process. Improper equipment calibration, software bugs, electrical interference, and equipment misuse can all introduce error into a data set. When a study involves use of observers, there is also the potential for recorded observations to vary over time and across conditions. The instrumentation threat can only be controlled by employing knowledgeable and careful use of the processes through which data are collected.

STATISTICAL REGRESSION

This threat becomes a possibility when groups are formed based on extreme scores. For example, if a large group were given a reaction time test and then divided into two groups consisting of the fastest 10% and the slowest 10%, a subsequent test of reaction time would likely show the fast group performing more slowly and the slow group performing more quickly. In such a case, we say that the group scores have regressed toward the average.

SELECTION BIAS

Whenever a study involves comparison of two or more groups receiving different experimental treatments, the groups must be highly similar for the variables being measured at the beginning of the study in order for any subsequent comparison of treatment effects to be valid. Suppose we wanted to compare the efficacy of two different quadriceps strengthening exercises. We might design a study with two groups of participants, with each group training with one of the two exercises over a period of 6 weeks. If we planned to do our comparison by testing the quadriceps strengths of both groups at the end of the experimental period, it would be rather important to know that the two groups started the study with similar quadriceps strengths. If we had randomly assigned our participants to the two groups, we could reasonably assume that the groups were likely to be highly similar. However, if we allowed the participants to choose which of the two exercises they wanted to train with, we would be in danger of selection bias. For example, if one exercise appeared to be easier or less time consuming, less fit participants might be more likely to volunteer to be in that exercise group. The single best way to control the selection bias threat is through random assignment of participants to groups.

EXPERIMENTAL MORTALITY

Experimental mortality refers to participants withdrawing from a study for any reason. If the number of participants dropping out is small and unrelated to the treatment, the threat is minor. However, large numbers of participants withdrawing from the protocol can result in the sample being too small to adequately represent the population and also in difficulty with appropriate comparisons of groups. Flu season is not the best choice of time to conduct a study if the participants are not able to miss a few days of the experimental treatment. The threat is worse if the reasons for participant withdrawal are related to the treatment. For example, if an exercise training protocol is resulting in stress injuries among participants, this would suggest that the study should be halted. (It would also suggest that the study was not well designed!)

SELECTION–MATURATION INTERACTION

This threat can arise when the maturation effect influences groups within a study differently. This is particularly the case when the study is designed to compare different age groups. Many studies on the characteristics of aging, for example, compare young adults in a certain age range to older adults in a certain age range. In such studies, if the treatment period extends over a length of time, there is the potential that the aging process may be affecting the older group differently than the younger group. Random formation of groups eliminates this threat, but sometimes, it is not possible or not convenient to form groups randomly.

EXPECTANCY

The design of some studies is such that the researchers tend to expect one set of scores to be better than another. For example, researchers would tend to expect that posttreatment scores might be better than pretreatment scores or that scores of one group would be different than scores of another group. Such would be the case for skilled versus unskilled groups, younger versus older groups, or trained versus untrained groups. The effect is the same thing whether the person who measures or rates the outcome variable is conscious or unconscious of the expectancy. Expectancy can therefore become a threat to internal validity if measures are not taken to ensure objectivity in the assessment and recording of data. Rater training and use of multiple raters are strategies for helping to minimize this threat.

✔ Check Your Understanding

List and, in your own words, briefly describe each of the threats to internal validity.

Threats to External Validity

Campbell and Stanley have described four common threats to external validity.[1] These are described in the following section of the chapter and summarized in Table 6.2.

INTERACTION EFFECT OF TESTING

This is a potential threat for studies involving a pretest prior to an experimental treatment. If the pretest in some way motivates the participants to respond differently to the treatment than if they had not had a pretest, this threat is in effect. For example, if a pretest made participants aware that they were functioning or performing at a low level, this might motivate them to be more attuned or dedicated to

TABLE 6.2 Threats to External Validity	
Threat	**Description**
Interaction effect of testing	The pretest changes the group's response to the experimental treatment
Interaction of selection bias and experimental treatment	A biased sample produces skewed results not representative of the population
Reactive effects of experimental setting	Some element of the setting causes modification of participant behavior
Multiple-treatment interference	Experiencing one treatment affects participant response to a subsequent treatment

following the treatment protocol. One way to minimize this threat is not sharing pretest results with the participants, although simply taking a pretest could also heighten participant awareness even in the absence of knowing the results.

INTERACTION OF SELECTION BIAS AND EXPERIMENTAL TREATMENT

This threat arises when the sample does not well represent the population. Suppose a high school health teacher is conducting a survey of the dietary habits of high school athletes. She extends an invitation to all athletes at her school to volunteer for participation. The tennis players, who all happen to be taking an advanced tennis class, receive extra credit from the teacher of that class if they volunteer to participate. Unbeknownst to the teacher conducting the survey, over half of the students who end up in the sample are tennis players. As you might expect, the survey results do represent the dietary habits of high school tennis players but are very different from those of football, baseball, basketball, and lacrosse players. This threat primarily becomes an issue when the sample is biased and/or the population to which the results are generalized is defined too broadly.

REACTIVE EFFECTS OF EXPERIMENTAL SETTING

This threat becomes an issue whenever the setting in which data are collected causes the participants to behave differently than they normally would. We have previously mentioned the fact that capturing observations of high-level athletic performance requires going to an actual competition, as opposed to filming in a laboratory setting because in the absence of the competitive environment and with the constraints of laboratory space, the performance is likely to be modified. Back in the 1950s, a researcher documented a specific type of reactive effect of an experimental setting. Known as the **Hawthorne effect**,[3] participant performances can improve simply due to the fact that they are participating in a study and being observed by researchers.

Hawthorne Effect
Phenomenon in which participants' performances during a research study improve due solely to the fact that they know they are being observed.

MULTIPLE-TREATMENT INTERFERENCE

When a single group of participants is exposed to more than one experimental treatment, the exposure to one treatment can affect participant response to subsequent treatments, with the effect being either positive or negative. For example, students in a research methods course might perform better on the second exam than on the first one because taking the first exam alerted them to the kinds of questions the instructor is likely to ask on subsequent exams. Alternatively, if the students thought the first exam was easy, they might not study as well for the second exam, causing them to perform less well. This effect can become an issue in research studies that test more than one experimental treatment on the same participants.

Check Your Understanding

List and, in your own words, briefly describe each of the threats to external validity.

EXPERIMENTAL RESEARCH DESIGNS

In designing a study, the researchers make decisions about things such as how many groups of participants are needed, what experimental treatments will be given, and how many times data will be collected (referred to as repeated measures). These decisions are based on the nature of the research question, controlling as many threats to internal and external validity as possible, and also practical considerations such as availability of appropriate participants, the time invested, and the cost of the data collections.

These practical considerations are perhaps especially important considerations for students, since you are investing a fair amount of time and other resources into your education. So although you may be fascinated by some aspect of performance by cyclists during the Tour de France, tennis players during the Australian Open, or triathletes during the Ironman Triathlon, your research budget may not allow for travel to these events for data collection. Similarly, you may be interested in the influence of the Mediterranean, South Beach, or Weight Watchers' diets on some aspect of health, but dietary studies typically involve providing prepared foods to the participants over a course of months, which also may not exactly be in your budget.

Sometimes, however, practical considerations may need to take a back seat to the internal and external validity of your study. For example, although it would streamline the data collection not to have to collect data on a control group, the inclusion of a control group usually improves the internal validity of a study by enabling a clear contrast to the effect of the treatment on the experimental group. Similarly, although it costs less time and potentially supplies to collect data on a small number of participants as compared to a larger group, it is critically important to ensure that you have a sufficient sample size that your statistical tests will show differences between groups when true differences are present in the population that your sample represents.

As you may discern from all this, there are a number of decisions to be made in designing a research study, with concomitant advantages and disadvantages for the outcome. This section of the chapter discusses a number of common research designs identified by Campbell and Stanley[1] that have been organized into three categories: preexperimental designs, true experimental designs, and quasi-experimental designs. In describing each design, we will use the following notation:

- Each line represents a different group of participants.
- R indicates random assignment of participants to groups. (The absence of R indicates that random assignment is not used.)
- T represents an experimental treatment.
- D indicates a data collection.
- The order of events is from left to right.

Preexperimental Designs

The preexperimental designs are weak designs that do not utilize random assignment of participants to groups and control few threats to validity. These designs do not allow conclusive determination of cause–effect relationships. Although sometimes one of these designs may be selected due to practical constraints, these designs are best avoided.

Preexperimental designs are often used in educational settings where the convenience of using participants enrolled in a class outweighs the control-related advantages of random selection of participants and/ or random assignment of participants to groups.

ONE-SHOT STUDY DESIGN

This design involves one group of participants that receives a treatment followed by data collection to assess the effects of the treatment:

$$\boxed{T}\ \boxed{D}$$

Nothing can be concluded from such a study, because there is no way to determine whether the treatment had any effect on the participants. If a research methods course instructor were to give only one exam (the data collection) at the end of a semester and, based on the results of that exam, draw conclusions about the quality of instruction in the course (the treatment), this would be an example of a one-shot study. The one-shot study design is clearly a very poor way to attempt to answer a research question.

ONE-GROUP PRETEST–POSTTEST DESIGN

The one-group pretest–posttest design improves upon the one-shot study in that the posttest data can be compared to the pretest data to determine whether change has occurred:

$$\boxed{D_1}\ \boxed{T}\ \boxed{D_2}$$

Unfortunately, however, using this design, we cannot conclude that any change reflected in the posttest data is based upon the treatment. History, maturation, and testing effects all threaten the internal validity of such a study. Using this design, an elementary physical education teacher might give a battery of fitness tests at the beginning and end of the school year as a test of the effectiveness of the physical education program. If the students improved, this could be construed as a good reflection on their physical education. However, there would also legitimately be some plausible rival hypotheses. Given that the students aged by approximately 9 months between the pretest and posttest, the students were older and therefore likely somewhat larger, stronger, and more neurologically mature at the end of the year. There also might have been a positive practice effect from the students having taken the pretests at the beginning of the year.

STATIC GROUP COMPARISON DESIGN

The static group comparison offers an advantage and a weakness compared to the one-group pretest–posttest:

$$\boxed{T}\ \boxed{D}$$
$$\boxed{D}$$

The advantage is that there is a second group, a control group, which does not receive the treatment so that the test results of the two groups can be compared. The weakness is that there is no pretest, and so we cannot be assured that the groups were equal to begin with. Had the groups been randomly formed, we could have much more confidence in the likelihood of equality across groups, but that is not the case with this design. Selection bias and selection–maturation interaction are always threats to the validity of the results of a study using this design.

This design is sometimes used of necessity when circumstances do not readily allow random assignment of participants to groups. An example might be comparison of two different sections of an activity course in soccer at a university. It might be of interest to compare the soccer skills of students from courses taught by two different instructors or perhaps courses taught by a single instructor who deliberately experimented with two different instructional philosophies. (Maybe one class emphasized drills on soccer skills, whereas the other prioritized participation in game situation play.) A drawback for this design, however, is that in the absence of a pretest, we cannot be sure that the students in one of the classes were not significantly more skilled than the students in the other class at the beginning of the semester. In the scenario described, however, it is often reasonable to assume that students in different physical activity classes for a given sport tend to have about the same skill level, making this a reasonable design for student research projects.

Variations of the static group comparison can compare two groups, with each receiving a different experimental treatment and can also be extended to comparison of three or more groups. The variation shown here includes two experimental groups and one control group:

T_1	D
T_2	D
	D

All of these variations are participant to the same threats to the validity of the results.

✔ Check Your Understanding

1. Why are these designs referred to as "preexperimental"?
2. Why is the static group comparison a stronger design than the one-group pretest–posttest?

True Experimental Designs

The **true experimental designs** are so-called because they embody the characteristics of good experimental research, controlling for most threats to the validity of the study results. These designs all require random assignment of participants to groups, which creates a strong probability that the groups will be similar at the beginning of the study on the dependent variables being measured. Random assignment of participants to groups controls threats for past history, maturation, testing, statistical regression, selection bias, and selection–maturation interaction. It remains the responsibility of the researchers to guard against differential influences on groups or the history threat over the course of the study, instrumentation problems, and experimental mortality.

True Experimental Designs
Designs that begin with random assignment of participants to groups, thereby controlling most threats to internal validity

Most designs can be expanded to include more than one experimental group.

POSTTEST-ONLY DESIGN

The posttest-only design is the same as the static group comparison design, with the important exception of random assignment of groups:

R	T	D
R		D

Because this design involves random assignment of participants to groups, the researchers can have a good measure of confidence that the groups are similar for measures of the dependent variables at the beginning of the study. The presence of a control group enables conclusions that any changes in the dependent variables for the experimental group were due to the effect of the treatment and not to extraneous variables.

Like the static group comparison, this design can also be modified such that there are two experimental groups and no control group, or such that three or more groups are included. The design shown here includes two experimental groups and one control group:

R	T_1	D
R	T_2	D
R		D

PRETEST–POSTTEST DESIGN

This design builds upon the posttest-only design with the addition of a pretest:

R	D_1	T	D_2
R	D_1		D_2

It can also be extended to include additional groups:

R	D_1	T_1	D_2
R	D_1	T_2	D_2
R	D_1		D_2

Although random assignment of participants to groups makes it unlikely that the groups will be substantially different, there is still some small possibility that the groups will be unequal despite having been randomly formed. The addition of the pretest gives the researchers the ability to conclusively demonstrate that the groups were equivalent at the beginning of the study for the variables being measured.

SOLOMON FOUR-GROUP DESIGN

This is a sophisticated design that always includes four groups:

Group 1	R	D_1	T	D_2
Group 2	R	D_1		D_2
Group 3	R		T	D_2
Group 4	R			D

Do not make the mistake of assuming that any study involving four groups of participants must be a Solomon Four-Group. Several designs discussed in the chapter can include three experimental groups and a control group.

The purpose of this design, beyond testing the effects of the experimental treatment, is to also specifically test for any reactive effects of testing. Notice that with this design among the groups receiving the treatment (1 and 3), only group 1 has a pretest as well as a posttest. Among the groups not receiving the treatment (2 and 4), only group 2 has a pretest as well as a posttest. Looking at the posttest scores for all four groups, the researchers can determine whether the treatment or the pretest had a greater effect on the participants. For example, if the posttest scores for groups 1 and 3 are greater than the posttest scores for groups 2 and 4, the treatment clearly had an effect on the variable(s) being measured. However, if the posttest scores for groups 1 and 2 are greater than the scores for groups 3 and 4, then the pretest had an effect on the dependent variables that outweighed the effect of the experimental treatment.

Researchers use this design in studies where they have a real concern that the pretest will exert a powerful influence on the posttest measures. This is often a potential concern with tests of skill. Although the design is effective in controlling the threat of reactive effects of testing, it also has disadvantages. Because there must be four groups, a large number of participants must be involved. The data set also does not lend itself to analysis by any single statistical tool, which complicates the interpretation of the results. Table 6.3 summarizes the controls to internal and external validity provided by the true experimental designs.

✔ Check Your Understanding

1. Why are true experimental designs considered to be stronger than other types?
2. What two factors does the Solomon Four design evaluate?

TABLE 6.3	True Experimental Designs Controlling Threats to Validity[1]			
	Threat	**Posttest Only**	**Pretest–Posttest**	**Solomon Four-Group**
Internal validity	History	Yes	Yes	Yes
	Maturation	Yes	Yes	Yes
	Testing	Yes	Yes	Yes
	Instrumentation	No	No	No
	Statistical regression	Yes	Yes	Yes
	Selection bias	Yes	Yes	Yes
	Experimental mortality	Yes	Yes	Yes
External validity	Selection–maturation X	Yes	Yes	Yes
	Expectancy	Yes	Yes	Yes
	Testing—treatment X	Yes	No	Yes
	Selection bias—treatment X	Depends	Depends	Depends
	Experimental arrangements	Depends	Depends	Depends
	Multiple treatments	No	No	No

Quasi-Experimental Designs

As previously discussed, when designing a study, researchers must often make a choice between optimizing internal validity in a highly controlled laboratory environment and optimizing external validity by collecting data in a field setting where there is less control but much more of a real-world setting. The quasi-experimental designs are specialized for the latter purpose. These designs are also employed when circumstances prevent random assignment of participants to groups.

TIME SERIES DESIGNS

This family of designs involves repeated measurements of the same dependent variable(s) taken on one group of participants over what are usually constant intervals of time. In order for the research to be experimental and not merely descriptive, there must be a treatment at some point among the observations. What is called an interrupted time series design inserts a treatment into the middle of the data sampling series:

$$D_1 \quad D_2 \quad D_3 \quad T \quad D_4 \quad D_5 \quad D_6$$

Despite whatever trend may appear across all observations, a comparison of the data sampled at D_3 and D_4 should demonstrate whether there was or was not a treatment effect.

This design is used when the researchers expect there to be incremental changes occurring over time, possibly due to maturation or testing effects. Although there may be steady improvements in the scores over time, the treatment effect is evaluated as the difference between the data samples immediately preceding and following the treatment. A time series design is commonly used in case studies of single participants, where repeated measures are recorded at regular time intervals. Such a design can also be used to study the effect of new rules or laws such as the effect of a ban on use of handheld cell phones while driving on a variable such as annual automobile accident death rate.

EQUIVALENT TIME SAMPLE DESIGN

A variation on the interrupted time series design involves at least two applications of the experimental treatment among the periodic data collections:

$$D_1 \quad D_2 \quad T \quad D_3 \quad D_4 \quad T \quad D_5 \quad D_6$$

This general arrangement is known as the equivalent time sample design. It enables testing not only the effect of the treatment but also to what extent there is a lasting effect of the treatment. If measures D_2, D_4, and D_6 are lower than D_1, D_3, and D_5, this would suggest that the effect of the treatment is not lasting, but fading. This type of design is often used in studies of the efficacy of a new drug.

NONEQUIVALENT CONTROL GROUP DESIGN

This design is like the pretest–posttest design, but without the random assignment of participants to groups:

$$
\begin{array}{ccc}
D_1 & T & D_2 \\
D_1 & & D_2
\end{array}
$$

It can also be extended to include additional groups:

$$
\begin{array}{ccc}
D_1 & T_1 & D_2 \\
D_1 & T_2 & D_2 \\
D_1 & & D_2
\end{array}
$$

Given all of the advantages of random assignment of participants to groups for controlling threats to validity, why would a researcher ever choose this design? The answer is that in some circumstances, random assignment to groups is either inconvenient or simply not possible. For example, if we wanted to study the effects of participating in a soccer class as compared to a swimming class on aerobic fitness, we could test students enrolled in university activity courses on mile run times at the beginning and end of a semester of instruction. Students in a lecture course could serve as a control group. Because students enrolled in the courses on a voluntary basis rather than being randomly assigned, this scenario would constitute a nonequivalent control group design.

EX POST FACTO DESIGN

The designation of ex post facto design is based not on the experimental arrangements but on the nature of the groups being compared. When the treatment is not controlled by the researchers, the design is ex post facto. Such is the case in studies measuring one or more dependent variables to compare men and women (where the treatment is gender), young and older age groups (where the treatment is age—see Chapter 7), or low- and high-skilled athletes (where the treatment is skill level). Most commonly, this design can be represented as follows:

$$
\begin{array}{cc}
T_1 & D \\
T_2 & D
\end{array}
$$

Table 6.4 summarizes the elements of all of the designs discussed.

✔ **Check Your Understanding**

1. In what types of settings are the quasi-experimental designs appropriate?
2. Under what circumstances is the independent variable not controlled by the researchers?

TABLE 6.4 Examples of Experimental Research Designs

Preexperimental Designs								
One-shot study							T	D
One-group pretest–posttest design						D_1	T	D_2
Static group comparison (*two or more groups*)							T	D
								D
True Experimental Designs								
Posttest-only design (*two or more groups*)						R	T_1	D
						R		D
Pretest–posttest design (*two or more groups*)						R	D_1	T_1	D_2
						R	D_1	T_2	D_2
Solomon four-group						R	D_1	T	D_2
						R	D_1		D_2
						R		T	D
						R			D
Quasi-Experimental Designs								
Time series (*several different versions*)		D_1	T_1	D_2	T_2	D_3	T_3	D_4
		D_1	D_2	D_3	T	D_4	D_5	D_6
Equivalent time sample design	D_1	D_2	T	D_3	D_4	T	D_5	D_6
Nonequivalent control group (*two or more groups*)						D_1	T_1	D_2
						D_1		D_2
Ex post facto (T not controlled by researcher)							T_1	D
							T_2	D

D, data collection; T, treatment or intervention; R, randomization.

CHAPTER SUMMARY

- The general goal of experimental research is to discover underlying mechanisms or processes that explain how something works.
- A cause–effect relationship can only be documented through carefully designed studies that first show a relationship between the cause and the effect, but then go on to show through logical interpretation that one factor is the cause and the other the effect.
- Strong internal validity requires that the study is designed such that only the manipulation of the independent variable(s) affects changes in the dependent variable(s) and that all plausible rival hypotheses are eliminated.
- Strong external validity requires that the sample is accurately reflective of the study population and that the conditions under which the data are collected are representative of the "real world."
- Categories of threats to internal validity include history, maturation, testing, instrumentation, statistical regression, selection biases, experimental mortality, interaction of selection bias and experimental mortality, and expectation.

- Categories of threats to external validity include the interactive effects of testing, the interaction of selection bias and experimental treatment, the reactive effects of experimental setting, and multiple-treatment interference.
- Research designs are grouped into preexperimental designs, which are weak in controlling threats to validity; true experimental designs, which are strong in controlling threats to validity; and quasi-experimental designs, which are used in situations when external validity is more of a priority than internal validity.

REFERENCES

1. Campbell DT, Stanley JC. *Experimental and Quasi-experimental Designs for Research.* Boston, MA: Houghton Mifflin 1963.
2. Rosenthal R. Sport, art, and particularity. *J Philos Sport* 1966;13:49.
3. Brown JAC. *The Social Psychology of Industry.* Harmondsworth, UK: Penguin, 1954.

RELATED ASSIGNMENTS

1. **Write a short paper explaining what characterizes experimental research, including the roles of independent, dependent, extraneous, and confounding variables.**

2. **Write a short paper explaining the concept of experimental control and why it is important.**

3. **Write a one-paragraph description of an example of five of the study designs explained in the chapter. Write another paragraph explaining which of the example studies you have described is best in thwarting threats to internal validity. Write another paragraph explaining which of the example studies you have described is best in thwarting threats to external validity.**

4. **Explain the difference between random selection of participants and random assignment of participants to groups. How does each of these processes contribute to the design of a research study?**

5. **What are the advantages and disadvantages of collecting data in a controlled laboratory environment?**

IN-CLASS GROUP EXERCISES

1. **Read the first scenario for a research study in Special Interest Box 6.1. Within your group, determine the design for this study, and list the threats to internal and external validity present.**

2. **Within your group, identify the independent variable and the dependent variable for each of the investigations described.**

   a. An athletic trainer wishes to study the effect of participation in a conditioning class on grip strength in elderly women. The grip strength of 25 participants in a conditioning class is measured and recorded at the beginning and at the end of a 16-week period.

   Ind. V. _____ Dep. V. _____

b. A researcher is interested in the effect of fatigue on running stride length in rats. A group of rats is run to exhaustion on rat treadmills. Every 2 minutes, a high-speed camera is turned on to enable measurement of rat stride length.

Ind. V. _____ Dep. V. _____

c. The effect of participation in a running class on VO_{2max} is studied. Members of a group of forty participants are matched as closely as possible on finish times for the mile run. The members of each matched pair are randomly assigned to groups. One group participates in a running class, while the other does not. Both groups' VO_{2maxs} are tested at the end of the semester.

Ind. V. _____ Dep. V. _____

d. A purveyor of ergogenic aids wishes to compare the effects of topically applied emu oil, ostrich oil, and snake oil on muscle strength gains. He convinces the instructors of three university weight training classes to have students rub one of these oils (one oil per class) over their triceps prior to performing bench-press exercises. At the end of the semester, he assesses maximum bench-press capability across classes.

Ind. V. _____ Dep. V. _____

e. An elementary school teacher investigates improvement in fitness over the course of the school year by giving a group of 300 students a battery of eight fitness tests at the beginning and end of the school year.

Ind. V. _____ Dep. V. _____

f. A clinician wishes to assess the effectiveness of two different exercises on patellar tracking in patients with chondromalacia. Patients assigned to one physical therapist do static quad sets, and patients assigned to a second physical therapist do straight leg raises with external femoral rotation. At the end of 3 months, all patients are evaluated and scored on a 10-point scale for proper patellar tracking during knee extension.

Ind. V. _____ Dep. V. _____

g. A hundred Labrador Retrievers are randomly divided into two groups and tested for obedience. One group is then trained using milk bone rewards, while the other group is trained using verbal praise. At the end of the 6-week training period, both groups are retested for obedience.

Ind. V. _____ Dep. V. _____

3. **Within your group, identify (1) the independent variable, (2) the dependent variable, and (3) the research design employed for each of the investigations described.**

a. A researcher wishes to assess the effects of 40% VO_{2max} training versus 70% VO_{2max} training on performance in the 12-minute run test. She randomly assigns 60 student volunteers to one of three groups: 40% VO_{2max} training, 70% VO_{2max} training, and control (no training). All three groups are tested on the 12-minute run at the end of a 6-week training period.

Ind. Var. _____ Dep. Var. _____

Design: _____

b. A professor wishes to evaluate the effectiveness of his lecturing at the end of a semester-long course in sport history. He decides to use student performance on the final exam for the course as the measurement of effectiveness.

Ind. Var. _____ Dep. Var. _____

Design: _____

c. A clinician wishes to assess the effects of a rehabilitation program on perceived pain level among low back pain patients. A perceived pain test is given to a group of patients who have just been referred to the clinic and to another group of patients who have been receiving therapy for a period of 6 weeks.

Ind. Var. _____ Dep. Var. _____

Design: _____

d. A tennis instructor wishes to study the effects of participation in a tennis class on self-esteem. He administers a self-esteem inventory to 25 students enrolled in his class and to 25 students not enrolled in a tennis class. At the end of the semester, he administers the same inventory to the same two groups.

Ind. Var. _____ Dep. Var. _____

Design: _____

e. The effect of participation in a conditioning class on grip strength is studied. The grip strength of 25 participants in a conditioning class is measured and recorded at the beginning and at the end of a semester.

Ind. Var. _____ Dep. Var. _____

Design: _____

f. The effect of fatigue on stride length during running is studied. The stride lengths of a group of 50 runners are measured and recorded at the end of each mile over the course of a half marathon.

Ind. Var. _____ Dep. Var. _____

Design: _____

g. The effect of participation in a running class on VO_{2max} is studied. A group of 40 participants are matched as closely as possible on finish times for the mile run. The members of each matched pair are randomly assigned to groups. One group participates in a running class, while the other does not. Both groups' VO_{2maxs} are tested at the end of the semester.

Ind. Var. _____ Dep. Var. _____

Design: _____

h. A researcher investigates the difference in undergraduate GPAs between male and female students entering a graduate program in Nutrition.

Ind. Var. _____ Dep. Var. _____

Design: _____

7

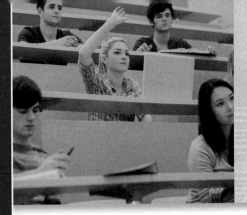

Descriptive Research

"Judge a man by his questions rather than his answers."—Voltaire

CHAPTER OUTLINE

Basic Descriptive Research

Correlational Research

Survey Research
Questionnaires

Interviews

Other Descriptive Approaches
Case Studies
Developmental Research
Observational Research

CHAPTER OBJECTIVES

After studying this chapter, you will be able to:

1. Define descriptive research in general.
2. Identify specific types of descriptive research approaches.
3. Describe correlational research approaches.
4. Create appropriate questions for surveys or questionnaires.
5. Recognize situations where developmental or observational research approaches should be used.

■ IN Chapter 6, we described the fundamentals of experimental research. Recall that when a researcher performs this type of research, he or she "manipulates" an experimental treatment in order to establish cause–effect relationships. Although commonly used in many disciplines, experimental research is not the only way in which to systematically acquire knowledge within the health sciences. In fact, descriptive research that focuses on the here and now can provide valuable insight into many issues that exist around us and is often a precursor to experimental research. Researchers who use descriptive research collect information related to their particular interests and then use that information to depict its current status. From this research, we can begin to describe and understand relationships in the important variables we hope to someday manipulate experimentally.

BASIC DESCRIPTIVE RESEARCH

When gathering descriptive data about participants, be sure to collect measures that help those who read the research understand important sample details.

Descriptive Research Studies that captures important characteristics of the participants without experimenter manipulation.

Imagine you are a researcher who investigates childhood obesity. You have been hired by a school system superintendent, Dr. Simpson, who is interested in determining if the elementary students in the Springfield School system are generally a healthy weight, or if they are overweight or obese. In addition, the superintendent wants to know how physically active the children are outside of school. How do you approach this type of research? Unlike experimental research described in Chapter 6, you will not manipulate anything, or try to see if an intervention causes change. Rather, you want to examine a group of individuals and carefully describe certain characteristics of that group as they are today. We term this type of research descriptive. In **descriptive research**, the research intends to capture thoughts, attitudes, behaviors, physical attributes, and other characteristics of groups so as to provide a characterization of the group at a certain point in time.

It's tempting to consider experimental research as "real" or more important than descriptive research. However, we need descriptive information to guide our decisions related to interventions. Think back to the earlier example of the school superintendent asking for help understanding obesity rates at her school. Without a better understanding of the physical characteristics of the children overall, it would be difficult to make any physical activity recommendations. In other words, it wouldn't make sense to put in place a program to fight obesity if we didn't know if the children are obese or not. So, descriptive research is an important step in the entire research process.

What are some basic characteristics that you might want to describe in this group of elementary school students? The most basic characteristic is the actual number of students. In Springfield Elementary, there are a total of 312 students at the school. Beyond the absolute number, consider the broad range of ages (5 to 11 years) represented in grades Kindergarten through 5th grade. Each grade level has two classes. In order to get descriptive information about overweight/obesity status, you need

Body Mass Index An estimate of body composition based on a ratio of height to weight.

to determine a measure or group of measures that capture this information. After looking over the relevant literature (as described in Chapter 3), you determine that **body mass index** (BMI), which is a ratio of height to weight, will provide you with a valid, accurate measure to estimate overweight/obesity status. You rationalize that the Centers for Disease Control and Prevention (CDC) uses it; therefore, it is good enough for you! Here is a link to the CDC BMI calculator: http://www.cdc.gov/healthyweight/assessing/bmi/. You can also calculate BMI (in kg/m^2) by hand using the following formula:

$$BMI = \frac{\text{Weight in kilograms}}{(\text{height in meters})^2} \qquad 7.1$$

Dr. Simpson wants information on children who are considered overweight and obese. The CDC reports that BMI levels of 25 to 29.9 are considered to be "overweight" and >30 are considered to be obese in adults, with lower BMI values representing overweight and obesity in children. The cutoff value for categories of overweight and obese differs as a function of age and gender, so BMI scores are often converted to percentile ranks to enable direct comparison. In percentile rankings, underweight is <5th percentile, normal BMI is 5th to 85th percentile, overweight is ≥85th percentile, and >95th percentile is considered obese. Table 7.1 provides descriptive information about BMI as a raw score and percentile rank.

You are making good headway describing the students of Springfield Elementary School! Next, you need to describe their physical activity levels. Again, you hit the books to determine what other

TABLE 7.1	Descriptive Data from Springfield Elementary School							
Grade Level	Total Number of Students	Age Range (Year)	Average Height (m)	Average Weight (kg)	BMI (kg/m²)	BMI (Percentile Rank)	Average Steps Per Day
Kindergarten	32	5–6	1.02	19.96	15.9	51.4	11,478
First	61	6–7	1.09	21.32	17.9	64.9	12,091
Second	63	7–8	1.13	22.68	17.8	77.2	11,293
Third	57	8–9	1.17	27.67	19.9[a]	92.1[a]	10,326
Fourth	60	9–10	1.19	29.48	20.8[a]	94.3[a]	10,192
Fifth	61	10–11	1.30	37,378	22.4[a]	95.5[a]	9,987

[a]Overweight according to CDC.

researchers have used, and you decide to go with a simple measure, steps per day averaged over a 7-day period as measured by a pedometer, for your first look at describing the children's physical activity.

Examine Table 7.1. This provides a pretty good snapshot of the basic characteristics of the children at Springfield Elementary School in relation to their overweight/obesity status and physical activity at this point in time. You could provide Dr. Simpson with an initial report that suggests, in general, younger children tend to be within a healthy range of BMI, whereas older children tend to be overweight. However, most researchers would most likely want to delve deeper into the description of these students. There are several different descriptive techniques that researchers can use to more clearly understand characteristics of groups. These most typically include correlational and survey, but also may include developmental and observational research as well as case studies.

Check Your Understanding

1. Explain how descriptive research differs from experimental research.
2. Why would a researcher want to perform descriptive research?
3. From the example in Table 7.1, what other descriptive information may be important to report?

CORRELATIONAL RESEARCH

You have just initiated your descriptive research at Springfield Elementary School. Dr. Simpson expressed an interest in understanding more about overweight and obesity levels within the school, as well the amount of physical activity the children get each day. Perhaps there is a relationship between obesity and the amount of after-school physical activity? Examining the relationship between or among variables such as these is called **correlational research**[1] (we will discuss the specific statistical methods used with correlational research such as the Pearson Product Moment correlation coefficient in Chapter 11). In this type of research, the research doesn't try to manipulate or change the relationship, but rather describe the relationship as it currently exists by measuring the variables of interest and determining if the variables change together (in which case, there is a relationship) or independently (in which case, there is not a relationship).

Correlational Research
Studies that examine relationships between or among important variables.

Relationships can be positive, where the variable increase or decrease together (e.g., there is a positive relationship between height and weight in growing children, which indicates that as they get taller, they get heavier), or they can be negative, where one variable increases as the other decreases (e.g., as cardiovascular fitness increases, time taken to complete a 1-mile run decreases). If relationships exist between or among variables, then correlational research can be used to predict the value of one variable when the others are known. The stronger the correlation, whether positive or negative, the better the ability to predict.[1,2]

Another important function of correlational research is to lay the foundation for future experimental studies by establishing an association between or among variables. As you may recall, the first condition for determining cause–effect relationships is to establish a strong correlation between the cause and the effect. Without a strong association, there would be little benefit to performing experimental research (no matter how well controlled it might be).

In our example, to examine the correlation between obesity and physical activity, you would have to find an accurate measure of obesity status (e.g., BMI) as well as an accurate measure of physical activity (e.g., average time spent in moderate to vigorous physical activity [MVPA] after

Make sure you collect the most accurate measures of the variables of interest.

school as measured by an accelerometer) and measure both variables in all of elementary school children (kindergarten through 5th grade). Next, you would plot the variables on an X–Y graph. Without getting into the statistical methods, you can determine something about the strength of the relationship between these variables by looking at the scatter of point on an X–Y graph. Basically, if you can see a pattern in the scatter, some sort of a relationship probably exists.

Figure 7.1 depicts the BMI versus MVPA data from the 5th grade children. Each data point represents one child's BMI score on the *y*-axis against MVPA on the *x*-axis. In this example, the arrow pointing from top left to bottom right sums up the pattern fairly well. This graph suggests there may be some sort of negative relationship between BMI and MVPA. That is, these two variables seem to change together (e.g., are related), and it looks like that as MVPA increases, BMI decreases. A positive relationship exists when both variables increase or decrease together; a graph of a positive relationship would start at the bottom left and point to the top right.

A key to identifying variable correlation is selection of appropriate measures. If a measure doesn't sufficiently represent the variable of interest, then the resultant relationship may look weaker than it actually is. For example, the use of BMI to represent body composition has come under some scrutiny,

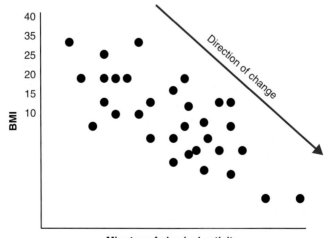

■ **FIGURE 7.1** Children's BMI plotted as a function of average minutes of physical activity outside of school. Notice that as BMI gets larger, MPA gets smaller, denoting a negative relationship.

since it tends to overestimate obesity in muscular individuals. In our example, BMI gives you a good estimate of body composition, but you would probably want to use a more precise measure of body fatness (perhaps estimated from skinfold equations specifically validated for children, or from a BOD POD or some other, more precise measure) if you were to continue with your research. In addition, both measures need to be independent of each other (see Special Interest Box 7.1).

SPECIAL INTEREST BOX 7.1

What Happens When Measures Are Not Independent?

A student wanted to examine the relationship between body composition and physical activity in middle school children and hypothesized that as body composition increased, physical activity decreased. She decided to use BMI as her measure of body composition. She rationalized this choice on the fact that it would be too difficult for her to be consistent with skinfold measurements in children. The student wanted an accurate measure of physical activity and decided to use an accelerometer to measure average energy expenditure (EE) over 4 days. After carefully screening children for any injuries or disabilities that might impede physical activity, she collected data on 31 children with an average age of 11.6 years. Next, she plotted BMI against EE, much like in Figure 7.2, and calculated a correlation coefficient. Much to the student's initial delight, there was a strong positive correlation between BMI and EE. Then, she looked at the correlation again. She had hypothesized that a negative relationship should exist! Her world turned upside down—was her sample different from the general population? Had she collected data incorrectly? Were all of the accelerometers broken? The published literature she had read all suggested that a negative relationship existed, so she decided to examine her data in greater detail to see what was happening with her correlation. After looking at her measures, she had an "Aha!" moment.

Can you see what the student originally missed in her measures? It isn't obvious without digging a little deeper. Both BMI (kg/m^2) and EE (kcal/min/kg) are calculated using each participant's body weight in kilograms, in which case they are not independent. This artificially increased the appearance of a positive relationship between the two seemingly independent variables. Fortunately, the student was able to solve the problem by using another accelerometer measure, activity count, which does not use weight in its calculation. The new correlation turned out to be negative.

While Special Interest Box 7.1 shows an example of how researchers can inadvertently find correlation because of a poor choice of variables, it's also true that researchers may want to look for correlation between variables that are supposed to measure the same thing. This is one way in which researchers validate items on questionnaires (look for a strong association between items that are supposed to measure the same thing) or assess new equipment (look for strong relationship between new and 'gold standard' equipment).

It is important to note that, as discussed in Chapter 6, although a relationship may exist between or among variables, we cannot assume that this implies causation or that one variable *causes* the other. It is tempting to conclude that lower physical activity after school might cause greater levels of obesity. However, correlational research does not allow us to make that conclusion—we can only say the variables are related. In other words, it is possible that increased obesity leads to lower levels of physical activity, perhaps due to psychological or other factors. At this point, we would need to follow up with an experiment to show that one causes the other.

Correlation does not equal causation.

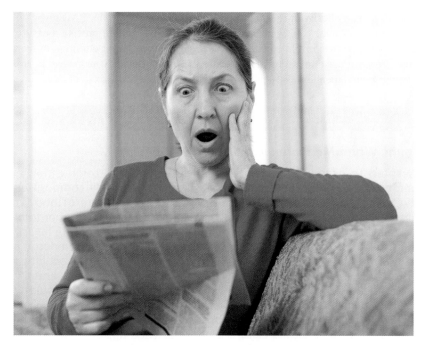

■ **FIGURE 7.2** A 10-year survey by the government that costs $3 million revealed that 3/4 of the people in America make up 75% of the population.

✔ Check Your Understanding

1. Why do researchers use correlational research?
2. What does it mean if two variables are correlated?
3. What is the difference between a positive and negative correlation?
4. A researcher claims that, based on a negative correlation between physical activity and obesity, an increase in obesity causes a decrease in physical activity. Can he make that claim?

SURVEY RESEARCH

In our previous example, we can see that "moderate to vigorous physical activity" is a very broad category that could include a variety of different activity types (e.g., free play, team sports, individual sports) at different levels of effort (moderate, vigorous) and ability (even young children can be on select sports teams!). In order to get at more specific information about the physical activity of these children, we need to use another descriptive research method called survey research. In the broadest sense, survey research allows researchers to get information that is more detailed from individuals by asking them questions about their activities, behaviors, or attitudes on the topic of interest. You can then look at the answers provided by groups of individuals or specific populations to determine if trends exist. Survey research is often used in social and behavioral sciences. Within the field of kinesiology, those interested in sport and

Surveys require planning in what questions to ask and how to ask them.

exercise psychology and biobehavioral health often use survey research. Often, surveys are collected in conjunction with quantitative measures of dependent variables so that the researchers can better interpret their results.

On the surface, it might appear that creating survey questions is simple. All you do is ask questions! However, as with any other type of research, you must carefully plan *what* you want to ask and *how* you want to ask it in order to maximize the validity of the response and minimize error. The way you ask a question can have a huge impact on how a person will respond. For example, if you are interested in determining the amount of time a child is involved in physical activity outside of school, you could ask in several different ways. You could ask, "How many minutes of physical activity outside of school does your child get each day?" At first glance, it appears as though this question gets right to the point. However, can you see some of the issues parents might have with that sort of question? First, each parent might interpret "physical activity" in a different way. One parent may interpret physical activity as structured play experiences, while another, as any time the child moves. Furthermore, there may be a great deal of day-to-day variability in time spent in activities: On Mondays, a child might have 60 minutes of soccer, and on Tuesday, 20 minutes of outside play. In this light, it makes sense to think through what the specific purpose of your question is—what do you want to determine exactly? Then, you can figure out the best way to ask that question. A better way to determine out of school activity might be to ask, "On average, how many days a week does your child get more than 30 minutes of physical activity," or "how many total minutes per week does your child engage in physical activity?"

Significant thought must go into how to ask each question. In addition, the researcher must consider the survey as a whole. Given the overall purpose or objective of the survey, what questions should be asked? How many questions should be included? At the same time, the researcher must consider *who* will take the survey: Who is the population of interest, and what is the most appropriate way to sample from this population?

There are many different survey techniques. We will discuss two of the most common types: questionnaires, and interviews. Both involve asking individuals questions. However, interviews usually involve open-ended questions that individuals (called "respondents") answer orally or in written form. Within interviews, more leeway exists for individual expression. Alternatively, questionnaires often come in a written format (or, increasingly, via websites such as SurveyMonkey or QuestionPro, where they can be administered electronically) and often provide respondents with a more narrowly defined choice of answers. Many questionnaires do include several open-ended questions that allow the respondents to make clarifications or describe related information.

Questionnaires

Questionnaires can provide a good, quick method of gathering data on behaviors, habits, or attitudes from a large sample of the population. A well-constructed questionnaire consists of a series of questions that will provide insight into some aspect of human nature. As a novice researcher, you should look for published questionnaires that have already been validated (we discussed the importance of validity in Chapter 6) rather than making up your own. Many published questionnaires exist, such as the Minnesota Multiphasic Personality Inventory (MMPI). Researchers can either administer the questionnaire at one time to a large group (such as during a class or at a clinic) or distribute it via mail or the Internet.

Don't make up your own questionnaire if a published one already exists.

We have stressed the necessity of planning throughout the text, and this holds true for the development of questionnaires as well. This includes deciding on the most appropriate question format. Occasionally, researchers will decide to use open-ended questions in their questionnaires. Open-ended questions do not have specific responses associated with them. Rather, they provide the respondents with an opportunity to formulate their own responses, such as, "How does exercise impact your everyday life?" or "How does your involvement at the Physical Therapy clinic make you feel?" Open-ended questions within a questionnaire can help the researcher identify themes in response. However, the downside of these types of questions is that they require both thought and action on the part of the respondent, which may make some people hesitant to take the questionnaire in the first place. Additionally, you need to consider how you can analyze or even summarize information from open-ended questions. The results of a good research study are repeatable, which can be difficult if all the questions are open ended and subject to interpretation.

More often, questionnaires use closed rather than open-ended questions. Closed questions provide an embedded answer that the respondent can circle, check, or list. To provide examples of the different types of closed questions that can be used, we will use an existing questionnaire designed to examine leisure time physical activity in older adults.[3] In particular, Orsega-Smith et al. were interested in the barriers or constraints (physical, psychological, economic, etc.) that exist to park and recreation use for an older population. The questionnaire has 12 different sections that focus on specific topics such as environmental effects on exercise, stress, health status, and use of park and recreation services. The first example is a multiple-choice question, where the respondent selects the most appropriate answer related to the use of park and recreation services.

3. During your most recent local park visit, how did you travel to the park?
Choose the *one* primary method:
A. *By car*
B. *Walked*
C. *Bicycled*
D. *By bus*
E. *Other (please specify)*

Note that with this question, the respondents must pick only one choice of transportation. Through pilot work, the researchers determined the types of transportation most frequently used in order to create the question. However, certain situations exist where the respondents may have more than one answer. To accommodate this, another way of structuring questions is to provide a list of responses from which the respondent can choice one or more. Here is an example from the same questionnaire.

8. In which of the following local park and recreation district programs have you participated in over the past 12 months?
Mark *all* that apply:
__*Sports programs (golf, tennis, etc.)*
__*Group exercise (yoga, tai chi, etc.)*
__*Dance classes (line, ballroom, etc.)*
__*Arts and crafts (knit, floral arrangement, etc.)*
__*Outdoor (gardening, floral arrangement, etc.)*
__*Clubs (books, walking, cards, tours, etc.)*
__*Self-directed exercise (lap swim, weights, treadmill, bicycle, etc.)*

Researchers often use another type of question, called a Likert scale,[4] that allows the respondent to provide an answer that falls along a continuum, which may have between 3 and 9 points that are equidistant apart. For example, in the section of the questionnaire examining the impact of environmental factors on recreation activities, the researchers asked the following question on a 6-point Likert scale:

	How much does your participation in physically active recreation *decline* during periods of bad air pollution?	Does Not Apply	Not at All	Declines a Little	Declines Somewhat	Declines Quite a Bit	Completely Declines
1.	Walking outside	1	2	3	4	5	6
2.	Light sport/ recreation activities (e.g., fishing, bowling, golfing with a cart)	1	2	3	4	5	6
3.	Moderate sport/ recreation activities (e.g., hunting, tennis, golf without a cart, dancing)	1	2	3	4	5	6
4.	Strenuous sport/ recreational activities (e.g., jogging, swimming)	1	2	3	4	5	6

Another type of Likert scale asks the respondents to subjectively evaluate their personal levels of stress.

Use the 10-point scale below to indicate your assessment of stress levels. There are no correct answers. Just give your best opinion for each of the questions.

	Least Stressed Life									Most Stressed Life
1. Right now, where do you say *you* are on this scale?	0	1	2	3	4	5	6	7	8	9
2. Where do you think *most people your age* are on this scale?	0	1	2	3	4	5	6	7	8	9
3. In 5 years, where do you think you will be on this scale?	0	1	2	3	4	5	6	7	8	9

As you can see, the type of question depends on what points you are trying to understand. If the participants find that they are forced into making one choice, but none of the answers apply, then the questionnaire will not provide valid information (see Special Interest Box 7.2).

Figure 7.3 provides an example of a validated questionnaire called the Park/Recreational use and Personal Health Inventory, created by collaborators from the University of Illinois, Pennsylvania State University, and University of Delaware. Note the professional design of the questionnaire. It is easy to read and follow, and the authors have taken care to space the questions so that there are

SPECIAL INTEREST BOX 7.2

Pitfalls in Questionnaire Construction: What Do You Mean?

You must develop the questions in your questionnaire so that any ambiguous words are operationally defined if necessary, or else modify your language for clarity. For example, a novice researcher recently constructed a questionnaire on physical activity in cancer survivors. One of the questions was, "were you physically active prior to diagnosis?" with a forced choice of "yes" or "no." The next question asked was, "how many minutes a day did you exercise on average?" The researcher administered the questionnaire to a small group of older women in order to pilot test it and was surprised to find that several of the women who answered "yes" to the first question could not answer the second. When asked why, one respondent replied that she was very physically active—she walked daily, took the stairs instead of the elevator, gardened, and did all of her own yard work—but she didn't monitor time or even try to stay active for a given time period. In essence, she lived a physically active lifestyle, but did not specifically exercise for any set period of time. Was she physically active or wasn't she? The novice researcher made several mistakes in constructing her question. First, she did not operationally define "physical activity" so that the respondents knew exactly what she meant. Second, she didn't provide a time context beyond "prior to diagnosis," which could have meant 1 month, 1 year, or 10 years depending on how the respondent chose to answer. Also, she provided a forced choice (yes or no), which left little room for respondents who were in between sedentary (a definite "no") and regular exercisers (a definite "yes"). Finally, the follow-up question specifically denoted exercise, which, as the respondents pointed out, does not necessarily equate to physical activity. In this case, the researcher revise the questionnaire so physical activities were placed into three categories of mild, moderate, and vigorous, and respondents could select as many activities as applied from a list within each category.

neither too many nor few on a page. The survey itself is 16 pages long, which could become discouraging for participants if the content is not optimally delivered. When developing questionnaires, students should have a knowledgeable professional check for both content and delivery at various stages.

Interviews

Investigators use interviews when they wish to obtain more detailed information from a smaller sample of participants. Just as with questionnaires, the data collected is only as good as the questions asked. Unlike a questionnaire, an interview is generally administered to one or a few individuals at a time, consists of open-ended questions, and may require transcription of the responses from audio or videotape.

There are several different types of interviews. In *structured interviews*, all respondents are asked the same set of questions in the same order, regardless of the response. For example, an interviewer may ask an adolescent male the following series of questions in a structured interview (with hypothetical responses):

Question 1. What sort of things motivate you to be more physically active?
Response 1. *"My friends motivate me a lot. We will play pick-up basketball at least once a week, maybe twice. During the rest of the week, I try to do things like running and lifting weights that will keep me in shape for basketball. I also love to eat, so if I exercise, I can eat a lot more!"*

Section A: Use of Recreation and Park Services

Instructions: Please answer the following questions about your park activities.

1. Is there a local park within walking distance of your home?
 ○ Yes
 ○ No

2. How often do you use your local parks areas or playgrounds during the summer months, June through September?
 ○ Never (Skip to Q. 8)
 ○ Less than 1 time per month
 ○ 1-3 times per month
 ○ 1 time per week
 ○ 2-3 times per week
 ○ 4 or more times per week

3. During your most recent local park visit, how did you travel to the park? Choose the one primary method.
 ○ By car
 ○ Walked
 ○ Bicycle
 ○ By bus
 ○ Other (specify below)

4. Who was with you during your most recent visit?
 Mark all that apply.
 ○ No one, I was alone
 ○ Friends
 ○ Family
 ○ Other (specify below)

5. Who suggested visiting the park?
 Mark the one best answer.
 ○ Self
 ○ Souse/Significant other
 ○ Friend
 ○ Children
 ○ Parent
 ○ Grandchild
 ○ Coworker
 ○ Other (specify below)

6. How long did you stay during your most recent visit to the park?
 ○ Less than 15 minutes
 ○ 15-29 minutes
 ○ 30-44 minutes
 ○ 46-59 minutes
 ○ 1 hour to 1 hour & 29 mins
 ○ 1 hour & 30 mins to 2 hours
 ○ More than 2 hours

2. If you walk as a leisure-time activity, where do you typically walk? Mark the one most likely place.
 ○ Neighborhood
 ○ Local park
 ○ Mall
 ○ Outdoor track
 ○ Indoor track
 ○ Other, specify: _____

3. Describe the people with whom you actually participate in physically active recreation. Physically active recreation is any activity that involves bodily movements (e.g., walking, gardening, exercise, sight seeing).

How often does the person participate with you?

	Most of the time	Some of the time	A little of the time	None of the time	N/A
Spouse/Significant Other	○	○	○	○	○
Friend/Co-worker	○	○	○	○	○
Child	○	○	○	○	○
Health Professional	○	○	○	○	○
Parent	○	○	○	○	○
Other (specify):	○	○	○	○	○

4. Describe how each person below encourages you to participate in physically active recreation:

	How often does the person encourage you?					How much does the person encourage you?			
	Most of the time	Some of the time	A little of the time	None of the time	N/A	Strongly	Moderately	Slightly	Not at all
Spouse/Significant Other	○	○	○	○	○	○	○	○	○
Friend/Co-worker	○	○	○	○	○	○	○	○	○
Child	○	○	○	○	○	○	○	○	○
Health Professional	○	○	○	○	○	○	○	○	○
Parent	○	○	○	○	○	○	○	○	○
Other (specify):	○	○	○	○	○	○	○	○	○

■ FIGURE 7.3 An example of a valid, reliable questionnaire.

Question 2. Are there any barriers to physical activity in your life?
Response 2. *"Barriers? Not really. Well, maybe money. I'd like to join a gym, but the ones around here are really expensive. I can use my brother's weight set at home for free. But other than that, I don't really think so."*

In *semistructured interviews*, the interviewer has a general framework of questions; however, the direction the interview goes depends on the answers made by the respondent. After a respondent answers, the interviewer may choose to "probe" more deeply into the response, getting at more detailed descriptions of thoughts, attitudes, experiences, or behaviors.

Use a semistructured interview if you want to probe more deeply into a response.

Question 1. What sort of things motivates you to be more physically active?
Response 1. *"My friends motivate me a lot. We will play pick-up basketball at least once a week, maybe twice. During the rest of the week, I try to do things like running and lifting weights that will keep me in shape for basketball. I also love to eat, so if I exercise, I can eat a lot more!"*

Question 2. So, you say your friends motivate you to play ball. Do they motivate you at other times? During the times when you are not playing basketball, do you lift weights or run with your friends or do you do that alone?

Response 2. *"Actually, I don't work out with them outside of basketball. We hang out, but we don't do anything else physical. I like to run alone—I think it gives me an edge out on the court."*

In this example, the interviewer probed more deeply to find out if the respondent's friends motivated him for all physical activities or just for basketball.

✔ Check Your Understanding

1. Under what circumstances should an investigator use survey research techniques?
2. When is a questionnaire preferable to an interview?
3. When is an interview preferable to a questionnaire?

OTHER DESCRIPTIVE APPROACHES

Researchers may use other types of descriptive research techniques besides those mentioned previously. In certain situations, researchers may want to focus their attention on only one or several persons, and provide a more complete description over a period of time or during an intervention. Alternatively, they may want to compare actions of individuals at different ages or closely observe individuals during activities. All of these represent different types of descriptive research techniques.

Case Studies

In certain situations, researchers want to know more detail about an individual or situation than a questionnaire or even an interview can provide. They may be interested in how a child with a disability responds to a particular movement environment, or how a diabetic responds in terms of nutritional choices before, during, and after a nutrition-based intervention. In situations such as these, researchers want to gather a large amount of information about the "case" for a variety of purposes. A researcher may want to describe an individual, situation, or therapeutic or educational setting as completely as possible in order to provide an accurate record for future reference, or to provide initial information from which to base an intervention. Another use of **case studies** is to evaluate the efficacy of a program or therapeutic practice. Again, because the research is descriptive, the researcher does not manipulate or change aspects of the program, but rather carefully details its impact on one or several individuals. Adaptive physical education is one area where case studies are frequently used, and it is easy to see why. Children with certain disabilities may have the same underlying condition (e.g., cerebral palsy, Down syndrome) that will present in a highly individualized manner. This makes experimental research difficult; at the same time, practitioners need evidence that interventions work. Researchers want to know "how does this technique work with this individual?" and use case studies to record both the intervention and the outcome.

Case Study A detailed description of an individual, group, intervention, or therapeutic or educational setting

In populations where large individual differences exist in response to interventions, case studies provide a way to document change.

Take, for example, your hypothetical research at Springfield Elementary School. Let's say you discovered that the children in two kindergarten classes had very different average values for BMI and physical activity, and in fact, the children in classroom 1 had average values that were much higher for BMI and lower for physical activity. You might want to examine this particular kindergarten class in greater detail, in order to get a picture of the children as a whole. Further, you may wish to study two children within the kindergarten class, to get a more in depth view of their physical activity over a week. You may even want to document these students as they go through a movement education program, as a way to determine if the program was effective for them. One of the drawbacks of this research is that there is no way to objectively assess causation with this descriptive format. In Chapter 9, we will discuss single-subject design research (SSDR), which also involves observing one or a small group of participants; unlike case studies, SSDR allows for statistical analysis and causal inference.

Developmental Research

Developmental researchers' interests lie in examining change over time, to examine the interacting influences that growth, maturation, and environment have on different aspects of physical activity or motor behavior. In general, age serves as the independent variable of interest, and one or more dependent variables are described at different ages. In fact, the previous example of Springfield Elementary is actually a type of developmental research, since the sample of children was subdivided by age groups! Clearly, age-related change occurs quite rapidly during childhood, and these changes are often the subject of developmental research. However, as numbers of individuals over the age of 65 years swell, researchers have an increased interest in understanding the aging process at the other end of the spectrum. Thus, many researchers use developmental studies to answer a huge range of questions about health, movement, and exercise across the life span.

Several different study designs fit within the framework of developmental research. Arguably, the longitudinal research design is the gold standard when an investigator is interested in developmental change.[5] With a **longitudinal design**, a researcher follows the behavior of one or several individuals over some meaningful time period, which could be months or even years. Within the field of motor development, Roberton and Halverson[6,7] followed seven children for over 15 years (from 3 to 18 years old). At each data collection session, they had the children perform fundamental motor skills, such as overarm throwing and hopping. Then, they carefully detailed how each child moved, providing descriptions of the qualitative changes in the action of the arms, legs, and trunk. Using this information, they could derive a developmental trajectory that mapped the changes occurring in these motor skills as children age on a year-to-year basis. As you might imagine, longitudinal research can be long and labor intensive, and for most researchers, such designs are not feasible.

As a shorter-term solution to describing developmental change, investigators may choose to use **cross-sectional designs** if they are interested in tracking change over time. In contrast to a longitudinal study (following a few individuals over long periods), a cross-sectional study includes groups of individuals within a narrow age range at one

Longitudinal Design
Describing a small group of individuals over a long time period, such as months or years.

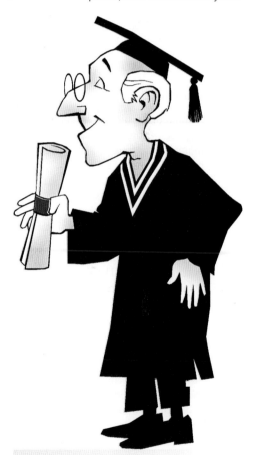

"It only took me 75 years to finish my longitudinal study on motor skill change across the life span!"

Cross-Sectional Design
Describing different age groups at one point in time to simulate the process of development.

point in time, thus simulating developmental change. In this example, instead of describing change in seven children each year for 15 years, Halverson and Roberton could have tested groups of 3-, 6-, 9-. 12-, 15-, and 18-year old children over a short period of time and then inferred a developmental change based on their observations of age group differences. The underlying assumption in a cross-sectional design is that each age group once acted like the preceding one (i.e., the 6-year-olds once hopped like the 3-year-olds) and will one day move like the later age group (the 6-year-olds will one day hop like 9-, 12-, 15-, and 18-year-olds). The benefit of a cross-sectional research design is that the investigator can complete developmental research in a much shorter time period (and a graduate student actually has hope of finishing a thesis or dissertation before retirement age). At the same time, this design has several problems of which researchers must be aware. First, historical events can differentially impact one of the age cohorts. These "events" could be something as simple as a new gadget that improves balance (like training wheels) or body mechanics (like a batting tee for baseball); younger groups may change as a result of the new gadget rather than as a function of development. The other problem, of course, is that we must infer (rather than observe) development from changes in the different age groups.

Observational Research

Although questionnaires and surveys can provide significant amounts of data, at times, researchers may desire more objective measures than self-report. Let's go back to Springfield Elementary for a moment and look at physical activity that was acquired through parental report. For a first pass, this measure provides a ball park figure of how much a child moves outside of school. However, consider a typical sport that a child may play after school: baseball. In baseball, 1 hour of game play may equate into little physical activity (depending on position played, skill of pitchers, number of hits, etc.). Parents could report that their children get several hours of physical activity each week while playing baseball when in fact the children were relatively sedentary! In such instances, observational research would provide a better measure of physical activity. Researchers observe systematically, in that they carefully define the behavior of interest, and then observe from specific points in time and from particular locations. They may even use video as a tool to enhance their ability to accurately observe more detail. Such research techniques are often used in educational research when researchers want to detail the on and off task behaviors of a classroom of students.

In our baseball game example, you might begin by listing the behaviors seen in a baseball game (sitting on a bench, running bases, standing in the field, batting, etc.) and rating those activities on a scale from 1 (sedentary) to 4 (vigorously active). Then you would head out to the field for a game, video camera in hand. After recording the game, you would watch the players of interest (those in 5th grade at Springfield Elementary) and code their behaviors every 4 minutes over the course of the game. You could convert these values into percent of time scores and then could say with confidence that Child A was vigorously active 12% of the game, whereas Child B was vigorously active 36% of the game. This would give you a far more accurate view of how active children were than parental report.

✔ Check Your Understanding

1. Under what situations would a researcher want to use a case study?
2. How do case studies differ from observational research?
3. What developmental research designs involve watching few participants over a long time? How about many participants of different ages over a short time?

CHAPTER SUMMARY

- Descriptive research involves documenting important characteristics of individuals, groups, interventions, and therapeutic treatments. It does not involve experimental manipulation.
- Descriptive research is often the foundation of experimental research.
- When researchers perform correlational research, they look for associations between or among variables.
- Both questionnaires and interviews are forms of survey research.
- Questionnaires must be carefully constructed so that respondents interpret questions similarly.
- Researchers can perform structured interviews, where each respondent receives the same list of questions, or semistructured interviews, where the interviewer modifies questions based on the respondent's response to the previous question.
- In a case study, a researcher describes a "case," which can be one or several individuals, an intervention, or a therapeutic or educational setting of interest.
- Developmental research can occur over a long time span (longitudinal) or at one time with participants of representative ages (cross-sectional).
- Observational research involves describing behaviors at specific time intervals and can be qualitative or quantitative.

REFERENCES

1. Field A. *Discovering Statistics Using SPSS*, 4th ed. Washington, DC: Sage, 2013, 12.
2. Pyrczak R. *Making Sense of Statistics: A Conceptual Overview*, 5th ed. Glendale, CA: Pyrczak Publishing, 2010:57–60.
3. Orsega-Smith E, Payne L, Mowen A. The role of social support and self-efficacy in shaping leisure time physical activity in older adults. *J Leis Res* 2007;39(4): 705–727.
4. Carifio J, Perla RJ. Ten common misunderstandings, misconceptions, persistent myths and urban legends about Likert scales and Likert response formats and their antidotes. *J Soc Sci* 2007;3(3):106–116.
5. Haywood KM, Roberton MA, Getchell N. *Advanced Analysis of Motor Development*. Champaign, IL: Human Kinetics, 2012.
6. Roberton MA, Halverson LE. *Developing Children: Their changing Movement*. Philadelphia, PA: Lea & Febiger, 1984.
7. Roberton MA, Halverson LE. The development of locomotor coordination: longitudinal change and invariance. *J Motor Behav* 1988;20:197–241.

RELATED ASSIGNMENTS

1. **Use the Internet to find surveys or questionnaires on the following topics that are valid and reliable:**

   a. Preschool children's physical activity
   b. Patient health and depression
   c. Patient health and cancer
   d. Perceived competence
   e. Additional questionnaire of your choice

Write a brief synopsis of each questionnaire. What is the purpose? For whom is it valid? How many questions are there and of what type? Finally, can you find a published research study that uses this questionnaire and cite it?

2. Write a 1-page paper that compares the purpose of descriptive research to that of experimental research (described in Chapter 6).

3. Compare and contrast developmental, observational, and case study research studies. Under what situations would you use each of these? Develop scenarios where each type of research study would be most appropriate.

IN-CLASS GROUP EXERCISES

1. Within your group, develop a 5-item questionnaire to assess physical activity in college students. Carefully consider wording and structure, and limit yourself to only five questions. Once you have finished, exchange your questionnaire with that of another group. Compare and contrast their questions with yours, then revise your questionnaire.

2. Within your group, determine two variables that may have an association that are readily available or easily collected (e.g., total SAT score and college GPA; height and weight). Collect these variables from the members of your class and create an X–Y plot of those variables. Next, compare your group's results to those of other groups. Discuss the difference.

8

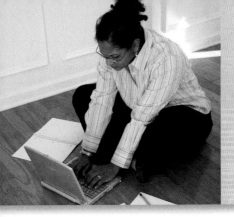

Qualitative Research

"Qualitative research is pragmatic, interpretive, and grounded in the lived experiences of people."—Marshall and Rossman, Designing Qualitative Research.[1]

CHAPTER OBJECTIVES

After studying this chapter, you will be able to:

1. Explain five characteristics of qualitative research.
2. Describe qualitative research traditions and perspectives.
3. Discuss four ways to increase the trustworthiness of qualitative research.
4. Identify data sampling and collection methods that match the research purpose.
5. Describe how qualitative research questions and designs evolve during the data collection and analysis process.
6. Identify data analysis techniques that lead to description and interpretation of phenomena that answer the research question.

■ QUALITATIVE research studies examine social situations that occur at a particular place and time. Researchers place people's lived experiences at the center of the research process. Although it is possible to enumerate or count things that people do or the number of people who participate, qualitative research permits the researcher to capture the richness of people's lives, their emotions, and their personal interpretations of what they see, hear, and feel. Statistical research designs often examine large, randomly selected samples to discern trends, means, and differences in group characteristics. These macrodesigns focus on generalizing findings from a sample to a larger population. Conversely, qualitative researchers work at the microlevel, using labor-intensive observations and interview techniques to develop in-depth understandings of the ways participants understand daily events in their world.

There are five characteristics of qualitative research that can help you to distinguish these research studies from other research designs.[2] First, qualitative research is typically conducted in natural settings. Researchers travel to the research setting or situation instead of bringing the research subjects to their laboratory. The researcher's role in qualitative research is to learn about the participants' world. The natural setting is considered the primary context in which all social interactions occur. The term **context** describes the social, historical, political, and temporal setting in which participants work, interact, and live.

Context The social, historical, political, and temporal setting in which participants work, interact, and live. In qualitative research, the context or setting is the framework for understanding how people relate, interact, and interpret their world

Second, qualitative researchers often employ many different data collection methods and techniques to delve deeply into participants' lives and to verify the trustworthiness of their findings. In this chapter, we will discuss a few of these data collection methods, such as observation, interview, and photo diary. Third, qualitative researchers study the complex settings in which people live their lives. Researchers do not attempt to control the setting or to limit or reduce the complexity. Instead, researchers employ research designs and techniques to capture complexity and work to communicate how phenomena blend to create participants' lived experiences. In qualitative research, the term **phenomenon** describes any fact, circumstance, or experience that is apparent to the senses and that can be scientifically described or appraised.

Phenomenon (singular)/ Phenomena (plural) Any fact, circumstance or experience that is apparent to the senses and that can be scientifically described or appraised

Fourth, qualitative research designs are fluid and flexible, unfolding as the researcher gains deeper insights into the complexity of the context. Researchers expect the design to become more complex as they identify key informants and key contexts within the research setting. As the situation evolves, researchers identify and follow **themes** that emerge as individuals interact within particular contexts. They consider each situation to be unique, perhaps one of a kind. If the situation occurs once, we know that it exists and work to understand how these phenomena emerge and evolve. Finally, qualitative researchers' primary emphasis is on interpretation of the lived experiences of their participants. Interpretive qualitative research, however, is more than a descriptive record of what occurred; it reflects a detailed interpretation of the what, when, why, and how of the situation as observed by the researcher and interpreted by participants.

Themes Organizing concepts, constructs, or patterns used to structure qualitative data. Themes may begin as a researcher's intuitive hunch and are then documented through observation, interview, or photography as organizing concepts. Themes typically represent abstract conceptualizations that can become key focal points when communicating results.

From these characteristics, we can deduce several assumptions that guide qualitative research.[2] First, qualitative researchers believe that social interactions are both holistic and complex. It is not adequate to record a sentence without understanding the situation in which it was expressed, including what events preceded it and the conversations and consequences that followed. Second, because the situation is real and evolving while the researcher is present, it is important to remain open to new possibilities. Certainly, qualitative researchers learn quickly to go with the flow. Since the situation is developing each day, it is impossible for researchers (or thesis and dissertation committee members) to anticipate every aspect of the research design prior to entering the field. Instead, the qualitative researcher develops the general timeline and selects the initial setting and participant sample, understanding that additional participants, settings, and research questions may be added as the researcher's understanding of the context deepens. Additionally, because the researchers' understandings are developing quickly, data analysis cannot wait until the researcher leaves the field but begins almost immediately to inform the design and alert the researcher to developing themes.

A third assumption of qualitative researchers is that their research perspective is **subjective**. The researcher is uniquely equipped with motivation, expertise, and skills to make sense of complex environments. The human brain functions more effectively to observe and analyze unique situations than most computers. Often qualitative researchers serve as both the data collection "instrument" and the data analysis "software." Thus, their personal histories, expertise, and previous experiences *will* influence the topic they choose to investigate, the site and participants they select to examine, and their interpretations of what they have learned. In other words, like all researchers, they make research and methodology decisions based on their own biographies and social identities. They understand that their personal histories shape their research questions and their interpretation and presentation of findings. Therefore, a responsibility of qualitative researchers is to foreground their biographies and their personal and professional connections with the research topic, participants, and setting. They explain these relationships clearly in research reports so the reader may, in turn, interpret and understand the researcher's perspectives. Further, qualitative researchers learn and practice techniques to increase their awareness of these influencing factors and use methods of triangulation, dependability, confirmability, and transferability to establish the trustworthiness and authenticity of the research findings. We will discuss these concepts in detail later in the chapter.

> **Subjective/Subjectivity** The personal perspective of the researcher that influences the selection of the research topic, research questions and methods. It is the responsibility of the qualitative researcher to discuss these influences and to explain their expertise and experience in the research setting.

Finally, qualitative researchers work both deductively and inductively to develop a deeper understanding of the situations and people in the research setting. At times, they work to examine how a social theory can be used to explain and predict individual relationships and the consequences of decisions that people make in crisis situations or in the daily workplace (deductive). At other times, researchers may enter the setting with minimal understandings of the participants or the situation. They spend an extended time period looking, listening, questioning, and reflecting to generate new theory that is grounded in the events and interactions of the people and places they have visited (induction/grounded theory). In each situation, however, the researcher's focus is on first capturing a rich description of the events and social interactions and then interpreting these from the participants' perspectives.

Qualitative researchers ask a range of research questions that represent many different philosophical and theoretical perspectives. In this chapter, we will first explore three qualitative traditions: naturalistic, interpretive, and critical. Next, we will map the preliminary steps in conducting a qualitative research study, creating a trustworthy research design, selecting the research site and participants, and entering the site. We then will discuss data collection and analysis techniques used to better understand and interpret social settings. Qualitative research traditions, methods, and protocols have developed extensively over the last four decades, becoming a central research paradigm for social scientists, educators, and researchers who seeks in-depth answers to social questions. Currently, it is a well-respected research method that has proven its value in understanding complex social settings.

QUALITATIVE RESEARCH TRADITIONS

Qualitative research provides a comprehensive approach to studying social settings and phenomena. Because social scientists have different purposes and assumptions, it is not surprising to find different philosophical streams of thought guiding different research categories. I will group these into three major categories of inquiry, naturalistic, interpretive, and critical, and then include a few examples of specific research topics and questions within each category of inquiry.

Naturalistic Inquiry

Naturalistic Inquiry
Research conducted in existing social settings. Researchers strive to preserve the existing context and minimize reactions or changes caused by their presence.

Although all categories or genres of qualitative research are conducted in naturalistic settings, scholars who assume an explicitly **naturalistic** stance attempt to preserve the natural setting of the school, community agency, hospital, fitness club, or camp with as little disturbance to the daily activities as possible. This is a significant challenge because most participants react when an outsider enters their organization or community. Naturalistic researchers, such as ethnographers and narrative researchers, understand that their initial presence in a setting will attract attention and comment. They work initially to communicate a reason or purpose for their presence and then, once participant curiosity is satisfied, attempt to blend inconspicuously into the setting. Additionally, they plan to spend an extensive time period in the setting, making friends and meeting key informants, participating in events of the specific community, and inducing participants to accept them and to act naturally in their presence. Scholars in two qualitative genres, ethnography and narrative inquiry, focus extensively on capturing and interpreting natural settings.

ETHNOGRAPHY

Ethnography is the earliest distinct tradition[3] in qualitative research. It was derived from anthropology and qualitative approaches to sociology. Anthropologists first employed these techniques as they sought

Culture   Commonly held ideas, customs, skills, and daily actions of a group of individuals

to understand how people collectively form societies and maintain their culture. Thus, the study of culture is central to all ethnographies. A **culture** is defined as the commonly held ideas, customs, skills, and daily actions of a group of individuals. Often, people clustered together to preserve and experience common beliefs, traits, or ways of understanding the world. Ethnographers investigating schools, businesses, and communities ask research questions such as "What is the culture of this group of people?" Ethnographers enter most cultural settings as outsiders who come to learn and document the beliefs, actions, events, and contexts of particular cultures. These settings can be as exotic as Margaret Mead's cultural anthropology of the Samoans in the 1920s to current educational scholars' studies of urban high school physical education programs.

Ethnographers typically study groups, communities, organizations, or social movements using prolonged engagement in the setting.[1] They may choose to participate with community members in daily activities, removing themselves briefly to a private place to record field notes and reflect on their experiences. Analyses of qualitative ethnographic field notes result in the identification of patterns in participant interactions, attributing meaning to ceremonies, rituals, and artifacts. Today, ethnographies take many forms from those that examine the culture of schools, hospitals, fitness facilities, and laboratories to investigations of interactions on the Internet such as Facebook (virtual ethnographies) and spontaneous public gatherings such as "flash mobs" (public ethnographies). Autoethnographers rely on their personal experiences within a culture to provide insight into the culture, situation, or events they are monitoring.[3] Critical ethnographers examine marginalized cultures with the purpose of raising individual or public awareness of discrimination.

NARRATIVE INQUIRY

Narrative ethnographers convey and interpret participants' stories of significant life events. Often, participants have lived in turbulent times, such as a war, or taught in schools during the implementation of a controversial new law, such as Brown vs. the Board of Education that integrated black students into formerly white schools. Teachers and students' stories of these historically significant events are useful in enhancing our current understanding of the event from the personal perspectives of those who struggled to create new cultural communities. Narrative researchers might ask research questions such as "What does this narrative or story tell us about this person or their world?" or "How can this individual's narrative be interpreted to illuminate the life and culture of this group of people?"

Narrative inquiry also can take the form of life histories in which the researcher may visit and interview a key informant many times over a lengthy time period. A **key informant** is an individual who possesses unique information or has lived through a special event and is willing to share their information and experiences with the researcher. Interviews are conducted over weeks or months providing respondents an opportunity to read and edit interview transcripts and reflect on these events. This process deepens their own understandings and interpretations of the outcomes and helps them to consider the event's impact on their life. Currently, narrative life histories are being collected from World War II veterans and black scientists who serve as role models and whose contributions provide roadmaps for new generations. These data cannot be collected with a paper and pencil survey or questionnaire. Instead, the richness of experience as captured on digital audio and video recorders communicates how these events and experiences changed participants' lives and contributed to the evolution of particular cultures.

> **Key Informant** An individual who possesses unique information or has lived through a special event and is willing to share his or her information and experiences with the researcher

Interpretive Inquiry

Interpretive inquiry evolved from ethnographies as researchers placed an even greater emphasis on the relevance and meaning that participants ascribed to life events and experiences. Although many people experience the same event within the same culture, each person makes sense of his or her experiences in different ways. Interpretive scholars attempt to construct specific individuals' interpretations to compare differences in perspectives within common experiences. Phenomenology and heuristic inquiry are forms of qualitative research that place the individual's experiences at the center of the research study.

> **Interpretive Inquiry** Qualitative research that examines participant's perspectives and interpretations of life events and experiences

PHENOMENOLOGY

Phenomenologists seek to understand the very nature of the experience—what makes a phenomenon, event, or experience what it is. Practical applications in research explore individuals' meanings and interpretations of their lived experiences and how they perceive, describe, judge, and remember it and how they talk to others about this experience or event.[3] Phenomenological researchers collect several extensive interviews from individuals who have experienced the phenomenon of interest. The focus of the analysis is on identifying the essence of the experience and how the individual perceives and interprets it. Research questions include "What are the meaning, structure, and essence of the lived experience for this person or group of people?"

Phenomenologists might focus on individuals' experiences as second language learners in schools or the experiences of a physical therapist working with Native American populations. Each phenomenological account begins with a description of the "turn" or a rationale for the research, for example, what turned or attracted the researcher to the topic of interest. Thus, the researcher's personal history becomes part of the story and facilitates the search for the essence of interpretation. As the story continues, the researcher's experiences become entwined with those of participants, forming a new, rich, and more compelling story.

Heuristic Inquiry

Interpretive research can take many forms in addition to phenomenology. For example, heuristic inquiry explores the researcher's personal experiences with a phenomenon and weaves it together with other individuals' experiences with the same phenomenon. The purpose is not specifically to compare the experiences, although this often is part of the exploration; instead, the focus is on the creation of shared meanings that deepen and extend the individuals' unique perspectives. Research questions include "What is my experience of this phenomenon and how can I better understand my experience by understanding others' experiences and interpretations?"[3]

Critical Inquiry

Critical Inquiry Research conducted to increase people's awareness of social injustices and to encourage both participants and future readers to commit to social justice and change

Researchers within the third broad category of qualitative research, **critical inquiry**, approach their research topics with a clearly articulated mission or political agenda. Critical researchers conduct research to increase others' awareness of social injustices and to encourage both participants and future readers of the research findings to become committed to correcting the wrongs revealed in their research. Some qualitative researchers conduct critical ethnographies to examine the culture of marginalized or underserved groups. Critical scholars often position their research from an orientational perspective. In other words, they study issues that affect groups of individuals because of their gender, race, ethnicity, sexual orientation, or some life circumstance (poverty, imprisonment, discrimination).

Orientational Inquiry

Orientational researchers assume a position of political advocacy with the goal of increasing awareness, commitment, and social change. They study topics, participants, and settings that reflect social injustices and frame their research questions to evoke an emotional reaction from the reader and, at times, from the participants themselves. Orientational researchers may approach their research from many perspectives, such as feminist, Marxist, Freudian, or capitalist theories. Feminist researchers, for instance, may seek to reveal and emphasize the centrality of gender in social relationships and societal processes. Feminist researchers use the lenses of social justice to value women's perspectives as a way of raising consciousness and enhancing women's roles as agents of social change. Research questions often involve the exploration of women's histories and culture as they impact and are impacted by politics (power structures) and economics. A feminist research study might explore questions such as "What are the barriers that prevent girls from participating on boys' athletic teams?"

Critical scholars examine topics associated with racism and ethnicity with the purpose of social change. Detailed studies of racist treatment and injustices are conducted both to increase awareness of these events and to simultaneously deconstruct the dominant assumptions and behaviors that contribute to injustice. Queer theory examines prejudices and discrimination based on sexual orientation. Researchers may question "What are the consequences when lesbian and gay athletes choose to reveal their sexual orientation/lifestyles to other team members?"

The purpose of critical inquiry often is to deconstruct the dominant social perspective and to (re) construct a more socially just and inclusive position. The focus of this research genre, however, is not just to study and understand the phenomenon but to critique and change society. Researchers may ask, "What are the dominant social positions that result in policies that foster and promote exclusion?" These critical researchers have come full circle from the purported objective stance of more traditional forms of research to use the inquiry process and research findings to advocate for social justice and change.

SECTION SUMMARY

Table 8.1 provides a summary of the qualitative traditions discussed in this section. It is important to be aware of the comprehensive nature of qualitative research traditions and genres as they are reflected in researchers' diverse philosophical and theoretical positions. Remember that all qualitative researchers study the context or situation that creates and shapes the phenomenon of interest. The context is central to defining and distinguishing the characteristics of all social phenomena. Researchers spend extensive

TABLE 8.1	Key Elements of Qualitative Research Traditions		
Tradition	**Genre**	**Description**	**Research Question**
Naturalistic		Studies of culture	"What is the culture of this group of people?"
	Ethnography	Studies of groups, communities, organizations, or social movements using long-term immersion in the setting[1]	"How do individuals within this community come together around a set of shared beliefs and ideals?"
	Narrative	Studies of participants' in-depth stories about significant life events	"What does this narrative or story tell us about this person or their world?" "How can this individual's narrative be interpreted to illuminate the life and culture of this group of people?"
Interpretive		Studies of the relevance and meaning that participants ascribe to life events and experiences	"How did this event influence these participants' perspectives?"
	Phenomenology	Studies of the nature or essence of experience	"What are the meaning, structure, and essence of the lived experience for this person or group of people?"
	Heuristic	Studies of the researcher's and participants' personal experiences and shared meanings	"What is my experience of this phenomenon, and how can I better understand my experience by understanding other's experiences and interpretations?"[3]
Critical		Studies of marginalized or underserved participants with the goal of promoting social justice	"What circumstances are responsible for the social injustices that have limited this individual's life?"
	Orientational	Researchers assume a position of political advocacy with the goal of increasing awareness, commitment, and action.	"How are community power structures organized to foster discrimination for this group of people?"
	Feminist, Marxist, capitalist, racist, etc.	Study topics, participants, and settings that reflect social injustices Frame research to deconstruct dominant social perspectives and evoke emotional reactions and responses from readers and at times from the participants themselves	"How have these people been oppressed within this community?" "What are the consequences of their exclusion for themselves and other members of the community?"

time periods embedded in a setting to understand the experiences more deeply. When researchers are investigating historical events, they may conduct an extensive series of interviews over a long time period to capture participants' unique perspectives and interpretations of their lived experiences.

Qualitative researchers reject the notion that a social context can or should be reduced to a few isolated variables. Instead, they explain that discovering the essence of most social phenomena requires in-depth understandings of multiple, complex interactions that occur within natural settings. Efforts to remove, reduce, or distill the phenomenon from its context diminish or remove these intricate relationships, invalidating the findings. These assumptions distinguish qualitative forms of research from other research designs such as those associated with quasi-experimental, controlled, or randomized research studies. Qualitative researchers seek rich, in-depth answers to complex social problems. They argue that research methods should reflect and illuminate the complexity of the setting, leading to comprehensive interpretations of social phenomena.

✔ Check Your Understanding

1. List three major categories of qualitative research.
2. Explain five characteristics of qualitative research.
3. Discuss four assumptions of qualitative researchers.

GETTING STARTED

Once you have selected a qualitative perspective and identified a research question, it is necessary to decide how comprehensive your qualitative research study will be. Unlike other forms of research that use a priori designs, qualitative studies *evolve* as researchers delve deeply into the context to answer the research question. As a rule of thumb, it is better to think small when envisioning the scale or your research. Rest assured that your study is likely to expand like exploding fireworks once you establish yourself within the research setting. In this section, I will discuss elements of qualitative research design, including sample selection and size, and suggestions to increase the trustworthiness of future findings.

Research Design: Sample Selection and Size

Qualitative research focuses on the study of social phenomena within a particular context or setting. Therefore, selection of the setting is a sampling decision of great importance both at the beginning as you plan your research design and latter when you justify the trustworthiness of your findings. Although it is efficient and easy to conduct your research in a place where you already have friends or acquaintances who will let you observe and interview, it is more difficult later to explain why this was the best site to answer your research question.

Instead, use a literature review to identify key factors or variables that appear to impact the setting or participants that you are studying. For example, if your question is "What instructional strategies and activities do middle school teachers use to keep students physically active in physical education?" use your literature review to confirm that students in experienced, expert teachers' classes exhibit greater time on task. Based on this knowledge, you know how to select a "purposeful" sample of expert, experienced teachers. National Board–certified physical educators must exhibit both characteristics, and thus, you would expect them to use effective strategies and activities to keep students engaged in activity. If all teachers you select are effective at engaging students in physical activity during the physical education lesson, you can then document the specific instructional strategies used and when, where, and how National Board–certified teachers use them to keep students physical active.

Purposeful sampling is a key element of qualitative research designs. Because the goal is in-depth understanding of a particular social setting, it is not useful to randomly sample schools. Likewise, because you will spend an extensive amount of time collecting data at each research site, it is not realistic to use a large sample size. Some researchers conduct case studies in one school spending a year or more in one site. Their findings are richly detailed, identifying a host of patterns and relationships that a casual observer or a survey researcher might not discover. Other researchers ask questions that are best answered by comparing the situation at several research sites. In these situations, purposefully sampling sites and participants optimally suited to answer the research question is the foundation for trustworthy research findings.

Other research questions require a comparison of some phenomenon across several research sites or participant groups. If your research question is "To what extent do teachers keep students physically active in physical education?" you might purposefully sample three schools with diverse characteristics and cultures to provide a range of situations in which to examine this question. Perhaps you know from the literature review that school location is important when examining student activity because the quality of school services often is impacted by the communities' real estate tax base. Schools located in affluent areas of the community may have a different school and physical activity culture than schools that service students who live in poverty. If location is a significant factor in your study, you may want to purposefully select schools that enroll students from families with high or low incomes. Additionally, if physical activity is impacted by teacher experience, then you may want to combine the location variable with teacher experience variables. In this case, you would purposefully seek opportunities to conduct your research in high- and low-income schools with teachers who represent greater than 15 years and fewer than 5 years of teaching experience. Clearly, it would not serve your purpose to select a random sample of schools and teachers because you are unlikely to satisfy the conditions that previous research has indicated make a difference in student levels of activity. You can answer your question more directly if you sample purposefully and selectively to match the unique characteristics of participants and the setting with key variables or phenomena in your research question.

While your research design might call for a specific number of sites, the selection of participants is also important. For example, if your research question is "How do personal trainers build trust with their clients?" you could use a qualitative design to shadow personal trainers to observe how they build trust. You may have contacted a site but found that only two of the seven personal trainers were willing to work with you. However, once you have been collecting observation and interview data with those two trainers at the fitness club for 3 weeks, all trainers relax and become more welcoming. Additionally, your two trainers have talked with the others about your research, and they now are willing to participate in your research. The personal recommendations from current participants in the site are an example of another form of sample described as "snowball" or "chain" sampling.[1] One contact leads to another, or a participant identifies a potential key informant that you did not realize had useful information. This process can help you to selectively sample key informants who can provide unique insights you are unable to gather from your original participants. A flexible, evolving qualitative research design permits snowball sampling of both research sites and participants. The purpose of snowball sampling is access to the sites and participants most influential in answering your research question.

Creating a Trustworthy Research Design

Trustworthiness is a reflection of the quality or soundness of the research design. We want others to believe and trust our research findings to be authentic and to accurately convey the essences of the phenomena and the patterns and themes we have identified in the natural research setting. Trustworthiness in qualitative research consists of credibility,

Trustworthiness The extent to which your research findings are believable. This perception is based on design factors associated with credibility, confirmability and transferability of qualitative research.

Credibility Research findings that are believable and that reflect an authentic and accurate portrayal of the research setting and themes

Prolonged Engagement The commitment of the researcher to spend an extended period of time in the research setting

Triangulation The use of multiple data sources to confirm or reject information. If a teacher suggests that the parachute lesson is the students' favorite, then researchers need to check with students to ask them specifically which lessons in the curriculum they like the best. Additionally, the researcher should observe the parachute lessons to gain first hand evidence of the lesson and to analyze the lessons to determine why students might select it as their favorite.

Transferability The extent to which the findings are useful to others in similar situations.[1] In qualitative research the burden of transferability exists with the reader of the research, not the researcher. Researchers, however, can increase opportunities for transfer by providing rich descriptions of the setting and participants.

dependability, confirmability, and transferability. **Credibility** involves the ability of the researcher to present believable findings. In qualitative studies, researchers plan to stay in a setting for a long period of time. This process described as **prolonged engagement** increases the opportunity for researches to observe many events, to interact with many individuals under a variety of settings, and to both confirm and refute developing themes.

Qualitative researchers also collect many different types of data (observational field notes, interview and focus groups, artifact) and can use these various sources of information to confirm and challenge the data. This process, described as **triangulation**, permits the researcher to examine each finding from several different perspectives. Triangulation contributes to the confirmability of the research. We have more confidence in the accuracy and authenticity of themes when the data can be confirmed by other participants or through other data sources. The researcher can check her findings with participants, described as member checks, to ensure she is representing and interpreting the situation in a manner consistent with participants' perspectives. The researcher also can discuss themes with peers knowledgeable about the setting and familiar with qualitative research procedures and protocols. During prolonged engagement, the researcher also searches for alternative explanations and instances or cases in which the situation occurs, but the meaning to participants is different. These instances, described as negative cases, reflect inherent inconsistencies found in most social settings and may add credibility to the description of the natural setting.

The researcher's commitment to collect rich, highly detailed, and descriptive field notes makes the setting come alive for readers of the research. Finally, although qualitative researchers are not focused on statistical generalizability, they are concerned with transferability. **Transferability** refers to the extent to which the findings are useful to others in similar situations.[1] Rich description of the research setting, participants, and themes assists other researchers to transfer findings from the original study and apply them to their situation. Although the burden of transferability exists with the reader, rather than the original researcher, the researcher can facilitate this process through selective sampling and the use of rich descriptions detailing each phenomenon in the research setting.

Entry into the Research Site: Explaining the Purpose of Your Research

Once your proposal and Institutional Review Board approval are in hand, you need to contact participants and gain access to the research site. Conceptualize and explain your research question and purpose broadly. This allows you to begin your data collection by looking generally at the setting and allows you to explore several alternatives before narrowing to specific research questions. For example, if your research question is "What opportunities and barriers impact implementation of a new curriculum?" you are free to ask questions about instructional time, lesson schedule, teacher philosophy, equipment, and resources. You also can observe how "faithfully" teachers implement the curriculum as part of this larger question. When you first arrive, you may not be able to judge the opportunities and barriers that impact this situation, but by phrasing your question broadly, you keep your options open.

✓ Check Your Understanding

1. Discuss how sampling decisions will differ based on the type of research question you ask.
2. Explain two factors you need to consider when selecting a qualitative research sample.
3. Describe three characteristics of a trustworthy qualitative research design.

DATA COLLECTION

Collecting qualitative data requires the use of different techniques, with each having a unique purpose and function. Developing a data collection timeline permits the qualitative researcher to plan the setting and time period in which to utilize different data collection methods. The timeline encourages the researcher to work deliberately while providing a sense of urgency to complete each phase and move to the next. The timeline also guides data collection by permitting the researcher to observe the setting, form hunches, and gradually collect data to refute a hunch or support the development of significant themes.

Data Collection Timeline

A data collection timeline is a roadmap to help the researcher and the participants understand the methods selected and the order in which they will be used. When observation is selected as a way of understanding the research setting, the researcher can build several weeks of observation into the beginning of the study to allow time to gradually become familiar with the setting. This also permits the researcher to become more accepted by participants and to observe events, behaviors, reactions, and consequences over an extended time period. As a researcher, you should avoid asking for participant explanations too early in the study because these can bias your perspectives, leading you to accept the participants' conclusions without searching for your own impressions. Participants often want to influence the observer. They want you to understand and affirm their rationales and not question their decisions. By observing without participants' input for a period of time, you look harder for patterns and begin developing your own explanations. Later, you can test these out by asking participants, as there will be plenty of time to do this later. At the beginning of the study, it is important that the qualitative researcher consider many alternatives, gathering support in the natural context for those that appear most logical. Table 8.2 presents a timeline for a research study in which answers to certain interview questions can influence or bias the researcher.

TABLE 8.2	Timeline for Data Collection								
Method	Week 1	Week 2	Week 3	Week 4	Week 5	Week 6	Week 7	Week 8	Week 9
Entry	X								
Observation		X	X	X		X	X		
Student/ client interviews					X			X	
Teacher/ trainer interviews									X

Notice in the data collection timeline that, after gaining entry into the research site(s) during week 1 (introductions, informed consent, parental permissions, assent forms), the researcher plans to spend 3 full weeks observing, collecting field note data, and forming her own opinions about the situation and the way individuals interact. Once her themes are beginning to form, she is ready to interview student or client participants to gather their impressions and insights into the research question while simultaneously testing her developing categories and themes. With these insights in mind, the researcher then returns to observations to view the research setting from these participants' (biased) viewpoint. Finally, the researcher is ready to talk with the teachers or trainers about their perspectives on the curriculum including their level of fidelity or faithfulness of implementation. As she asks the interview questions, the respondents refocus their attention from a more general topic (e.g., satisfaction with the program) to level of implementation. Teachers who are implementing the curriculum explain how they use it in their lessons, while teachers who are not using the curriculum are more likely to describe reasons why they do not like it and have chosen not to implement it. We will discuss data collection methods in more detail in the next section.

Data Collection Methods

Qualitative researchers employ many different methods to collect different types of data. Each method has advantages and disadvantages, and there is no perfect data collection tool. Therefore, it is critical to understand each tool and match it to the requirements of the research question. **Data sources** in qualitative research include the setting or context described during the observation, the perspectives of the participants elicited during interviews, and written or virtual documents gathered from participants or online that provide insights into the mission and goals of the organization. Gathering data representing several different perspectives enables the researcher to check and cross-check findings contributing to data credibility and triangulation. The researcher often begins the data collection by watching and listening to become familiar with the setting. Observation or field note data are collected early in the study and then periodically throughout the data collection time period to better understand the situation. Once the researcher has identified the key informants in the setting, he can arrange additional interviews with individuals or groups to expand his understanding based on their perspectives.

Data Sources Aspects within the context, including participants, behaviors, events, and artifacts, that can be used as separate sources to triangulate findings

OBSERVATIONS

Observations provide an opportunity for the researcher to learn about the research setting or context where the social interactions occur. These include the physical characteristics of the building including the equipment, layout, size of the offices, and how much space is allocated to each component of the program or agency. Observations also permit the researcher to watch how people interact and note what they say, their voice tone and inflection, gestures, and facial expressions that accompany conversations. Special Interest Box 8.1 includes an excerpt from observation data collected in a study describing strategies teachers use to present content in high school physical education.[4]

The longer the researcher is in the setting, the more comfortable the participants become with his presence. Although the first weeks often involve helpful introductions and explanations, as the observations continue, the researcher becomes a partner in the process and is allowed to hear and see more of the actual daily interactions.

The observer's role can range on a continuum from a nonparticipant to a participant in the research setting. Nonparticipants often sit at the side of the room taking notes and observing without interacting with participants during meetings, lessons, or appointments. Conversely, participants become involved in many aspects of the setting, participating with children in physical education classes, working out with clients, or asking questions in meetings. Depending on the level of researcher participation and the qualitative research tradition selected, observation periods can assist researchers to fade into

SPECIAL INTEREST BOX 8.1

Observation Data

Students are seated at desks in a classroom for the introduction to their personal fitness class. Several students are talking quietly; two have their heads down on their desks. Two are flipping pencils across the room. Ms. Davenport enters the classroom and gives the pencil shooters a hard look. They quickly retrieve their pencils, tap their chests, and quietly say, "My bad." Ms. D. returns an assignment in which students recorded and graphed their heart rates during three physical activities: rope jumping, basketball shooting, and volleyball blocking. She explains that today they are going to calculate target heart rates so that students can regulate the intensity of activity to avoid exhaustion and still receive health benefits from their workout. Students discuss their intensity for each task and comment on "how hard" they thought they were working. Ms. D. emphasizes the importance of personalizing the experiences that no two people have to feel the same or need to compare themselves with others. She distributes a worksheet with instructions and formulae needed to calculate target heart rates and then works through each using Damien's (one of the pencil shooters) age and scores from the previous class. Damien is attentive and works through the calculations with the class. Ms. D. then encourages students to insert their own scores and work through the problem independently. She walks around the room asking and answering questions. All students are engaged in the math problems, although a few are struggling and appear to need help. Ms. D. assists and then asks other students to pair with the strugglers to help. When all have completed the assignment, she says, "Now we are going into the gym and participate in three different activities. We will use the heart rate monitors to help you stay in your target zones. I should not need to tell you to work harder or rest a bit. You will know based on the upper and lower boundaries of your target heart rate zone that you just calculated. Set your heart rate monitor and evaluate yourself accordingly. OK, please walk to the gym" (p.160).[4]

the background or become a trusted participant in the research setting. In Special Interest Box 8.2, I described the evolving data collection protocols I used when collecting observation data in an elementary physical education program.[5]

The data collected as field notes become an important backdrop to understand, confirm, and interpret data collected from other sources (interviews, artifacts). By triangulating field note, interview,

SPECIAL INTEREST BOX 8.2

I collected observation field note data for one full school day each week for 22 weeks during the 2001–2002 school year, arriving 15 minutes before the first fifth-grade class and staying until the last first-grade class was on the buses. I arrived the same day each week and, therefore, observed the same five classes (grades 1 to 5, n = ~215 students). Early in the observation period, I sat unobtrusively at the side of the gymnasium, moving as necessary to avoid flying objects and moving children. During the third observation, Jill [teacher] invited me to participate in the lesson, which I did, leaving my notebook on the side. This fortuitous event seemed to help the children feel more comfortable with me, and they willingly chatted about the activities and stations as we rotated together around the gym. In subsequent classes, I typically spent parts of each class taking notes about class structure, content, and lesson focus and the remaining time participating with the children. I reconstructed the events and conversations that occurred during my participation time either prior to the beginning of the next class or immediately on leaving the school in the afternoon. (p. 73–74)[5]

and artifact data, the researcher can cross-check or compare data from one data source with others. Data triangulation is critical to affirm the trustworthiness of your findings.

Interview and Focus Groups

Whereas field note data focus on participants' observable behaviors and actions, interviews and focus group data reveal their thoughts, expectations, emotions, and understandings. Data from carefully structured interviews can add depth and meaning to participants' actions and provide a rationale for their behaviors. Often, data from interviews and focus groups are critical to developing a more comprehensive picture of the phenomenon of interest. In qualitative research traditions, such as phenomenology and narrative inquiry, that examine individuals' lived experiences and interpretations of life events, interviews are the primary data collection source. This is particularly true in life histories and historical narratives where there is no longer an opportunity to observe critical events.

Interviews are typically conducted individually or with two or three participants who know each other well. Interview data can be used to confirm or triangulate information the researcher already possesses, to reveal new facts, or to help the researcher interpret data from observations or from other interview responses. Special Interest Box 8.3 reports data from an interview with the two physical educators who created Scooter City, a unit integrating fitness and social responsibility, in their gymnasium.[5]

Conversely, focus groups are typically conducted with groups of individuals who may or may not know each other. A skilled focus group leader can structure questions to encourage participants to talk with each other as well as the interviewer, respond to other focus group members' comments, and reveal information that is immediately confirmed or refuted by other focus group members. At times, members can come to a deeper understanding of the problem or issue during a focus group. Critical qualitative researchers use focus groups to guide group members to a new awareness of injustices in their lives.[6] They can build confidence and provide strategies to empower individuals to question and ultimately initiate change in their situation.

SPECIAL INTEREST BOX 8.3

Jill and Pam described the Scooter City unit as a tremendous amount of preparatory work with extensive student-related record keeping. They saw the content as an opportunity for students to learn to make decisions and choices associated with physical activity and to practice and apply skills learned in other units during these guided choice tasks. Both teachers also pointed out connections to other activities that students valued and found meaningful:

Pam: I have done Scooter City at my old school in conjunction with my bicycle safety unit. The first year, I would have my Scooter city inside for a lesson, and then we would take those rules we had learned about right-of-way, signaling and pedestrian safety outside to our bicycle course.

Jill: I have done Scooter City in the past with less of a focus on riding the scooters and with more about what skill and fitness activities were going on. For example, 1 year I tried to tie it into fitness, like, I named a street Hamstring Highway and we did things on Hamstring Highway that had to do with legs.

Pam: When Jill and I started teaming together, we made some necessary changes because of the number of students in the double classes. We can build it even more next year to have more "eye" content. Is that a word? I mean more eye-attracting appeal that gets kids' attention and holds them throughout the period. (p. 79)[5]

Learning to conduct interviews is a skill that requires training and practice. Interview questions are carefully planned and positioned in the interview to gain the respondent's confidence and guide them to reveal information that is critical to the researcher's understanding and interpretation of the study. Carefully planned interviews are choreographed in sections or stages, each with a unique purpose. Think of the shape of normal curve that gradually rises through a series of topics to prepare the respondent for a series of crucial, perhaps even sensitive, questions and then using a series of less emotional questions to gradually return to a more neutral tone, ending the interview on a positive note. Figure 8.1 demonstrates this process, emphasizing stages that can be used to structure interviews.[4]

Photo Diary

Although there are many methods and techniques that can be used effectively to collect qualitative data, one of the most interesting involves asking participants to take photographs or videos of events or experiences important to themselves and the researcher. For example, to understand what physical activities children chose after school, researchers can give them a single use camera to take pictures of themselves and their friends participating in these activities. As this data collection method has become more sophisticated, researchers have asked participants to create videos of experiences they have had either in schools or in other parts of their lives that reflect their understandings and lived experiences with the phenomena of interest. Participants also can cut out pictures from magazines; make scrapbooks, posters, and wikis; and write blogs to help researchers understand factors that are most salient and meaningful in their lives. Qualitative researchers are utilizing a number of novel and creative data collection approaches to interpretive research. These hold promise to provide additional insights into social interactions and institutions that are central to individual's lived experiences.

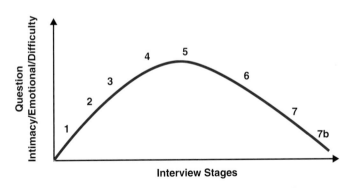

Stages of an Interview
1. Creating natural involvement
2. Encouraging conversational competence
3. Showing understanding
4. Getting facts and basic descriptions
5. Asking difficult questions
6. Toning down the emotional level
7. Closing while maintaining contact
7b. Informal follow-up

With your Partner
A. Imagine a future conversational partner
B. Draft/Preview your Main Questions (1-3)
C. Consider which of the 6 types of probes you might use
D. Will you frame interview as a Tree or a River?
E. Begin to organize and plan your interview using protocols, checklists, or outlines.

■ **FIGURE 8.1** Interview stages.

✔ Check Your Understanding

1. How can a data collection timeline be used effectively to structure a qualitative research design?
2. List three methods to collect qualitative data.

DATA ANALYSIS

Qualitative data consist of rich descriptive field notes that paint a picture in the reader's mind of the setting and the social situation in which participants interact. Data also consist of interview and focus group transcripts that provide rationales and explanations of participant behaviors and decisions and assist researchers to understand phenomena from the participants' perspectives. Today, data also can consist of a variety of artifacts from lesson plans to client's charts and workout records. Photo diaries, videos, scrapbooks, and wikis are used to develop the qualitative picture of diverse social and situational interactions that occur surrounding the research question. Certainly, analyzing these diverse data sources requires expertise in a variety of techniques and methods. Computer software such as NVivo, MAXQDA, and ATLAS.ti can assist the researcher to organize, code, categorize, and retrieve data. However, there is no substitute for an experienced data analyst who can identify and triangulate complex themes across multiple data sources.

Themes

One objective of qualitative research is to identify comprehensive themes that assist the researcher to make sense of the data. Themes are reoccurring structures that explain or describe participants' thoughts, situational issues, and patterns in the context. Researchers construct themes by first becoming very familiar with the data and then coding and categorizing it to reflect coherent concepts or constructs present in the situation.

OPEN, AXIAL, AND SELECTIVE CODING

Coding An increasingly complex strategy to assign common categories and properties to textual and artifactual data. Codes represent key words or phrases that link concepts across different data sources. Codes facilitate triangulation and are the foundation or the building blocks for themes.

Coding can take many forms depending on the data type and format. Usually, researchers begin by using a process described as open coding[5] in which words, phrases, sentences, and paragraphs are highlighted and assigned a name that reflects the major topic discussed. For example, if teachers are discussing their concerns that, "many urban students cannot play outside after school because of dangers in their neighborhood," analysts might code the phrase as "physical activity," "after school," and "safety." The computer software programs can be used to copy and store the phrase in files for each of these three codes, permitting the analyst to search and retrieve coded phrases across all data sources and place phrases reflecting each code in a central file.

Open coding is descriptive. The codes represent salient behaviors or topics that a colleague or anyone familiar with the data would be likely to understand and accept as a reasonable description. Researchers begin the process of open coding very early in the data collection process, and each new interview transcript or observational field note file is coded soon after the data are collected. Open coding involves the identification of categories and properties of each phenomenon. The coding process influences the researcher's perspective early in the data collection process. Being familiar with data helps researchers realize when they are asking irrelevant questions or interviewing individuals who simply do not possess or understand the situation adequately to inform the research question. Rather than waiting until the conclusion of the data collection and analysis process to realize these problems, the qualitative researcher can respond quickly by changing the setting, selecting additional informants to interview, and reshaping the research design to address his evolving understanding of the situation. This flexibility could not be achieved without the qualitative assumption that the research design and themes evolve and emerge within the research process. Each change requires justification and a clear rationale, but ultimately the research question is better answered through this evolutionary approach to data collection and analysis.

Axial coding occurs simultaneously with and following the opening coding process. Axial coding seeks more abstract interpretations of descriptive open codes. Axial codes begin as hunches and, with substantial support from multiple data sources, become themes that organize and make sense of complex cultures and settings. Most scholars agree that qualitative research themes emerge from the axial coding process. Qualitative analysts examine data categories and properties and search for interpretive explanations of lived experiences that are central to social research. Axial coding reveals themes that are interpretive, not descriptive. Themes represent key understandings that motivate individuals to act in certain ways or patterns that lead to particular consequences within the settings. Axial coding of themes is often followed by selective coding in which researchers return to the research setting after the axial coding process is completed to verify themes and seek new data to support these abstract constructs. In selective coding, the researcher returns to his original theoretical framework and literature review to clarify and confirm themes that emerged during the study. This third coding level assists the researcher to compare themes with those found in other research (review of literature) and to place new findings within the existing body of knowledge on the topic.

With practice, each qualitative researcher develops protocols and ways of examining data for descriptive codes and interpretive themes. The findings are always subjective and situationally situated in a particular context. Qualitative researchers are not concerned with generalizability or objectivity. Qualitative research emerges from a different paradigm that does not adhere to the rules of statistical research designs. Instead, qualitative research offers scholars a different lens to examine a few research sites in great detail. These labor-intensive research methods are critical for understanding and interpreting social interactions in ways that are grounded within a specific setting or situation.

✓ Check Your Understanding

1. List three types of analysis techniques used to describe and interpret qualitative data.
2. How is qualitative research different from other types of research traditions?

CHAPTER SUMMARY

- Qualitative research is notable for its focus on complex, natural settings; the use of flexible, evolving research designs; multiple data sources and methods; and an interpretive focus on individual's lived experiences.
- Qualitative research is subjective. Because the researcher is the primary research instrument, it is critical that she reveal her background, biases, and personal reasons for engaging in the research.
- Qualitative researchers assume that social interactions are holistic and complex. Because social systems are evolving, it is critical to remain open to new possibilities and to adjust the research design as necessary. This may include adding or omitting settings or participants, increasing/decreasing time in settings, and refocusing the research purpose and questions to emphasize events or phenomena that are critical to participants and to reflect their perspectives.
- Qualitative research forms or genres continue to evolve to reflect diverse sociological and educational perspectives. These range from traditional ethnographic to sociocritical, phenomenological, and hermeneutic.

- Currently, most qualitative genres can be organized within naturalistic, interpretive, and critical categories.
- Researchers select the research genre based on the purpose and research questions.
- Similar to all forms of research, qualitative research is evaluated based on criteria specific to its characteristics and assumptions. Criteria for sample selection, data collection/analysis, and trustworthiness require careful attention to research questions and protocols.
- Triangulation (comparison of data from different sources) is one method used to establish trustworthiness.
- Data triangulation and trustworthiness are enhanced by attention to issues of credibility, dependability, confirmability, and transferability.
- Data analysis may include open (descriptive), axial (interpretive), and selective (literature/theoretical) coding.
- Qualitative research provides an in-depth look at social and cultural issues grounded within a specific setting, time, and place. Qualitative research genres are particularly sensitive to historical, political, social, and cultural phenomena, issues, events, and concerns.

REFERENCES

1. Marshall C, Rossman GB. *Designing Qualitative Research*, 5th ed. Thousand Oaks, CA: Sage, 2011.
2. Rossman GB, Rallis SF. *Learning in the Field: An Introduction to Qualitative Research*, 2nd ed. Thousand Oaks, CA: Sage, 2003.
3. Patton MQ. *Qualitative Research & Evaluation Methods*, 3rd ed. Thousand Oaks, CA: Sage, 2002.
4. Ennis CD, McCauley MT. Creating urban classrooms worthy of student trust. *J Curr Stud* 2002;34(2):149–172.
5. Ennis CD. Examining curricular coherence in an exemplary elementary school program. *Res Q Exerc Sport* 2008;79(1):71–84.
6. Rubin HJ, Rubin IS. *Qualitative Interviewing: The Art of Hearing Data*, 3rd ed. Thousand Oaks, CA: Sage, 2012.

RELATED ASSIGNMENTS

1. **Select a topic of interest, and develop eight interview questions that follow the diagram in Figure 8.1. Select a person who is knowledgeable about your topic, and ask permission to interview him or her and to record the interview. After the interview, listen to your questions, tone, and interview style. Critique your questions and the answers your respondent provided. Who did the most talking during the interview? Did your questions elicit the responses you expected? How could you revise your questions to guide the respondant to provide the information you were seeking?**

2. **Pick a busy place at a nearby park or shopping mall to practice your observation skills. Assume the role of a nonparticipant observer to record the events that occur in your setting. Select a place to sit where you can see and hear interactions between individuals. Are there patterns of activities that are repetitive? After observing the pattern several times, can you close your eyes and describe it to someone else? Next, write a "thick description" of the setting. Be sure to include the colors, smells, and sounds that are occurring around you. Try to avoid making judgments about the intentions, reasons, feelings, or emotions that you witness. Instead, simply describe what is occurring. For example, instead of saying "the people are happy and enjoying the beautiful day," explain what they are doing or saying and how they are behaving that leads you to believe they are "happy" and "enjoying" themselves. Describe their facial expressions, how they walk, and what they are saying to each other. Let your reader make the judgment from the descriptions you provide.**

IN-CLASS GROUP EXERCISES

1. Transcribe the interview that you recorded in #2 in the "Related Assignments" section above, and bring two copies of the transcript and two yellow highlighting markers to your research methods class. Ask the person beside you to read the interview transcript and highlight parts of the respondents' answer that pertain to the topic you were discussing. You do the same with the second transcript. Still working separately, both you and your partner review the transcript again and write a word or short phrase in the margin that describes the main point or subtopic of each highlighted section. Then, make a list of these categories or open codes, and compare your list with your partners. How many similarities did you find? Discuss any differences in the highlighted sections and codes, and come to an agreement about the best descriptors for each highlighted sections. Review the transcript once more to be sure that you have highlighted and coded every phrase or sentence that has meaning in the context of your interview. You now have a working list of key ideas or categories that your respondent perceived was most relevant for the topic you discussed.

2. For the course instructor: Take a class field trip to a busy place in the student union on your campus to make a group observation. Situate class members in different locations around the area being sure that everyone is viewing the same central location but from different viewpoints. During the next 15 minutes, ask each student to describe the setting from his or her viewpoint, and then return to your classroom. In the classroom, ask students to spend the next 10 to 15 minutes writing a paragraph describing their observations at the student union.

Questions for students: What was the purpose of the activities in the setting? What patterns, meanings, or interpretations can be made about the activities in the student union? Working in groups of three or four, compare paragraphs. What similarities and differences did the observers in your group record? What meaning or interpretations did individual observers give to their observations? Did everyone in your group agree on the nature and purpose of the activities in the union?

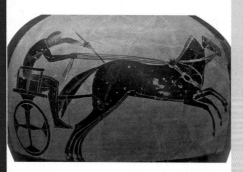

Other Research Approaches

9

"Athletes live a life quite contrary to the precepts of hygiene, and I regard their mode of living as a regime far more favorable to illness than to health"—Galen *(Philosopher, 200–129 BC)*

CHAPTER OBJECTIVES

After studying this chapter, you will be able to:

1. Identify alternative research designs that have been performed in kinesiology and health-related sciences.
2. Describe the general tenets of historical and philosophical research designs.
3. Explain the similarities and differences between experimental and epidemiological research.
4. Compare and contrast types of single-subject design research.
5. Explain the concept of effect size in relation to meta-analysis.

■ To this point, we have described methods of research that 21st century researchers within kinesiology and the health sciences use most frequently. Visit any exercise physiology or biomechanics laboratory, and you will likely find the researchers there actively recruiting and testing participants to examine the effectiveness of an intervention or comparing groups of similar individuals on some health-related measure. Although researchers commonly use experimental and descriptive techniques, other types of research also provide valuable information about human health and movement. These include historical and philosophical, epidemiology, single-subject, and meta-analysis research. Although the methods vary dramatically, all serve to answer important questions, involve logical research designs with systematic data collection, and represent valid areas of inquiry.

HISTORICAL AND PHILOSOPHICAL RESEARCH

As you can see from the quote from the Roman philosopher Galen at the beginning of the chapter, our notions of the role of physical activity and athletics to general health have evolved drastically over time. Another point you might garner from this quote is that historical and philosophical research may have common elements—you cannot understand the philosophies of an ancient Greek without examining historical context. However, historical and philosophical researches remain distinct lines of inquiry used to solve different types of problems in kinesiology and health.

Historical Inquiry

Those who perform historical research delve into the past with two purposes. First, they attempt to capture the thoughts and attitudes about health and physical activity during different periods in recorded history. This research leads us to the origins of the study of kinesiology and other health-related sciences and helps us understand why certain practices or belief systems came into being. Through this research, historians can uncover the prevailing viewpoints and perspectives of people during different eras. A common saying among sport historians is that sport is a microcosm of society. This suggests that studying sport within a given culture can provide valuable insights into the values, morals, and beliefs of persons living within that culture. Of course, good historians always remember that they interpret historical artifacts, such as books, artwork, or tools, using their own frame of reference. That is, they see the past through modern eyes.

A second purpose of historical research is to provide a framework for understanding issues and attitudes about health in the present by looking at the past. That is, the study of history provides historical context for our current values, morals, and beliefs and helps us understand where health-related policies and laws come from. Further, it can help us avoid problems encountered in the past. Were certain past cultures or societies organized such that they facilitated the spread of disease? Alternatively, how did others slow disease transmission and deal with other health-related issues? For example, politicians often discuss the virtues of globalization in a positive sense, but throughout history, this spread of goods, capital, information, and people has also been accompanied by the spread of devastating diseases, such as measles, venereal diseases, or tuberculosis, or, more recently, West Nile virus or H1N1 ("swine flu"), or HIV/AIDS. Historians play a role in understanding the antecedents of disease transmission during earlier time periods.

In 1903, J.B. Bury famously proclaimed, "History is a science, no less and no more…history is not a branch of literature" in his inaugural speech as the Regius Professor of Modern History at the Divinity School in Cambridge, England.[1] Bury made the point that historical research should be approached as a science, and historians must apply scientific rigor to their methods of data collection. As with experimental and descriptive research, specific methods of data (or, as historians refer to it, **evidence**) collection and analysis should be used that result in the best possible interpretation of the results. Historians note that, like other areas of inquiry, they have to start with a question (see Special Interest Box 9.1). Simply recording facts from earlier times is not historical research—the researcher starts with a question and then designs a method for answering that question. As part of this process, historians gather evidence, just as other types of scientists do.

Evidence Historical data or artifacts

Historians collect evidence from a variety of sources. **Primary sources** come from the time under study, including original books or writings, as well as physical evidence such as tools or medical equipment. If a researcher's interests lie in recent history, then people can provide primary sources of information, through personal interviews or recorded descriptions of events. When possible, researchers should use primary sources. The reasoning is

Primary Sources First hand evidence from the time under question, such as photographs, journals, and official records

---

SPECIAL INTEREST BOX 9.1

Developing Historical Research: Asking the Question

Consider the following example:

> Steve grew up near Cooperstown, NY, had visited the Baseball Hall of Fame many times, and had always found the history of baseball fascinating. He thought it would be a great idea to research baseball in the 1950s, since his favorite players were Mickey Mantle and Yogi Berra. While home for winter break, he went back to the Baseball Hall of Fame and studied the archives for information about this time period. He went through some artifacts and developed a 10-page narrative that described this time period. His History of Sport professor, after reading the report, suggested he begin again, stating "Your research has to start with a question. Find the question!"

What is wrong with Steve's approach to historical research? As we have discussed throughout the book, research involves asking a specific question and then gathering data in an attempt to answer that question. This is precisely what Steve is missing: a question to drive his research. Steve lets easily accessible data drive his research rather than letting his question drive his data collection! How can Steve rectify this situation?

> Steve spent some time reading newspaper articles from the 1950s. He recognized that two big events made a big impact on baseball around that time period. The first was the end of World War II, and the second was the introduction of television to American homes. He decided to focus on the later point and started to develop his question. He asked "Did widespread television ownership and mass marketing on TV change professional baseball from sport to commodity"?

Now that Steve has a question, he can move on to data collection, and it's clear he will need to go beyond the Baseball Hall of Fame to collect data.

---

similar to that of using primary sources in literature reviews (see Chapter 3) because they reflect a first-person glimpse into the time or event under study rather than someone else's reinterpretation of that event. Historians can find primary evidence in places like archives, libraries, public holdings, or collections. For example, researchers interested in health and medical history could start their search at a place like the College of Physicians of Philadelphia, "the birthplace of American medicine," which is home to both the Mütter Museum and the Historical Medical Library. The Internet is invaluable for determining where primary sources of evidence exist.

Material culture in the form of historical artifacts can also be primary sources. In these instances, the artifacts are objects created in the period under study. For example, the cigar boxes seen in Figure 9.1 (from the John and Carolyn Grossman Collection) depict (A) women involved in recreational sport and (B) sporty girls smoking cigars. Keeping in mind the historical context with the United States at this time—during the late 1800s, the popularity of light physical activity for women came into vogue—these artifacts provide evidence of several prevailing notions of the day. First, participation in recreational activities for college women was seen as positive as long as the women remained feminine and the exercise was not strenuous.[2] Second, smoking was a favorable choice for "sporty girls." Certainly, these attitudes have changed since those times! Compare primary to secondary sources of evidence. **Secondary sources** provide information about history from someone who did not witness it, but (like a

Researchers should confirm that historical artifacts are both authentic and credible before using them to address the research question.

Secondary Sources Evidence based on primary resources, such as books, magazines, and journal articles

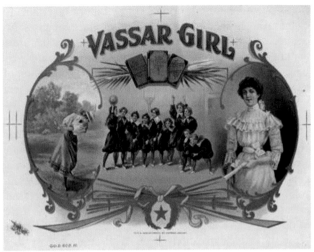

A

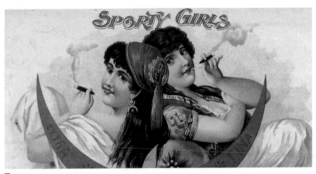

B

■ **FIGURE 9.1** Primary sources of historical data from cigar boxes in the 1800s depicting **(A)** Vassar girls and **(B)** sporty girls.

historian) gathered evidence about events. Encyclopedias and other Web-based information databases have entries that summarize multiple sources to provide an overview of historical events. Newspapers can also be secondary sources because they may reflect journalists' interpretations or recounting of events (i.e., describing others recollections of events) rather than the events themselves. In certain circumstances, newspapers can be primary sources, if the written article contains the authors' first-person account of an event. Historians often use secondary sources, but do so with caution—they must be sure to take into account any subjective biases that the authors may have had in creating the secondary source.

A good example of bias within newspaper journalism occurred during the 1928 Olympic games, when the International Olympic Committee first allowed women to participate in the modern Olympic games. Strong opposition to women's participation came from multiple sources (including the founder of the modern Olympics, Frenchman Pierre de Coubertin), including many sportscasters of the time. Controversy ensued after the 800-m run, where several women "collapsed" after the race. Newspaper accounts at the time suggested that not only women were unable to run such distances but that women's reproductive health would suffer for doing so. In the New York Times, one reporter said " even this distance makes too great a call on feminine strength". Similar stories in the world press created controversy and ultimately led to limiting the distances women were allowed to run in the games for the next 60 years. Later that century, historian Lynne Emory determined from primary sources of evidence that all of the women finished the race. Further, the "collapses" were racers lying down on the ground disappointed and winded after the race (rather than a mass display of exercise-induced cardiorespiratory failure). Had historians relied on the reporting of the event in newspapers from the time, they would have had an entirely different (and incorrect) conception of the event.

After historians begin to collect primary sources of evidence related to their question, they begin the process of external and internal criticism, which involves looking critically at the evidence to check its validity. A historian uses *external criticism* to establish the authenticity or legitimacy of the evidence. In short, is the evidence real or has it been forged or altered? This can be done through many different means, such as carbon dating with ancient artifacts, a comparison of signatures or handwriting, or even checking the consistency of writing style and language use. Once the historian establishes authenticity, the process of internal criticism begins. *Internal criticism* involves the determination of credibility of the evidence. Is a piece of evidence consistent with other pieces of evidence and what is known about the time period? Historians must also be aware of the context under which the evidence came into being. The final part of historical research is piecing together the evidence to create a "story" that provides the best possible answer to the original question.

✔ Check Your Understanding

1. What makes historical inquiry "research"?
2. Compare and contrast external and internal criticism.
3. What is "evidence" for a scientist interested in historical research?
4. What is the difference between primary and secondary sources in historical research?

Philosophical Research

Another type of research that is sometimes associated with historical research is philosophical research. At first glance, philosophical research seems to be the antithesis of experimental research. Stemming from the ancient Greek words "phileo," which means "love," and "sophia," meant "wisdom" (love of knowledge), philosophy entails a scholarly pursuit of the nature and meaning of knowledge, existence, morals, and reality. However, unlike experimental research, the philosopher does not physically test anything and quantitatively assess the results to determine causation. Rather, philosophers look to understand meanings through reflection, which is the process of actively thinking through a problem using logic and reason to explore it.

Philosophers do not gather "data" per se, nor do they use statistics to provide objective interpretations of results. A novice empirical researcher may debate the value of philosophical research in kinesiology and health sciences and then ultimately realize that the debate itself was philosophical research! However, Kretchmar[4] argues that in fact, philosophical and empirical research both involve the search for knowledge and differ primarily in how that search is undertaken, as the primary tool of philosophical research is reflection.

In addition, we can trace much of what we know empirically to basic philosophical points of view, which suggest certain questions are important to pursue. In fact, health professions in general owe their existence to the philosophical position that health is important to human existence. Different philosophies guide the study of health and disease as well as their treatment. For example, in Chapter 5, we discussed ethics in human research, and one of the primary principles is that the researcher must put the safety and protection of human participants above all else. This is a philosophical position that guides the ways in which we can study human beings, by positing that the benefits to humans must outweigh the risks (beneficence). The guidelines put forth in the Belmont report that guide the ethical treatment of human beings were developed through philosophical research and debate by a group of individuals with diverse backgrounds such as medicine, law, and bioethics and provide a clear set of rules for empirical researchers to follow.

The process of performing philosophical research entails a general, three-step process designed to allow for systematic reflection[4]:

1. Developing a thesis. This is similar to creating a hypothesis in empirical research.
2. Clarify the problem.
3. Search for arguments.

Two common ways in which researchers analyze philosophical problems are inductive and deductive reasoning. In general, reasoning is the process of forming conclusions or inferences based on premises or facts. **Inductive reasoning** is reasoning that goes from specific to general. That is, it is the process of building theories based on a small number of specific observations or examples. A clinical example of inductive reasoning illustrates the process well; clinicians examine a series of symptoms (small set of specific facts) in an attempt to determine a general diagnosis of injury or disease. In the sport sciences, a philosopher may be interested in trying to formalize the definition of "sport" in an attempt to decide if cheering is a sport (a question relevant to institutions trying to comply with Title IV in the United States). The process of inductive reasoning involves examining a number of activities considered "sports" (e.g., soccer, tennis, rowing), examining characteristics of these activities (e.g., elements of competition, use of physical or cognitive skill), and then making a general conclusion about what a sport is. In philosophical research, a scientist begins this process by looking at observations to see if common principles emerge.

Inductive Reasoning
Deriving general conclusions from specific observations

Just as inductive reasoning could be thought of as a bottom-up approach, **deductive reasoning** could be described as a top-down approach. In this form of reasoning, the scientist starts with a theory or principle and uses that to formulate a set of expected outcomes or observations. Again, in a clinical example of deductive reasoning, a clinician starts with the premise that a patient has a particular condition or disease and then looks for specific symptoms to confirm that. In our sport example, the philosopher would start with the premise of what sport is and then evaluate whether an activity such as cheerleading meets that definition.

Deductive Reasoning
Reasoning from a general theory to derive expected outcomes

An excellent example of philosophical research (with a strong historical base) is Hwang and Kretchmar's 2012 paper entitled "Aristotle's golden mean: Its implications for the doping debate."[5] The basis for the research is the ongoing, still relevant debate on the ethics and morals of drug use as performance enhancers in sport, which, at the philosophical level, is an open question. The authors attempt to reframe the question in light of Aristotle's golden mean:

Aristotle argues that we act from three attitudes: from the mean (or average), from excess, and from deficiency. Two of them, behaving from excess and deficiency, are vices, while acting at the mean is a virtue. He suggests that we apply this principle not only generally but also to particular cases including those involving some risk to the actor. In dangerous situations, we should act courageously because this is the mean between cowardice and rashness... Based on these notions...the golden mean itself is neither extreme nor deficient. But neither is it unrelated to the indefensible poles of behavior on each side. Thus, virtue, as understood in relationship to the golden mean is a "middling disposition" in human behavior.

The authors reflect on this position and provide a sophisticated philosophical argument too intricate and detailed to recount here (but definitely worth a read). They ultimately conclude that, in keeping with the golden mean, a doping ban follows to reason.

Accordingly, in our rough and ready world of contemporary big-time sport, the better part of reason suggests that the bans on performance enhancing pharmaceuticals be retained and enforced. However, because the wisdom of this decision is contingent on the variable nature of

TABLE 9.1   Relative Risk Formula for Cohort Studies

Exposure	Outcome		Total
	Yes	No	
Yes	a	b	a + b
No	c	d	c + d
Total	a + c	b + d	a + b + c + d

developing the disease. For example, suppose you hypothesized that low levels of physical activity during early childhood are a risk factor for overweight/obesity status in young adults. You sampled a population of preschool children, some of whom had low levels of physical activity and some of who had high levels, and followed with percentage body fat tests at specific time intervals and at the end of high school. In order to calculate relative risk, you would find incidence rate of obesity in those participants who were exposed to low levels of physical activity in preschool and divide by the incidence rate of those who were not. From this, you could determine the likelihood of becoming obese by 12th grade based on preschool structured physical activity. If you calculated a relative risk of 2, this indicates that children with low levels of physical activity in preschool are twice as likely to be obese as a senior in high school than those who had higher levels of physical activity.

In *case–control* studies, researchers look at the characteristics of individuals now, focusing on varying levels of the health state of interest, and then look back in time at exposure levels of different risk factors. The group who exhibits the health or disease state is considered the case, making the group without, the controls. The researcher examines both groups, with an eye toward those risk factors to which the case group was differentially exposed. We can examine the same problem we discussed above (do low levels of physical activity in preschool impact obesity status in young adults?) using a case–control design. Here, you would start with a population of obese (case) and average-weight (control) high school seniors. Then, you would survey them and determine their levels of physical activity as preschoolers. Next, you would compare the cases to the controls and calculate a measure called an **odds ratio**. In an odds ratio, the number of people exposed who do have the disease state is multiplied by the number who aren't exposed who don't get the disease, and this number is divided by the number exposed who don't get the disease times the number of people not exposed who do get the disease. Equation 9.2 shows how to calculate the odds ratio of a case–control design. Odds ratios are interpreted in the same way that relative risk is.

Odds Ratio Ratio of the odds of developing a health condition in the case versus control group

$$\text{Odds ratio} = \frac{a \times d}{b \times c}$$

Equation 9.2

where

a = those exposed who do get the disease (case group)

b = those exposed who do *not* get the disease (control group)

c = those not exposed who do get the disease (case group)

d = those not exposed who do *not* get the disease (control group)

The final type of analytic design is a randomized controlled trial. You may recall that in Chapter 6, one of the hallmarks of a true experimental design was the randomization of participants. Randomized controlled studies use this process as well, and further, the researcher provides an intervention and uses a control group to examine the long-term effects of a treatment (hence, the name). Again, an important distinction exists between true experimental and randomized controlled designs. In the former case, small numbers of participants with similar characteristics are used in order to improve internal validity. In the latter case, large numbers of participants with divergent characteristics are used in order to provide generalizability or external validity. In both cases, these represent the best method of assessing cause–effect relationships.

In a randomized controlled design, the researcher randomly assigns the population under study to either a treatment or control group. Upon admission to the study, the experimental group receives the treatment, whereas the control group receives a placebo. Alternatively, the treatment group may receive a novel treatment, where the other group receives traditional treatment; this is done in cases where it is not ethical to provide no treatment whatsoever or when the research question relates to a comparison to current practice rather than no practice at all. The effect of the treatment occurs naturally over time, and outcomes are measured at different meaningful points in time after exposure to the treatment. These outcomes are compared between groups to determine how exposure impacts outcome.

Figure 9.2 compares the different types of analytic designs in epidemiology. Exposure and outcome are represented at the top of the figure, and the arrows represent the direction in time that a study progresses. In a cohort study, researchers take measurements and then follow the participants over a period of time to see who develops a disease. In case–control studies, researchers match participants who do (case) or do not (control) have a particular disease and then look back and examine the history of exposure to the disease risk factors. Finally, a randomized controlled study randomly assigns individuals to either a treatment or intervention group or a control group and compares outcomes of these groups at specific time intervals.

Establishing causation requires a number of epidemiological studies with similar results along with clinical trials, complemented with experimental research in specific samples. At the same time, this body of evidence can have a large impact on public health in terms of clinical practices and public policy. Consider the Healthy People[7] initiative within the United States, initiated in 1979 based on the Surgeon General's Report, "Healthy People: The Surgeon General's Report on Health Promotion and

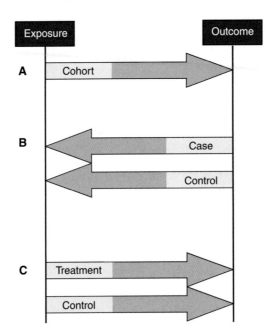

■ FIGURE 9.2 Time progression between exposure and outcome in epidemiological studies. *Arrows* from left to right indicate prospective studies. *Arrows* from right to left indicate retrospective studies. Number of arrows indicates number of groups compared. **A:** Cohort. **B:** Case–control. **C:** Randomized controlled.

Disease Prevention". Every 10 years from that point, the Department of Health and Human Services has collected epidemiological data on health in the US population and generated a series of objectives from the information coming from the previous 10-year "Healthy People" initiative. Over the past 30 years, the growing health crisis related to obesity has been tracked, and evidence-based physical activity guidelines have been promoted to help address that crisis. Healthy People 2020 focuses "on identifying, measuring, tracking, and reducing health disparities through a determinants of health approach" (www.healthypeople.gov/2020). In short, the Healthy People initiative represents ongoing epidemiological research used to improve people's health and guide public policy in the United States.

✔ Check Your Understanding

1. In what key ways do epidemiology and experimental research differ?
2. Describe how an epidemiologist would do cross-sectional research when looking at the impact of tobacco on incidence of lung cancer.
3. What are the three analytic designs in epidemiology? How is data collected in each instance to establish cause–effect relationships?
4. What do relative risk and odds ratios indicate?

SINGLE-SUBJECT RESEARCH

With a traditional experimental design, a researcher may examine two groups of participants, pretest on an important dependent measure, apply a treatment to one group, and then posttest on that measure and look for statistical differences. Such research comes with some assumptions, one of which is that the groups initially "look" similar and that the treatment causes a relatively uniform effect. However, in some fields such as rehabilitation, special education, and social sciences, the questions under study do not lend themselves to experimental research due to a high degree of variability in individual performance. Examining group scores will rarely lead to statistical differences in groups because so much interindividual difference exists that it masks group change. In these cases, the researcher may opt to use a different type of research called *single-subject design research (SSDR)*. As the name suggests, single-subject design research involves examining either a single or small group of participants.

It is easy to confuse SSDR with another form of research we discussed in Chapter 7 called *case studies* because both types are performed on single or small groups of participants. However, there are dramatic differences in the two. As you may recall, case studies are a type of descriptive research where researchers carefully describe the details in a certain setting, such as a patient's response to a treatment over time. Case studies are descriptive, however, and do not inform us about cause–effect relationships or allow any inferences to be made from the results. Here is where SSDR differs from case studies. A single-subject design is an experimental design, similar to the group design described in Chapter 5, used to establish causal relationships between independent and dependent variables.[8] This means that researchers use randomization and controls within the study, and in some cases, the participants, the researcher, or both may be blinded to the intervention phases, and the results are evaluated statistically. In SSDR, a baseline must be established for the dependent measure under study prior to intervention. In this way, participants act as their own controls, not unlike within-subject designs. After establishing baseline, the researcher provides the intervention and then looks for evidence of change in the dependent measure between baseline and postintervention. The researcher will most likely repeat this process in several "phases" of intervention and baseline or nonintervention in an attempt to determine if the intervention "causes" baseline change.[9] As you can see, this is quite different from case study research, where the researcher describes what occurs but does not attempt to randomize treatment order, establish baseline, or repeatedly manipulate the independent variable.

Single Baseline and Reversal Design

Researchers using SSDR have a variety of study designs from which to choose. The simple baseline design, notated as A–B, is the most basic. In an A–B design, the researcher establishes a baseline of the dependent measure of interest. This time period is called the "baseline phase." In experimental research, this is analogous to a pretest, where the researcher identifies what the group does on average prior to any intervention. In order to establish baseline, researchers have to test and retest a participant a number of times and show consistency in the results. That is, the baseline behavior is stable across the different observations. Generally, the researcher can test no fewer than five times, and the results of these tests shouldn't show any trends, such as scores creeping up or down.[8] Next, during the "intervention phase," the intervention is provided, and the participant is retested to see if any change occurred. Here, researchers look for consistency in the outcome measure as well as a clear-cut difference between the baseline and intervention phase.

Although both single study research design research and case studies involve one or several participants, SSRD also uses statistical methods to determine differences.

In instances where removing an intervention is impossible or unethical, multiple baseline designs should be used.

The simple baseline design will not allow for the assessment of causality; therefore, researchers often use designs that provide stronger evidence of the effect of intervention. One commonly used design is a withdrawal design (A–B–A), where, after the intervention phase (B), the intervention is removed (A). Researchers look for another change, either a return to baseline or a change from the intervention phase. Another iteration of this is the reversal design (A–B–A–B), where the researcher provides and then withdraws the intervention in four phases.[10] We discussed this briefly in Chapter 7. In order to interpret data from these types of studies, researchers visually inspect the data and look for a clear difference from the baseline observations to the intervention trials. When a reversal design is used, researchers look for a well-defined change from baseline and intervention and then a return to baseline after the intervention is removed (see Special Interest Box 9.3).

Several issues exist within reversal designs. The first and perhaps most obvious is this: What if the effect can't be reversed? Imagine an educational setting where an intervention results in improvements in learning. Taking away the intervention will not lead to a return to baseline! Also, what if the intervention leads to such positive change that it would not be in the best interest of the participants (or, perhaps even ethical) to take the treatment away?

Multiple Baseline Designs

Another type of design that avoids some of the issues with reversal designs is the *multiple baseline across subjects*, which uses the simple baseline design on more than one participant at the same time. This design allows for individualization of establishing baseline and also of treatment. With this design, the researcher needs to examine at least three participants. All of the participants are tested on the dependent measure, and baseline is established. The first participant who shows a stable baseline then receives the intervention, while the other participants continue at baseline. After different amounts of time at baseline, each participant is given the intervention and then followed for a period of time. The way in which a researcher demonstrates the effectiveness of the intervention is to show the effect across different participants. Figure 9.3 presents a hypothetical graph of a multiple baseline study.

As an example of a multiple-baseline-between-subjects research, Nicholson et al.[12] wanted to determine if children with ASD would benefit from a physical activity intervention prior to classroom activity. Specifically, they hypothesized that antecedent physical activity would improve academic engagement in four elementary school children diagnosed with high-functioning ASD, and, if so, would the effect continue after the intervention ended? The physical activity intervention included 12 minutes of jogging followed by 5 minutes of walking and stretching. As a dependent measure, they used Shapiro's Behavioral Observation of Students in Schools (BOSS),[13] which measures on-task or academically engaged behavior into the components of passive and active engaged time. Nicholson and colleagues collected baseline data for 2 weeks, and after which time, one student began the

SPECIAL INTEREST BOX 9.3

Using a Reversal Design to Study Children with Autism

Imagine that you want to investigate the use of therapy dogs in clinical settings to see if their use will calm children with autism spectrum disorders (ASDs), which, in turn, may improve on-task behaviors as well as the clinical experience for children, parents, and clinicians (note that people can pet and interact with therapy dogs, unlike service dogs). If true, physical and occupational therapists could benefit from the use of therapy dogs during clinical testing. How could this effect be established? Children with ASD have large individual differences, so any differences in performance with and without the dog present would be masked by the large variability between participants. On the other hand, a reversal design on several participants would be ideal. In this case, the independent variable is presence of a therapy dog, and the dependent measures are (a) a score on test designed to measure motor skill deficits in children and (b) on-task behaviors. First, a participant is tested on the movement test without the therapy dog present during the baseline phase in order to establish consistency. In this case, that means the participant should score similarly on each administration of the test. Then, the child is tested again during the intervention phase, and at each test, the dog would be present. The intervention is withdrawn for a nonintervention phase and then presented in another intervention phase. This is an A–B–A–B design.

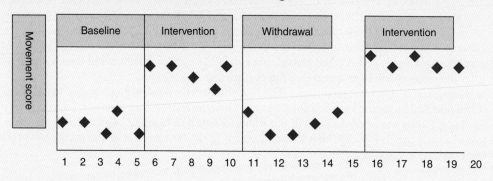

In this case, you can visually inspect differences between the phases with and without the dog present in that the scores consistently improve when the therapy dog is present. This design is similar to the one used by Miccinello.[11]

physical activity intervention, while the others stayed at baseline. Each week, another student received the physical activity intervention until all four received the intervention. This process was repeated until the fourth student finished 2 weeks of intervention. Finally, follow-up data were collected 4 weeks postintervention for a period of 2 weeks. Based on these results, particularly, the large effect sizes for academic-engaged time for all four students, the authors concluded that the physical activity intervention had an effect on active engagement in academics and may help students with ASD improve academic performance (Fig. 9.4).

✔ Check Your Understanding

1. Under what circumstances might a researcher choose a single-subject design?
2. How does SSDR differ from case studies?
3. Differentiate between reversal and multiple baseline designs.

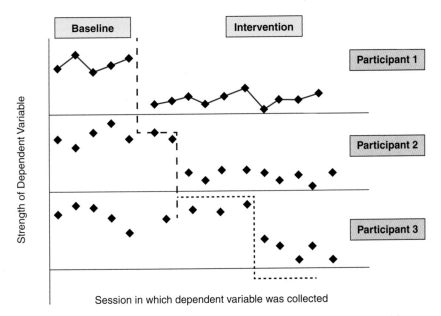

FIGURE 9.3 A hypothetical multiple-baseline-across-subjects design with three participants. Participant 1 receives treatment after establishing baseline in five observations. Participant 2 receives treatment after seven observations, and participant 3, after nine observations.

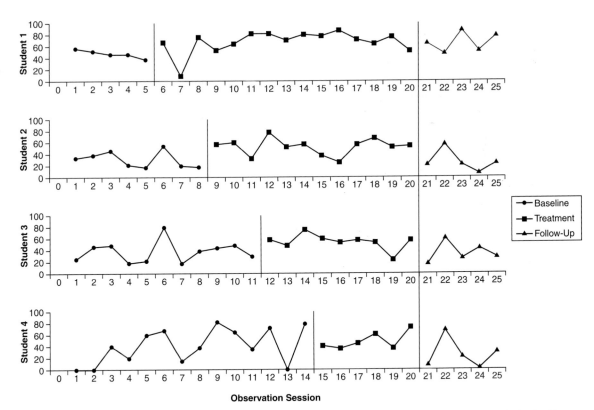

FIGURE 9.4 Results from the Nicholson et al.[12] study on the effect of physical activity on on-task classroom behavior. Note the improvement in on-task behavior in the measurements taken during treatment.

META-ANALYSIS

In Chapter 3, we discussed the importance of reviewing the literature as a part of the research process in order to determine what is already known about a health-related topic of interest and what gaps still exist in the research. Some topics are surrounded by scanty empirical evidence, with few studies devoted to them. On the other hand, some topics have dozens of related studies devoted to them! This may lead a novice researcher into a quandary: What exactly do the results of multiple studies tell me, and how do I summarize them? To add to the confusion, not all studies are created equal. Some may have impeccable methodology leading to strong internal validity. Others may be a little sketchy in their design or measures or some other aspect of the methodology. How can a research objectively assess all that information? Fortunately, a type of research called *meta-analysis* exists that allows for an objective approach to synthesizing the results of multiple existing research studies. A meta-analysis goes beyond a review of literature by systematically evaluating all existing studies on a particular topic using a number of criteria and then making conclusions on the effect size of the independent variable based on the results and about the generalizability of the effect. Because this is a type of research, a meta-analysis can be published in a research journal, and the results provide data just as any other research study does.

When looking for codes for data in meta-analysis, consider any factors that could have an impact on the outcome of the study.

The need for meta-analysis becomes clearer when considering problems that have a vast array of empirical methods used to examine them. Take, for example, a relatively simple question: Do existing studies indicate that diet, exercise, or diet and exercise interventions work best for weight loss? When Miller et al.[14] asked this question in 1997, they discovered that a whopping 700+ published studies existed in peer-reviewed journals! Within this group of studies was a broad array of methods. Intervention lengths and types varied, as did number of participants in each study. Participants also ranged in indexes of body fatness, among other measures. Even after providing minimal criteria for inclusion, such as requiring the study to report change in percentage body fat and to provide an exact duration of the intervention, they only whittled the total down to 493 studies, still a daunting number to summarize.

The previous example highlights the first two steps of meta-analysis. First, the authors must determine the inclusion criteria for studies of interest. Next, they determine all the published research on the particular topic. We described the techniques used in data searches in Chapter 3. Researchers must cast a wide net and therefore use several different databases that may have published research on a topic. Furthermore, specifications of the search should be noted and expressed in the write-up of the meta-analysis so that others can easily replicate the process. What key terms were used? What language should the articles be in? How many years back did the search go? For an example, we will use the study of Logan et al.,[15] who wanted to determine the effectiveness of motor skill interventions on motor performance in young children. Their first step was to identify the extant literature:

> *The following databases were searched for relevant articles: Academic Search Premier, PsycArticles, PsycInfo, SportDiscus and ERIC. No date range was specified and each search was conducted to include all possible years of publication specific to each database. Key terms for the search included motor, skill, movement, intervention, programme, or children. Searches were conducted using single and combined terms. Pertinent journals and article reference lists were also manually searched.*

This search yielded a pool of 22 studies.

Once researchers find all the research studies on the topic that they can, they must decide which of these studies to review more thoroughly. As we said earlier, studies can vary drastically in methodology so can descriptions of variables (in how they are either operationalized or measured) or reporting of results. There must be some standard by which studies can be compared. Thus, researchers must develop and clearly articulate specific inclusion and exclusion criteria for the studies they have found as their second step. What sort of things *must* be in a study in order to include it in the analysis? One critical component for inclusion is the presence of **effect size**; either effect size must be provided, or the researcher must be able to calculate it from the information given. Remember, meta-analysis synthesizes information in order to determine how large a treatment or intervention effect is present across a large number of similar studies. Without an effect size for each study included in the analysis, this is impossible to determine. Other inclusion criteria can include participant characteristics, date of publication (in some fields, rapidly changing technology can make older publications obsolete), and types of interventions—really, the authors may include or exclude anything that makes logical sense to their overall purpose.

Effect Size A measure of the strength of a treatment.

Again, here is an example from Logan et al.,[15] whose inclusion criteria were

1. Implementation of any type of motor skill intervention
2. Pre- and postqualitative assessment of fundamental motor skills (FMS) competence
3. Availability of means and standard deviations of motor performance

Criterion 1 allows for any type of motor skill intervention at all, which is fairly broad. However, criterion 2 limits the studies to process-oriented assessments, which will exclude any studies that provide quantitative values such as running speed or throwing distance as dependent measures. The final criterion ensures that the researchers can calculate effect size if not provided. Using these criteria, Logan and colleagues could narrow the field of published articles down to 11, which is a very manageable number.

The next step in performing a meta-analysis is coding the data. Prior to coding, the researcher must determine what the key components are that could influence effect sizes reported across the studies. Let's consider Logan and colleagues' problem again: the effectiveness of motor skill interventions on improving motor performance in young children. What components of a study could impact effect size? Certainly, the age and developmental status of the children under study would be important, so would the type and duration of the intervention. Other considerations are the intervention provider (teacher or researcher). In terms of the dependent measures, the assessment tool is important. In all, Logan and colleagues coded 10 variables plus effect size.

If you have read many research studies in the past, you may recall that within some studies, the researchers may not report effect size. Over the past decade, more and more journal editors require that authors include effect size when reporting their results. Nonetheless, plenty of published research exists with no mention of effect size. In Chapter 12, we will discuss the notion of effect size at length, but for now, you should know it represents the strength of a treatment. You can think about this in another way: How meaningful is the difference between two groups? If the treatment has a big influence on the dependent measure, then highly meaningful differences exist between treatment and control.

Within a study, effect size can be calculated using the following formula:

$$ES = \frac{\text{Mean score of treatment group} - \text{mean score of control group}}{\text{Standard deviation of control group}}$$

Equation 9.3

Let's look at an example that might illustrate this concept. Imagine you wanted to determine if using "exergame" interventions actually improve balance. In one of the studies you find, Nintendo Wii Fit was used as an intervention in older adults, and balance was measured using a stabilometer. Pretest scores were 10.0 ± 2.3 for the treatment group and 11.3 ± 1.9 for the control group. Posttest scores were 14.2 ± 3.1 for the treatment group and 12.1 ± 2.4 for the control group. Using the formula above, the following effect size was obtained:

$$ES = \frac{14.2 - 12.1}{2.4} = 0.875 \qquad \text{Equation 9.4}$$

As a rule of thumb, an effect size of 0.2 is considered small, 0.5 is moderate, and 0.8 is large.[16] So, in the previous example, we would consider this a large effect size.

Once the effect sizes have been calculated, they are included in a table with the other coded materials. Once all the studies have been coded and the effect sizes calculated, then a mean of the effect sizes for all of the studies is calculated. This tells us what the average effect size is for the particular problem under question. Sometimes, several effect sizes will be calculated within the group of studies. For example, in Logan et al.,[15] they examined pre- and posttest scores and looked at effect size for treatment groups (i.e., how much did the children change from pre to post), control groups, and also within the subsections of the motor skills test they saw most frequently, the Test of Gross Motor Development II. This allowed them to determine if, across the studies, children improved differently in locomotor or object control (e.g., throwing, catching). They found an effect size for treatment groups ($d = 0.39$, which is moderate) and that locomotor ($d = 0.41$) and object control ($d = 0.45$) skills were affected similarly. On the other hand, the effect size of the control groups was much smaller ($d = 0.06$), suggesting little change from pre- to posttest across the studies. Figure 9.5 shows these data graphically.

The final part of a meta-analysis involves interpreting all the columns and the effect sizes. One of the conclusions that Logan and his colleagues made was that motor skill interventions do improve fundamental motor skills in young children. Although that finding may seem to be common sense, only seven states in the United States mandate structured physical activity for preschoolers! Logan and colleagues recommended that, as an evidence-based practice, preschools should include motor skills interventions as part of their curriculum.

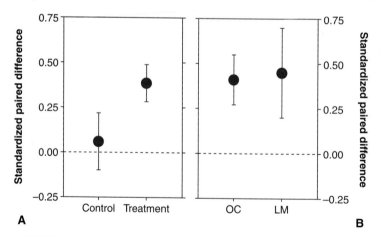

■ **FIGURE 9.5** Results from Logan et al.[15] showing the overall effect size of **(A)** treatments versus controls and **(B)** object control versus locomotor skills. The standardized paired difference scores were derived from the results of 11 studies in a meta-analysis.

✔ Check Your Understanding

1. How does a meta-analysis differ from a literature review?
2. Why is effect size essential in a meta-analysis?
3. Why do researchers need specific inclusion and exclusion criteria for studies?

CHAPTER SUMMARY

- Both historical and philosophical researches are important to the field of kinesiology and health sciences.
- Historical research involves developing a pertinent question and then answering it through an exploration of primary and secondary evidence.
- Philosophical research involved developing a thesis and then searching for logical arguments through inductive or deductive reasoning that will support or refute the thesis.
- Epidemiological research involves investigation populations for determinants of disease and health.
- Cross-sectional designs look at a cross-section of the population at one point in time in order to determine current relationships among determinants.
- There are three types of analytic designs. Cohort designs start with a population and follow over time to see who does and does not develop a disease state. Case–control designs examine a population retrospectively. Randomized controlled designs provide an intervention to a sample within the population and compare outcomes with control groups.
- SSDR provides a means for determining causation when the population under study is highly variable.
- Single baseline and reversal designs involve adding an intervention one or several times and comparing dependent measures to those of the baseline. In these studies, individual participants (rather than groups) are compared and act as their own controls.
- Multiple baseline designs involve providing an intervention just one time but at different time intervals for each participant.
- Meta-analysis is the process of examining a relatively large group of studies that have similar independent and dependent variables and determining a general effect size for all of the studies.

REFERENCES

1. Bury JB. The Science of History: An Inaugural Lecture: Delivered in the Divinity School [of] Cambridge on January 26, 1903.
2. Hult JS. The story of women's athletics: manipulating a dream. 1890–1985. In: Costa DM, Guthrie SR, eds. *Women and Sport: Interdisciplinary Perspectives*. Champaign, IL: Human Kinetics, 84–100.
3. Welch P, Costa DM. A century of Olympic Competition. In: Costa DM, Guthrie SR, eds. *Women in Sport. Interdisciplinary Perspectives*. Champaign, IL: Human Kinetics, 1994:123–138.
4. Kretchmar RS. *Practical Philosophy of Sport and Physical Activity*, 2nd ed. Champaign, IL: Human Kinetics, 2005.
5. Hwang CH, Kretchmar RS. Aristotle's golden mean: its implications for the Doping debate. *J Philos Sport* 2010;XXXVII,1:102–121.
6. Vankim NA, Laska MN. Socioeconomic disparities in emerging adult weight and weight behaviors. *Am J Health Behav* 2012;36(4):433–445.
7. Healthy People: The Surgeon General's Report on Health Promotion and Disease Prevention. 1979.
8. Horner RH, Carr EG, Halle J, et al. The use of single subject research to identify evidence-based practice in special education. *Except Child* 2005;71:165–180.
9. Logan L, Hickman R, Harris S, et al. Single-subject research design: recommendations for levels of evidence and quality rating. *Dev Med Child Neurol* 2008;50:99–105.
10. Tankersley M, McGoey KE, Dalton D, et al. Speaking of research: single subject research methods in rehabilitation. *Work: J Assess Prevent Rehabil* 2006;26:85–92.
11. Miccinello D. The effects of animal assisted interventions on children with autism during the Movement Assessment Battery for Children-2 (MABC-2). Unpublished Thesis, University of Delaware, 2011.
12. Nicholson H, Kehle TJ, Bray MA, et al. The effects of antecedent physical activity on the academic engagement of children with autism spectrum disorder. *Psychol Sch* 2011;48(2):198–213.
13. Shapiro E. *Academic Skills Problems: Direct Assessment and Intervention*. New York, NY: Guilford Press, 2004.
14. Miller WC, Koceja DM, Hamilton EJ. A meta-analysis of the past 25 years of weight loss research using diet, exercise or diet plus exercise intervention. *Int J Obes Relat Metab Disord* 1997;21:941–947.
15. Logan SW, Robinson LE, Wilson AE, et al. Getting the fundamentals of movement: a meta-analysis of the effectiveness of motor skill interventions in children. *Child Care Health Dev* 2012;38:305–315.
16. Cohen J. *Statistical Power Analysis for the Behavioral Sciences*, 3rd ed. New York, NY: Academic Press, 1969.

RELATED ASSIGNMENTS

1. Collect three peer-reviewed studies on a topic within kinesiology and health sciences that ask the same question and use similar methodologies. Calculate the average effect size across these studies using Equation 9.3.

2. Use the Internet to investigate the different sorts of questions that historians in the field of kinesiology ask. Create a list of three different studies, and describe the primary and secondary sources used by the researchers.

3. Epidemiological studies may relate to the determinants of disease but also of health. Using PubMed or a similar search engine, locate one of each type. Compare and contrast the methods, results, and conclusions of these studies.

IN-CLASS GROUP EXERCISES

1. Within your group, develop a historical question based on gender and health or physical activity within the 19th century. Use the Internet to help guide you in understanding the historical context at that time. Develop a list of both primary and secondary sources, and write one to two paragraphs that summarize your findings.

2. Divide the class into two large groups (one inductive, one deductive). Further subdivide the groups into smaller groups of three to four students. Earlier in the chapter, the philosophical question was posed "what is sport?" to determine if cheering can be considered a sport. Within each group, use either inductive or deductive reasoning to answer this question. After a period of time, regroup into the larger "inductive" and "deductive" groups and discuss. Finally, compare the discussions of the inductive and deductive group as a whole class.

3. As a group, develop a single-subject study experimental design to examine the influence of cell phone usage on reaction time, using an A–B–A design. Test two students within your group. Graph the data, and then visually analyze it for clear differences between baseline and reversal, and again back to baseline. Write up the results and your conclusions based on your study. Compare these among the different groups in the class.

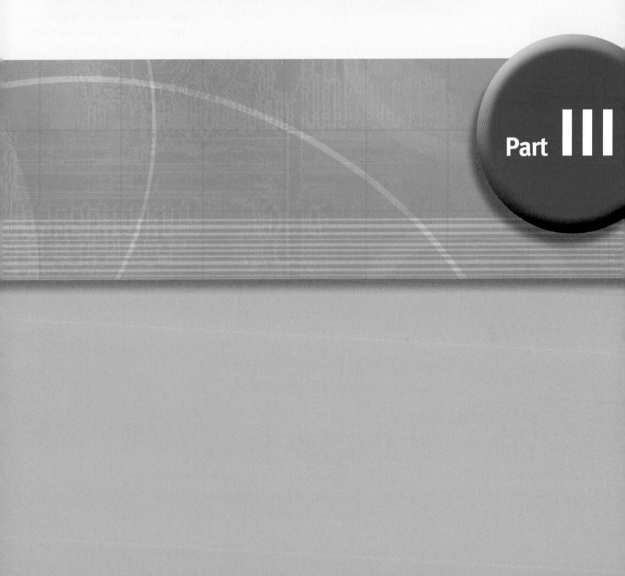

Understanding Statistics and Measurement in Research

Part **III**

10

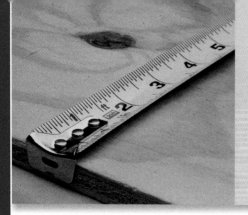

Basic Statistical Concepts

"To measure is to know."—*Lord Kelvin*

CHAPTER OBJECTIVES

After studying this chapter, you will be able to:
1. Explain how statistics can be used for description and inference.
2. Discuss the concept of statistical significance in defining the results of a study.
3. Describe the interrelationships among type I and II errors and statistical power.
4. Explain the advantages and disadvantages of different sampling techniques.
5. Describe common measures of central tendency and variability.
6. Differentiate between appropriate uses of parametric and nonparametric statistical tests.

■ STATISTICS are your friend! You may be entirely unconvinced of this right now, but after reading the next several chapters, you may be willing to consider this notion. Within the realm of research, statistics are tools that bring order to irregular-looking data sets and enable legitimate comparisons to be made and conclusions to be drawn. Use of statistics in research is not an option; it is essential. And, as will become increasingly apparent, there is an inexorable, logical link between statistics and research design. Fortunately, you need not become trained as a statistician in order to appreciate and understand the value of statistical analysis in the research process. Also of good fortune is the current-day widespread availability of statistical software packages, so that calculating a statistical analysis by hand is largely outdated. You need not be good in math to become competent in running many of the more common basic statistical analyses that you are likely to need for analyzing research data. It is common (and advised) for trained researchers to consult with statisticians in designing studies that are more complicated. However, a working knowledge of basic statistics is essential for being able to productively communicate with statisticians, as well as for understanding the research process and interpreting research results.

You may have already had an introductory course in statistics, in which case the material in this chapter will serve as a review of basic statistical concepts. Alternatively, this chapter introduces basic statistical concepts from the perspective of what the beginning researcher needs to know.

USES OF STATISTICS

Statistics is a subfield of mathematics that deals with procedures for collecting, analyzing, interpreting, and presenting data. Broadly speaking, statistics are used for two general purposes: description and inference. Suppose you have a data set consisting of reaction times on a computerized test for 300 sixteen-year-old girls. **Descriptive statistics** can give you several measures of what we call **central tendency**, or different ways of looking at representative times for the whole group, along with measures of **variability**, or the extent to which the times within the data set are spread out. **Inferential statistics** can give us insight into how well these scores are representative of reaction times for all 16-year-old girls who have the same characteristics as the 300 measured.

Descriptive Statistics

Descriptive statistics are used to characterize a group with regard to a set of measurements, or data, taken on all members of the group. As mentioned, descriptive statistics include measures of central tendency and variability, both of which are critical for characterizing the distribution of a data set. If you have had a course in measurement, this section will serve as a review for the commonly used measures of central tendency and variability.

Descriptive Statistics
Indicators of central tendency and variability of variables of interest

Central Tendency The extent to which values cluster in a data distribution plot

Variability The extent to which values are spread out in a data distribution plot

Inferential Statistics
Mathematical approach to deducing the probability of the occurrence of a characteristic in a population based on the measured characteristics of a sample

Datum *is singular for* data *(plural).*

MEASURES OF CENTRAL TENDENCY

A measure of central tendency is the one numeric value that represents the entire data set. Depending on the context, however, the choice of that measure of central tendency is calculated differently.

Mean Arithmetic average

The **mean** is the arithmetic average of a group of numbers, calculated as the sum of all the numbers divided by the total number of values in the data set:

$$M = \left(\sum X\right) / N$$

For example, the mean for the data set including 2, 4, 7, 8, 9 (totaling 30) is 6. Note that the mean must be calculated. In other words, it is not necessarily one of the numbers that lies within the data set. The mean is overwhelmingly the most commonly used measure of central tendency for research applications because it is the number that lies in the arithmetic center of the data set.

Median Value in the center of the data set, with 50% of the data values being larger and 50% being smaller

The **median** is always a **datum**, or a single data value, that resides in the middle of the data distribution, such that half the scores fall above it and half below it. If there are an odd number of values in the data set, the median is the central number within the data set. If there is an even number of values in the data set, the two central numbers are averaged to yield a single value for the median. For example, the median of the data set 1, 4, 17, 65, 80 is the number 17. Note that in this case, the median (17) is very different from the value for the mean (33).

Datum A single data point

Mode Most frequently occurring data value

The third and least precise indicator of central tendency is the **mode**, which is the most frequent score in a distribution. In a score distribution including 3, 4, 4, 4, 6, 8, 11, 17, 20, the mode is 4. Note that the mode (4) is different from both the median (6) and the mean (9). Should there be two scores occurring with the same frequency higher than the frequency of all other scores, the distribution is termed "bimodal". The distribution 3, 4, 4, 6, 7, 11, 11, 15, for example, is bimodal. The mode is of interest to clothing manufacturers in determining how many garments to produce in which sizes. However, it is seldom a measure of interest in research.

MEASURES OF VARIABILITY

Measures of variability provide an indication of the distribution of measures within a data set. Depending on the nature of the data collection, the scores might clump toward one end of the data distribution, clump toward the middle of the data distribution, or be evenly distributed.

Range High score minus the low score

As the name suggests, the **range** is the difference between the high and low scores. Researchers can report the range in two ways. If a data set includes the numbers 10, 23, 45, 61, and 88, the range can be reported as 10 to 88, identifying the low and high extremes, or it can be reported as a single number, in this case 78, which is the difference between the high and low scores. Note that the range provides no information about the distribution of any scores between the extremes of the data set.

Standard Deviation Numerical indicator of the spread of data values within a data set

The **standard deviation**, which serves as an estimate of the spread of scores away from the mean, is by far the most commonly used indicator of the variability of a research data set. There are several different approaches and formulas for calculating standard deviation, none of which we present here because calculators, spreadsheets, and statistical software all readily generate values for the standard deviation. A more important issue is proper interpretation of the standard deviation. Generally speaking, the larger the standard deviation, the greater the distribution of scores away from the mean. In a normal distribution, approximately 68% of scores fall within 1 standard deviation of the mean, with about 95% falling within 2 standard deviations of the mean and around 99% falling within 3 standard deviations of the mean.

Another indicator of variability often reported is the **standard error of the mean**, which is an estimate of the expected difference between the sample mean and the population mean. It is calculated as the standard deviation divided by the square root of the sample size:

$$SEM = S / \sqrt{N}$$

Note that as the standard deviation gets smaller, SEM gets smaller and that as the sample size gets larger, SEM gets smaller. The smaller the value of the standard error of the mean, the more confidence we have that the sample mean is an accurate representation of the population mean. For this reason, the SEM is a very useful statistic in research.

> **Standard Error of the Mean** Numerical indicator of the expected difference between the sample and population means

> *Descriptive statistics are commonly used at the beginning of the Methods section of research papers to describe the sample of participants*

COMMON USES OF DESCRIPTIVE STATISTICS IN RESEARCH

In papers reporting research in which human participants were tested, it is common for the section of the paper describing the participants to begin with identification of the means and standard deviations of participant ages, heights, and weights. Note that these statistical descriptions include both a measure of central tendency (the mean) and a measure of variability (the standard deviation). Following this, means, standard deviations, and often the standard errors of the means and ranges are presented for each variable measured. Descriptive statistics can be used to characterize any variable of interest with regard to central tendency and variability within a discrete group.

✔ Check Your Understanding

1. Why is the mean and not the median or the mode the most common measure of central tendency reported for research data sets?
2. Describe the purposes of each of the three measures of variability.
3. Which descriptive statistics would be important to report to characterize the SAT scores of all freshman students entering a college or university?

Inferential Statistics

Statistics are also used when the goal is to take data, or measures of certain characteristics, from a research study and from these make generalizations or inferences about the same characteristics of a larger group. The ability to accurately predict the characteristics of a very large group based on measurements from a small subset of the large group is quite a powerful leveraging tool. Let's say we would like to know what percentage of undergraduate US college students take a course in research methods. We could survey every program in every college and university in North America and compile the information. This would be quite tedious and time consuming. Alternatively, we could take data from a few representative colleges and then generalize our findings to the United States and Canada. How would we know that we could legitimately generalize such findings? We could do this by making sure that our sample of representative colleges was truly "representative" and by using inferential statistics. There are generally two types of questions that can be answered when using statistics for purposes of inference—is there a relationship between variables, and is there a difference across conditions?

RELATIONSHIPS BETWEEN VARIABLES

One important use of inferential statistics is determining whether a relationship exists between two or more variables of interest within the population. For example, it might be of interest to know if there is a relationship between GRE scores and grades among students in graduate programs. If indeed GRE scores can be used to predict performance in a graduate program, they then become a valuable screening tool for predicting which students will and will not be successful in the program. However, if there is no relationship between GRE scores and grades, then a graduate program need not require that students submit GRE scores prior to admission.

Researchers have used inferential statistics extensively to document a relationship between test outcomes in situations where it is desirable to be able to use a simple test in place of a test that is more troublesome or more expensive. For example, researchers consider an arduous treadmill test involving collection of expired respiratory gases as the "gold standard" for assessing maximum oxygen consumption capability, or VO_{2max}. Studies demonstrating the relationships between the results of laboratory tests of VO_{2max} and performance scores on field tests have led to widespread use of tests such as the 12-minute run, where the goal is to cover as much distance as possible within the allotted time, and the 1.5-mile run, where the goal is to complete the prescribed distance as fast as possible. Established relationships between the results of these field tests and the traditional treadmill test enable close estimates of VO_{2max} from the field test results. Chapter 11 includes further discussion of uses of statistics for evaluation of relationships.

DIFFERENCES ACROSS CONDITIONS

The second general question answered by inferential use of statistics is whether true differences exist between conditions. Sometimes, the question of interest is whether there are differences between groups, as between males and females, young and old, or trained and untrained, on some variable of interest. Another common research question is whether there are differences in a variable of interest before and after a period of time, which may include an intervention of some sort. The intervention may involve diet, training, a therapeutic drug, or a medical treatment. Some studies are designed to compare two different types of intervention, such as two different diets. Chapter 12 addresses a variety of statistical tests designed for evaluation of differences across conditions.

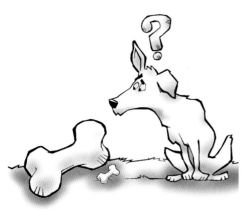

The null hypothesis, a statement of no difference between conditions, is often incorrect.

HYPOTHESES

Each statistical test for a relationship or difference is founded upon a hypothesis or prediction about the outcome of the test. Whereas the research hypothesis, as discussed in Chapter 6, is a statement as to what the researcher actually expects the outcome of a study to be, statistical tests are conducted to test statistical hypotheses. These statistical hypotheses can take two forms: null and directional. The

Null Hypothesis Statement indicating expectation of no relationship or difference between conditions for purposes of statistical testing

null hypothesis is always a statement that no correlation between variables or difference between conditions is expected. Examples of null hypotheses are the following:

There is no relationship between gender and ability in math.

There will be no difference in quadriceps strength before and after a 6-week lower extremity training protocol.

The research hypothesis may be the same as the null hypothesis, or it may be the opposite. For example, the researcher may or may not believe that there is a relationship between gender and math ability. The research hypothesis, however, is usually based on logical assumptions made from an understanding of published research papers related to the question, as opposed to a hazarded guess. Alternatively, a **directional hypothesis** is the statistical equivalent of the research hypothesis, indicating that either a correlation or a difference in a particular direction is expected. Because it is easier to test using statistical procedures, it is usually the null hypothesis, rather than a directional hypothesis, that is tested.

Directional Hypothesis Statement indicating an expected direction of a relationship or a difference for purposes of statistical testing

Check Your Understanding

1. How, generally, are inferential statistics used? Provide an example.
2. What is the relationship between the research hypothesis and the null hypothesis?

PROBABILITY

A question that remains is what degree of correlation or amount of difference is necessary in order for there to be support for a hypothesis? If we were to flip a coin 100 times, with a 50% probability of the toss coming up heads, we would expect exactly 50 of 100 tosses to come up heads. In reality, however, 100 coin tosses might yield 53 heads or 46 heads. In such cases, we would say that our results were different from those predicted because of error due to chance.

Statistical Significance

Before conducting a study, the researchers make a decision as to what amount of error due to chance they are willing to accept. (This represents the chance that the results of the study are not accurately representative of the situation present in the population at large). This level of tolerable error due to chance is known as the **alpha (α) level**. The alpha level is also referred to as the **level of significance** or criterion for accepting or rejecting the null hypothesis. The alpha level most commonly selected in studies in kinesiology and the health sciences is $\alpha = 0.05$, or a 5% level of confidence, indicating that the odds of the study results being an error due to chance are 5 in 100. In some studies such as large clinical trials involving testing of drugs with major health implications, the alpha level may be set at a more stringent level such as 0.01 or even 0.001. Why the difference? Although we might be comfortable with a 5% chance of the results of a study on the efficacy of a new diet for weight loss being wrong, we would likely not be comfortable with the results of a drug study resulting in 5 deaths for every 100 participants.

Alpha Level Margin of error due to chance deemed acceptable for erroneous rejection or acceptance of the null hypothesis within a given study

Level of Significance Same as alpha level

Whereas the alpha level is the level of acceptable error due to chance set by the researchers when planning a given study, what is reported after the study has been conducted and the results statistically analyzed is the exact probability (p) associated with the likelihood of the results erroneously being due to chance. Statistical software generates the p value. When the p value is smaller than or equal to the alpha level, the null hypothesis is rejected, which means the results of the study show a "significant relationship" or a "significant difference" between variables or conditions being compared with the statistical test. When the p value is larger than the alpha level, the null hypothesis cannot be rejected, and the findings are considered to be "nonsignificant."

Many a researcher has tried to make a case for the results of a study with $p = 0.06$ when $\alpha = 0.05$ as being "almost significant," "close to

The results of statistical tests are either significant or nonsignificant.

Statistic Value representing a characteristic of a sample

Parameter Value representing a characteristic of a population

in the last Olympic Games. In all cases, however, the researcher's goal in selecting participants for inclusion in a study sample is to ensure that the sample is representative of the population. Using research terminology, we refer to a measurable characteristic of a sample as a **statistic**, whereas the corresponding characteristic within the population represented by that sample is termed a **parameter**.

Sample Size Determination

A question that typically occurs early on in the process of planning a study is "how many participants will we need?" This question has obvious practical implications because the larger the number of participants, the longer it will take to collect and analyze the data and the greater the associated expenses. From this standpoint, it may seem like the fewer the participants, the better. However, we would typically place much greater confidence in the results of a study conducted on 1,000 participants than in the results of a study conducted with only 10 participants. Although this might suggest that it is desirable to include as many participants in a study as possible, this is not necessarily the case, particularly given the reality of the constraints of time and expense associated with data collection.

The balance that researchers hope to achieve in determining the appropriate sample size for a given study is based on arriving at a sample that will accurately represent the population for the variable being studied. The more closely a sample reflects the characteristics of the population it represents, the less the likelihood of both type I and type II errors. The probability of making a correct decision with regard to avoiding type I and II errors is known as **power**. The greater the power of a study, the greater the odds of arriving at statistically significant findings that accurately reflect the population. From a practical perspective, we can think of power as the degree of confidence we can have in the results of a study.

Power Probability of correctly rejecting or accepting the null hypothesis

With this in mind, it is clear that having an optimal sample size is important. Fortunately, it is possible to use commercial software, as well as software available at no cost on the Internet, to calculate the number of participants needed in order to have an appropriate level of power for a given study. Depending on the study design, the information you will need to calculate an acceptable level of power will vary. It is likely to include your predetermined levels of alpha and beta, an indication of the variability of the measures of interest within your sample, and identification of the size of the relationship or difference in the conditions you are investigating that you consider to be meaningful. Generally, the smaller the effect size between conditions and greater the variability of measures of the variable of interest, the larger the sample size needed. It is typical in most research on human participants in kinesiology and the health sciences to calculate the number of participants needed to arrive at a power level of 0.8. Special Interest Box 10.1 presents an example of sample size calculation.

✔ Check Your Understanding

1. What are the advantages of a small sample size?
2. What are the advantages of a large sample size?
3. How should sample size for a given study be determined?

Sample Selection

Another important question that must be answered during the early planning stages for a research investigation is "where will the participants come from?" There are several systematic approaches for selecting the sample for a study, with the approach of choice typically depending on practical considerations.

SPECIAL INTEREST BOX 10.1

Calculating Sample Size

Jill's plan for her senior thesis was to compare pretest and posttest measures of time on a half-mile run in children participating in physical education classes at an elementary school where she would be doing her student teaching and had been given the opportunity to plan the course of instruction for 12 weeks. Jill estimated that participation in her planned activities would improve student running time by an average of 10%. Her committee directed her to a paper by Kadam and Bhalerao[1] to assist her with sample size calculation so she could make sure that she tested a sufficient number of students to be able to detect the difference she hypothesized. Jill learned that the information she would need in order to calculate sample size for the study using the procedure of Kadam and Bhalerao included the following:

- Acceptable level of significance
- Power of the study
- Expected effect size
- Standard deviation in the population

Jill's committee directed her to use $\alpha = 0.05$ for the acceptable level of significance with power set to 80%, since these are the typically selected values for research on human subjects in kinesiology and the health sciences. However, she would need to either come up with estimates or consult related studies from the literature to determine reasonable values for effect size and standard deviation. Jill estimated that student running times would improve by 15% (her effect size). She looked at a number of studies published in the literature and selected a standard deviation of 0.5. The formula for calculating sample size presented by Kadam and Bhalerao[1] is

$$n = \frac{2\,(z_\alpha + z_{1-\beta})^2\,(SD)^2}{ES^2}$$

where n is the number of participants, z_α is a constant equal to 1.65 based on $\alpha = 0.05$ and the fact that student running times were expected to improve (known as a "one-sided test"), $z_{1-\beta}$ is the constant of 0.8416 based on the power level of 80%, and the standard deviation (SD) and effect size (ES) Jill selected are, respectively, 0.5 and 0.15.

So, substituting into the formula, we have

$$n = \frac{2\,(1.65 + 0.8416)^2\,(0.5)^2}{(0.15)^2}$$

$$n \approx 138$$

Jill was pleased to be able to report back to her committee that using the procedure they had recommended, she was able to calculate a sample size of 138 students needed for her study.

However, then one of Jill's friends informed her that there are a number of automatic calculators readily available online for determining sample size. Being a math whiz, Jill was just as happy to have had the opportunity to do the sample size calculation by hand using a formula. But looking online, she quickly realized that depending on the design of the study, different formulas are used for appropriately calculating sample size. One free online tool for calculating sample size for different types of studies is G*Power.[2]

RANDOM SELECTION

Random Sampling Procedure for selection of participants for a study that provides an equal chance of selection for all members of the population

Keeping in mind that we want the sample to accurately represent the characteristics of interest within the population, the theoretically optimum approach for determining the sample is **random sampling**. With a process of true random selection, every member of the population has an equal chance of being selected into the study sample. Thus, using a process of random selection, so long as the sample size is adequate, the sample should also be accurately representative of the population. If the entire population of interest is either small enough or sufficiently geographically constrained, a process of true random selection may be possible. For example, if we wanted to conduct a study about opinions within a national professional organization related to federal legislation on physical activity in K-12 education, we could run the membership numbers of individuals belonging to the organization through software containing a random number generator that would randomly sort the desired number of members into the selected sample. Members of the randomly selected sample would then be sent a questionnaire.

Sampling Error Inclusion of participants in a study that result in a sample not representative of the population due to chance error

As a cautionary note, however, it is important to recognize that random sampling does not guarantee that the resulting sample will be fully and accurately representative of the population from which it was selected. There is always some possibility that **sampling error**, or inclusion of chance variations resulting in a nonrepresentative sample, may occur. Nevertheless, random sampling is the approach most likely to result in a representative sample.

STRATIFIED RANDOM SELECTION

Stratified Random Sampling Selection procedure for participants in a study that provides an equal chance of selection for all members of purposeful divisions of the population

In situations where it is deemed important that a randomly selected sample also be appropriately representative of different subgroups that the population could be divided or stratified into, we could use a process known as **stratified random sampling**. Using our example of the national professional organization we wish to survey, if we wanted representation in the sample proportional to the size of the membership from each state, we could first identify what percentage of organization membership comes from each state and set up the software to randomly choose the appropriate percentage of the sample from each state. So if 8% of the organization's members were from California, 8% of the sample would randomly be selected from among Californians belonging to the organization. In a more complicated scenario, if stratification based on multiple characteristics were deemed important, we could also stratify the sample based on gender, age range, and job classification of members.

SYSTEMATIC SELECTION

Systematic Sampling Procedure for selection of participants for a study in which every nth individual on a list is selected.

If we needed to sample from an extremely large or, in some other way, unwieldy population, another sampling approach we might choose is termed **systematic sampling**. This consists simply of selecting every 100th or 500th or nth name on a list. This approach is commonly used for "public opinion" surveys. Although not truly random, this approach should yield a random sample so long as all of the population is on the list and the list is randomly ordered. If either of these stipulations is not the case, then the sample may be **biased**. A biased sample is one in which the variability within the sample is different from the variability within the population. Choosing names from a phone book, for example, eliminates the possibility of selection for anyone not having a phone or a listed phone number. In this case, the sample would be biased against those without listed phone numbers.

Biased Not representative of a population

CONVENIENCE SAMPLING

In practicality, true random selection of participants is not often possible. If you wish to study caloric expenditure during activity bursts in preschool children aged 3 to 5 years in preschool settings in Australia, it is obviously not going to be possible for you to draw in participants for your study from all over the country. Instead, you will use what we term a **convenience sample** of children from one or more local settings that you can conveniently access. When using a convenience sample, it is important to designate **inclusion criteria** for the study such that your sample will be adequately representative of the large population to which you hope to be able to generalize your results at the end of the study. The inclusion criteria should include all those characteristics that the children should possess in order to be included in the population. Another approach is to designate **exclusion criteria**, which can be used instead of or in addition to the inclusion criteria. If your population is defined as "apparently healthy children aged 3 to 5 years," your exclusion criteria would include having had no diseases or serious injuries within the recent past.

Convenience Sample Group of participants for a study selected because of readiness of opportunity

Inclusion Criteria Characteristics individuals must possess in order to qualify for participation as participants in a study

It is important when using a convenience sample to describe the sample characteristics as fully as possible, so that those reading about the study can evaluate the extent to which the study results are or are not likely to also pertain to a population or other subgroups of the population. For example, in our study of preschool children, it would be important to describe the profile of the sample in terms of socioeconomic, rural–urban, and racial or ethnic status mixes of the children.

Exclusion Criteria Characteristics individuals cannot possess in order to qualify for participation as participants in a study

RANDOM ASSIGNMENT TO GROUPS

A concept that students sometimes confuse with random selection is random assignment of participants to groups. If your study design involves three groups of participants, all of whom should have the same characteristics at the beginning of the study, it is important to use a random process for assigning participants to groups. Random assignment of participants to groups is the single best way to ensure that the groups are likely to be equal on the variable(s) of interest to begin with. As discussed in Chapter 6, allowing participants to choose which group they will participate is typically a good way to destroy the internal validity of a study. Suppose you were conducting a training study where you planned to have a high-intensity exercise group, a low-intensity exercise group, and a control group that did no exercise. Your "in-shape" participants would likely be choosing one of the exercise groups, while the "couch potatoes" would unquestionably choose the control group. Your results would be biased before you ever started the intervention.

✓ Check Your Understanding

1. What sampling approaches are best for enhancing the external validity of the study?
2. Explain the difference between random selection of participants and random assignment of participants to groups. Which of these is a major contributor to the internal validity of a study?

LEVELS OF DATA

Before a statistical tool can be chosen to analyze a set of data, we need to know the nature of the data set because there are categories of statistical tools that are legitimate only for certain types of data. As you may recall from a course in measurement, we classify data into one of four types.

Nominal Scale

Nominal Data Nonnumerical measures labeled by name

The type of data regarded as most basic is termed **nominal data** (coming from the word *name*). These data do not have numeric value; they are identifiable only by name or label. Sorting a basket of fruit into apples, oranges, grapes, etc., and then counting the numbers of each type of fruit would be constructing a nominal data set. Generally, a study involving nominal data involves sorting the data into categories and then doing a **frequency count** of the number of data in each category. For example, a nutritional analysis might involve counting items in different food groups consumed during a meal. Within the field of **epidemiology** or the study of health issues within large populations, many studies involve frequency counts of individuals exposed versus not exposed to diseases or environmental health hazards as compared to frequency counts of individuals presenting with a disease or other pathological health condition versus those who are not presenting.

Frequency Count Summation of nominal data within categories

Epidemiology Study of health and disease status of populations

Ordinal Scale

Ordinal Data Ranked measures

Ordinal data (from the word *order*) inherently provide more information than nominal data because they are ranked. We might construct a set of ordinal data by listing, in order, the student with the top score on a research methods exam through the student with the lowest score. It is unlikely that the scores are evenly spaced, but that is irrelevant when we are dealing with ordinal data. Only the rank order is of interest. Quantitative numbers can be rank ordered, in which case, although we can see how much difference there is between the numbers, all that matters is their rank order. Small quantitative data sets are often treated as ordinal data for purposes of statistical analysis, because, being small, they are unlikely to meet the requirements for use of a statistical test on higher levels of data.

Suppose, for example, we were interested in the correlation between GRE Verbal Reasoning scores and research methods course grade averages for a graduate class of nine students. We might be looking at the following data set after it has been rank ordered by GRE Verbal Reasoning score:

GRE Verbal Reasoning Score	Course Grade Average
160	92
158	94
153	92
151	90
150	90
149	88
145	85
143	83
142	80

Chapter 11 describes a statistical tool for ordinal data sets that could be used to determine if the correlation between these two sets of scores is significant.

Interval Scale

The next step up in data precision is **interval data**, which are true numeric data with adjacent numbers being equally spaced. With interval data, however, the number zero does not mean that the quantity being measured is completely gone. Degrees of temperature are classic examples of interval data, since a temperature of neither 0°F nor 0°C translates to the absence of temperature, but only to very cold temperatures. This means that quantitative ratios using interval data cannot be constructed. A temperature of 10° is 10° colder than a temperature of 20°, but it is clearly not half as cold.

Interval Data Numerical measures of quantities for which zero does not indicate complete absence of the quantity

Ratio Scale

The highest order of data is **ratio data**, which are equally spaced numeric data measuring quantities for which there is a true zero that signifies the absolute absence of the quantity being measured. Age, height, weight, distance, and time are all examples. Legitimate ratios can be constructed with ratio data. A person aged 40 years is twice as old a person aged 20 years.

Ratio Data Numerical measures of quantities for which zero indicates complete absence of the quantity

Check Your Understanding

1. List an example of each of the four data levels other than the ones cited in this chapter.
2. Explain why ratio data are most commonly used in quantitative research.

PARAMETRIC AND NONPARAMETRIC STATISTICS

All statistical tests fall into one of two broad categories: **parametric** and **nonparametric**. In order for a parametric statistical test to be appropriate for use on a given data set, the data must be either ratio or interval in level, and additionally, the following assumptions must be met:

Parametric Category of statistical tests used for sets of interval and ratio data that meet certain assumptions related to distribution

- The variable of interest must be normally distributed within the population.
- The variable of interest must have the same variance within samples drawn from the population.
- Scores or measures for the variable of interest must be independent.

Accordingly, all nominal and ordinal data sets must be analyzed using nonparametric statistical tests. It is also the case that some small sets of ratio or interval data must be analyzed using nonparametric statistical tests because they do not meet the requisite distribution requirements for parametric tests. How can you determine if a set of ratio or interval data do or do not meet the assumptions for parametric statistical tests? These assumptions can be verified from estimates of **skewness** and

Nonparametric Category of statistical tests used for nominal and ordinal data, as well as for sets of interval and ratio data that fail to meet certain assumptions related to distribution

Skewness Term characterizing a horizontal shift in a normal curve such that the largest frequency distribution is away from the middle

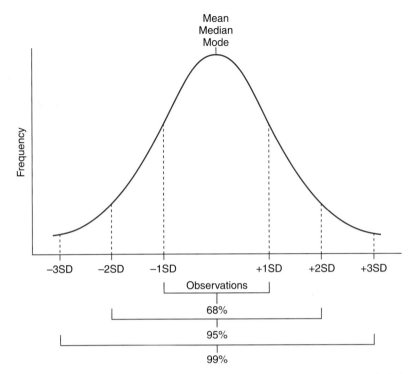

■ **FIGURE 10.2** The normal curve. Sixty-eight percent of the area under the curve is within ±1 standard deviation, 95% is within ±2 standard deviation, and 99% is within ±3 standard deviation.

Kurtosis Term characterizing a vertical shift in a normal curve such that the middle of the curve is elevated or depressed

---

Normal Curve Bell-shaped frequency plot for which the mean, median, and mode are coincident and centrally located and with 68% of the measures fall within 1 standard deviation, 95% of the measures fall within 2 standard deviations, and 99% of the scores fall within 3 standard deviations

kurtosis, which are generated by the more commonly used major statistics software packages. Skewness and kurtosis are descriptive terms applied to variations in the **normal curve,** displayed in Figure 10.2. The normal curve is a frequency plot of what is termed a perfectly normal distribution of scores. Note that the curve is bell shaped and horizontally symmetrical, and that the mean, median, and mode for the curve are all the same identical point in the center of the distribution. When the frequency of scores is normally distributed, the resulting graph yields the normal curve. The area under the normal curve includes 68% of scores within 1 standard deviation, 95% of scores within 2 standard deviations, and 99% of scores within 3 standard deviations of the mean.

Figure 10.3 shows curves that display positive and negative skewness, such that the highest frequencies of scores do not fall centrally but are shifted toward positive or negative extremes. Such a data set might be generated if we were measuring a group including a preponderance of high-skilled performers or a preponderance of low-skilled performers. Curves with a positive skewness are also termed *right skewed, right tailed,* or *skewed to the right.* Curves with a negative skewness are also termed *left skewed, left tailed,* or *skewed to the left.*

Figure 10.4 displays curves with nonnormal vertical characteristics or kurtosis. Such curves might arise when there are more or fewer "average" performers being tested. We would expect

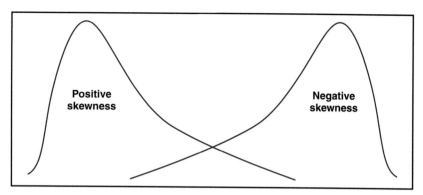

■ **FIGURE 10.3** Curves demonstrating positive skewness (with trailing end in positive direction) and negative skewness (with trailing end in negative direction).

corresponding changes in the size of the standard deviation with such curves, with a higher peak representing a larger value for the standard deviation and a flatter peak representing a smaller standard deviation.

✓ Check Your Understanding

1. Explain the conditions under which parametric statistics may be used and the conditions under which nonparametric statistics may be used.
2. Using your own words, explain how curves with positive and negative skewness and curves with accentuated and diminished kurtosis deviate from the normal curve.

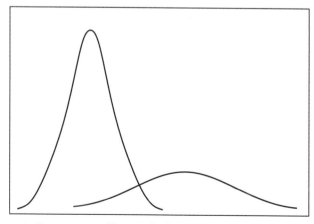

■ **FIGURE 10.4** Curves demonstrating accentuated kurtosis (high peak) and diminished kurtosis (shallow peak).

CHAPTER SUMMARY

- Statistics are a set of tools that can be used for objectively analyzing data.
- Globally speaking, statistics are used for two main purposes: description of a sample (a subset of a population) and inference or generalizing measures from the sample to the population.
- Statistical tests determine whether a null hypothesis or directional hypothesis is accepted or rejected at a particular level of significance, which is usually set at $\alpha = 0.05$ for research in kinesiology and the health sciences.
- Type I and II errors result when the null hypothesis is erroneously rejected or accepted, respectively. Increasing statistical power reduces the likelihood of type I and II errors.
- Determining appropriate sample size for a study enables conservation of resources and provides the level of power needed for a given study.
- The choice of a parametric or nonparametric statistical tool is based on the level of data (nominal, ordinal, interval, or ratio) as well as on whether the data set meets the assumptions upon which parametric statistics are based.

REFERENCES

1. Kadam P, Bhaleraol S. Sample size calculation. *Int J Ayurveda Res* 2010;1:55–57.

2. G*Power: http://www.softpedia.com/get/Science-CAD/G-Power.shtml

RELATED ASSIGNMENTS

1. **Explain the use of statistics for inference.**
2. **Select a published research paper on a topic of interest, and identify the α level and the p values for all statistical tests. Explain why the results of each statistical test were significant or nonsignificant. Discuss how the results of the statistical tests affect the conclusions from the study.**
3. **How does statistical power influence the likelihood of type I and II errors?**
4. **Determine the mean, median, mode, range, standard deviation, and standard error of the mean for the following scores on a research methods exam:**

81	85	79	63	91	88	77	72	85	83	93	84
76	85	72	71	94	81	80	79	89	90	87	86

5. **Explain what determines the selection of a parametric versus a nonparametric statistical test.**
6. **Explain the key features of the normal curve.**

IN-CLASS GROUP EXERCISES

Directions: Perform each of the following exercises working within your group:
1. **Flip a coin 10 times, and record the number of heads. Assuming that your null hypothesis is that there will be no difference in the number of heads and tails and your alpha level is 0.05, do the following:**
   a. Explain whether your results support or fail to support the null hypothesis.
   b. Construct a truth table that displays your results.
   c. Do your results represent a type I or a type II error? (Explain.)

2. Construct a table that lists the advantages and limitations of random, stratified random, systematic, and convenience sampling.

3. Design a study that will involve collection of nominal data. Write a null hypothesis and research hypothesis for the study. Will this study require use of parametric or nonparametric statistics? Repeat this exercise for ordinal, interval, and ratio data.

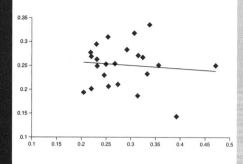

11

Finding Relationships among Variables

The object of statistical science is to discover methods of condensing information concerning large groups of allied facts into brief and compendious expressions suitable for discussion
—*Sir Francis Galton (1822–1911).*

CHAPTER OBJECTIVES

After studying this chapter, you will be able to:
1. Explain the concept of correlation.
2. Discuss the difference between positive and negative relationships.
3. Interpret both the significance and meaningfulness of an *r* value.
4. Differentiate between correlation and regression.
5. Describe multiple correlation techniques.

■ WHEN examining the world around us, we often notice relationships. Some relationships are easy to detect: "If I stay up studying past 3:00 AM, I won't make it to my 8:00 AM class," or "The more dormitory food I eat, the more weight I gain." Others may be weaker or more subtle, or not directly observable. Within the health sciences, the fact that relationships exist between and among different parameters has helped practitioners and scientists alike better understand factors that impact human health. Of course, many individuals may detect relationships, and therefore, we need a way in which to quantitatively assess their strength as well as their meaningfulness in an objective way. The study of relationships is termed correlation analysis. We briefly discussed correlation research in Chapter 7. Once relationships are established, this information can be used to predict future outcomes based on the initial values of the variables (e.g., predicting body composition from different skinfold sites). This is called regression analysis. In this chapter, we will cover the ways in which you can statistically measure relationships.

UNDERSTANDING CORRELATION

The key to understanding **correlation**, which is a statistical technique, is to remember the word at its foundation: relation. Correlation is all about finding out how two or more entities *relate* to each other. That is, is there some sort of connection among the entities? Inherent in the definition is the notion of coexisting change. If entities are correlated, they change together in a predictable fashion. Typically, in research, we call these entities "variables," which broadly defined means of measurable factors (e.g., strength, IQ, body composition) that are subject to change. So, correlation is an objective measure of how variables change together or of the relationship between two or more variables. Remember we stated in Chapter 7 that correlation does not imply causation. This means that even if we

Correlation A measure of the relationship among two or more variables

SPECIAL INTEREST BOX 11.1

Selecting appropriate variables is essential for correlational analysis—as a researcher, you must attempt to select the most representative variables. Consider the following example. Imagine you decide to investigate the phenomenon of the "Freshman 15," which refers to the hypothetical 15 lb that college students gain in their first year away at school. You begin with a hypothesized relationship "the more dorm food you eat, the more weight you gain." Sounds reasonable! As we described in chapter 10, you need to define and operationalize your variables. In this case, you need to find a measure of dorm food that can be quantified.

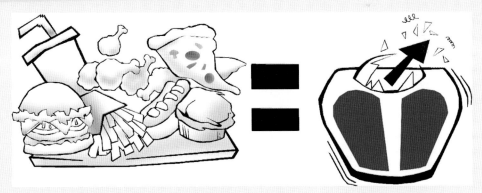

This is not as easy as it seems—you could pick "number of meals per week," which is not so precise, but measurable; "volume of food," which would be difficult to measure, but may be more precise; or "number of calories in consumed dorm food," which is probably the most accurate measure, but is directly related to the amount of food you put on your plate at each meal, so will change from one person's scoop of mashed potatoes to the next. Whew! This is harder than you thought, and you haven't even gotten to the measure of "weight" yet! In reality, the anecdotal observation that increased consumption of dormitory food leads to increased weight gain is a relationship that is not easily measured.

find a correlation between two variables, we cannot say that one causes the other. Let's look at cigarette smoking and lung cancer; research has shown a correlation between the two such that they both increase (change) together. As tempting as it is to say "increased smoking causes increased lung cancer," we cannot make that statement based on correlational analysis. We can only say that "increased smoking is associated with increased chance of developing lung cancer." The following example may be even clearer. A strong correlation exists between height and weight during childhood. However, height changes do not cause weight changes (or vice versa); these change as a function of normal growth and development. Other types of experimental designs and statistical analyses are required to establish causation (see Chapters 12 and 13).

✔ Check Your Understanding

1. When performing correlational analyses, what are researchers attempting to determine?
2. If a researcher finds that two variables are correlated, what conclusions can and cannot be made?
3. Why is the selection of appropriate variables so critical for correlation?

SIMPLE CORRELATION

Correlational analysis in its most basic form involves quantifying the relationship between two variables.[1,2] Exercise physiologists might look at the relationship between intensity of training and VO_2max. Biomechanists might look how changes in lower extremity contact joint forces are related to changes in gait kinematics. Researchers in sports medicine might investigate the relationship between ultrasound frequency and recovery time. Across the health sciences, researchers examine all sorts of relationships between variables. The statistical measure or value of that relationship is called the coefficient of correlation, which is a number between −1.0 and +1.0, with 0 indicating no relationship and ± 1 indicating a perfect correlation. The positive or negative sign indicates the direction of the relationship, as we explain below.

Positive Correlation

Positive Correlation A correlation where one variable increases as the other variable increases

In a positive correlation, the scatter plot runs from bottom left to top right

When two variables have a **positive correlation**, they are increasing or decreasing together. Look at Figure 11.1A for an example of a positive correlation. The scatter in a positive correlation will visually look like it is going from bottom left to top right, as this one does. If the first variable has a small value, then the second variable will have a small value as well. Alternatively, if the first value is large, the second value is also large. Each participant has one pair of values (variable 1 and 2), and these are plotted along an X–Y or scatter plot graph (we first presented this idea in Chapter 7). For example, you might have an interest in the relationship between cardiovascular fitness, using VO_2max as measure, and the distance traveled in a 6-minute run. You test 25 individuals of varying fitness levels, test their VO_{2max}, and then time them on the 1-mile run. Figure 11.1A shows this hypothetical scatter graph for this relationship. This relationship makes intuitive sense, since you would expect that people who have higher levels of fitness can generally run farther in 6 minutes than those with lower levels.

Negative Correlation

Negative Correlation A correlation where as one variable increases as the other variable decreases

In Figure 11.1B, a **negative correlation** is shown. Notice that the points tend to move from the top left to the bottom right. Negative correlation indicates

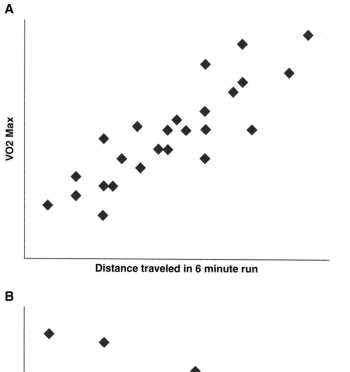

Distance traveled in 6 minute run

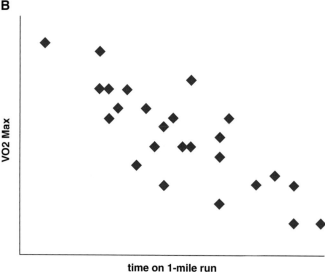

time on 1-mile run

■ **FIGURE 11.1 A,B.** Positive and negative correlations. Note that on the scatter plot, a positive correlation **(A)** starts at the bottom left and moves to the top right. A negative correlation **(B)** starts at the top left and moves to the bottom right.

that small values of one variable are associated with large values of the other variable, just the opposite of positive correlation. In other words, as values of X increase, values of Y tend to decrease on the scatter graph. For example, if you were to plot cardiovascular fitness as measured by VO_2max against time on a 1-mile run, you would most likely find a scatter graph similar to that presented in Figure 11.1B.

Strength of Correlation

As we said, correlation values can run from 0 to +1.0. This value provides an indication of the strength of the relationship. The closer the number is to either 1.0 or −1.0, the stronger the association is

TABLE 11.1   Data from an Undergraduate Research Methods Class Including Left and Right Grip Force, Grade Point Average (GPA), and Mass in Kilograms

Grip Force (left)	Grip Force (right)	GPA	Mass (kg)
250	240	3.21	57
350	310	3.14	77
340	320	2.89	57
300	280	3.90	59
350	250	2.98	64
370	300	2.86	66
310	320	3.65	52
320	270	3.12	56
350	410	3.50	56
400	380	2.01	71
780	840	2.77	68
650	600	3.48	84
380	370	3.24	68
370	270	3.29	57
470	480	3.47	77
900	900	3.30	89
620	550	2.56	102

between the variables. Here is an experiment you can try within your own class to demonstrate strength of correlation. In Table 11.1, we have provided data from one of our research methods classes, where the students measured their grip strength on a hand dynamometer and compared their left and right hand grip strengths. After we calculated the correlation coefficient, we determined there was a positive relationship between left and right grip strength of $r = 0.97$ (see Fig. 11.2A). In a positive correlation, the strength of the relationship is indicated by the proximity of r to 0.0 or 1.0. In this case, 0.97 is very close to 1.0, so the association between right and left grip strength is strong. In general, we don't expect to see relationships that are 1.0, which would indicate a perfect correlation, because some variability exists in almost all human characteristics.

For the same group of students in Table 11.1, we also took their mass in kilograms and their grade point average. We will use these to demonstrate what different values of r look like on a graph. In Figure 11.2B, left grip force and body mass are graphed. As you can see, the relationship is still positive, but it is not as strong. In fact, the r value is 0.71. Just below this in Figure 11.2C, right grip force and GPA are graphed and correlated, with a resultant r value of 0.125. All three of these relationships are positive correlations, meaning that small scores on one are associated with small scores on the other variable. However, as you might have suspected, the association between grip strength and GPA is much weaker than between the other two. This should be of no surprise, since students are not admitted to college based on how forcefully they can grip a dynamometer!

The farther a correlation is from 0.0, the stronger it is (up to 1.0).

It is important to keep in mind that a positive or negative sign has nothing to do with relationship strength; it merely indicates if the variables increase in the same or opposite directions. So, an r value of -0.87 indicates a stronger relationship than an r value of 0.75 because 0.87 is farther away from 0.0 than 0.75 is.

Check Your Understanding

1. Describe the relationship between variables in a positive correlation.
2. Describe the relationship between variables in a negative correlation.
3. Which relationship is stronger: -0.75 or 0.72? Explain your decision.

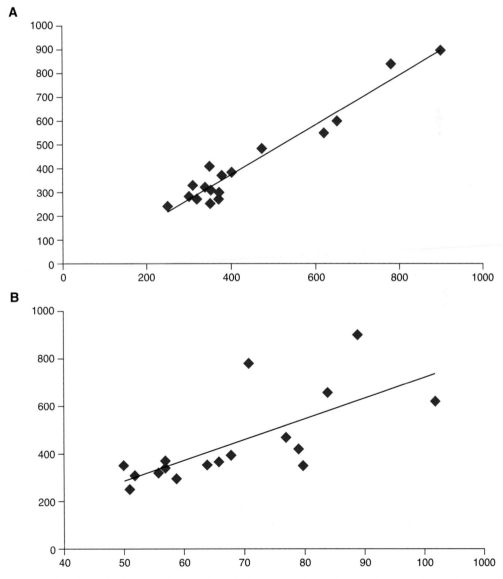

■ **FIGURE 11.2** The relationship between right and left grip force **(A)** is strong at $r = 0.97$. The relationship between left grip force and body mass **(B)** is moderate at $r = 0.71$. The relationship between right grip force and grade point average

C

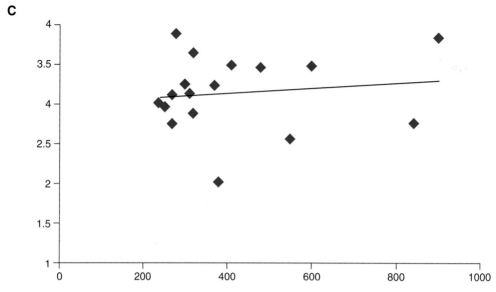

Calculating *r*

Pearson's r Pearson's Product Moment correlation, the parametric statistical test for strength of relationship between two variables

Although it is possible to calculate Pearson's r by hand, it is much quicker to use a spreadsheet.

We have used the letter *r* to indicate correlation values. This comes from a statistical test used to calculate correlation values, which is called the Pearson's Product-Moment Correlation Coefficient, or **Pearson's** *r*. Pearson's *r* allows us to quantify the relationship we can visually see in the X–Y plots. As you may suspect, *r* is a valuable statistic! In fact, the notion of *r* was developed around 1800s by Sir Francis Galton (see opening quotation) and, at the turn of the century, mathematically formalized by Karl Pearson,[3] who is considered by many to be the father of statistics.[4] The formula for calculating *r* is as follows:

$$r = \frac{\sum_{i=1}^{n} (X_i - \bar{X})(Y_i - \bar{Y})}{\sqrt{\sum_{i=1}^{n} (X_i - \bar{X})^2} \sqrt{\sum_{i=1}^{n} (Y_i - \bar{Y})^2}}$$

Equation 11.1

We are sure you look at that and think "oh, no!" and really, we don't blame you! So we will use a data set to demonstrate how to use this formula. We will use the data in Table 11.2, which includes the first 10 data points from Table 11.1. This table shows you the step-by-step process for calculating *r*, through summing, squaring, and cross multiplying the numbers. You can insert these numbers into Equation 11.1 if you want to calculate r. Of course, a quicker way of calculating Pearson's *r* is to use a spreadsheet such as Excel. Special Interest Box 11.2 provides you with the steps you need to calculate *r* using Excel.

TABLE 11.2	Calculating Pearson's *r* between Left and Right Grip Strength				
	Left Grip Strength	**Right Grip Strength**			
Participant	X	Y	X²	Y²	X–Y
1	250	240	62,500	57,600	60,000
2	350	310	122,500	96,100	108,500
3	340	320	115,600	102,400	108,800
4	300	280	90,000	78,400	84,000
5	350	250	122,500	62,500	87,500
6	370	300	136,900	90,000	111,000
7	310	320	96,100	102,400	99,200
8	320	270	102,400	72,900	86,400
9	350	410	122,500	168,100	143,500
10	400	380	176,400	144,400	159,600
N = 10	ΣX = 3,340	ΣY = 3,080	ΣX² = 1,131,000	974,800	1,040,900

Interpreting *r*

Of course, once you have calculated *r*, you need to figure out what it means! We have alluded to some of the ways you can interpret Pearson's *r*. As we said in Chapter 10, statistics allows us to provide an objective interpretation of a series of observations. In terms of correlation, we want to be able to reject the null hypothesis that states no relationship exists between a pair of variables. This indicates that, within a level of confidence, a significant relationship exists. Most researchers use the term *significant* sparingly outside of statistics so that they are not misinterpreted as meaning something is statistically significant when, in fact, statistics haven't been used. So, you can be fairly sure that if you read something is significant, the authors refer to statistical significance. Once we determine a relationship is significant, we need to know if it is positive or negative. Finally, we want to know how strong that relationship is; how tightly are the variables associated? Note that the first step is always determining significance; if a Pearson's *r* is not significant, there is no point in determining direction or strength of association. This is a logical but sometimes overlooked point.

DETERMINING SIGNIFICANCE OF *R*

In the case of correlation, the term "significant" means that the *r* value is significantly different than zero. What does that mean? We interpret this to mean that a real relationship exists between the variables, and we can most likely rule out error or chance as the reason for the *r* value. Just because a researcher discovers *r* = 0.70, which seems far away from 0.0, it does not mean that the researcher can conclude significance. The researcher must compare the *r* value obtained (called r_{actual}) with a critical cutoff value of *r* (called $r_{critical}$). $r_{critical}$ is not a constant number; it changes based on the number of participants in a study as well as the alpha level chosen before the study begins. From these numbers, you can calculate a critical value of *r* ($r_{critical}$), which is the cutoff value for determining significance. If your value is greater than the critical value ($r_{actual} \geq r_{critical}$), then you can reject the null hypothesis that *r* = 0.0, and you can say the relationship is significant.[5] For many students, the previous procedure of calculating $r_{critical}$ is unnecessary, since computer software will provide the critical *r* value as well as the

r_{actual} Pearson *r* calculated from the data set

$r_{critical}$ The significance cut-off value of *r*; only values greater that this are significant

If the p value is less than alpha (often 0.05), then the Pearson's r is significant.

SPECIAL INTEREST BOX 11.2

Calculating *r* Using an Excel Spreadsheet

Calculating Pearson's *r* using Excel is a straightforward task. We will assume you have already generated X and Y data on two variables of interest (we will use the 10 values of left and right grip strength from Table 11.1 above).

1. After opening Excel, label column 1 as the X variable and column 2 as the Y variable. Place each participant's data in these columns.

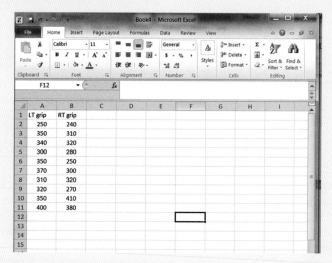

2. Next, go to the tab marked "data analysis" and click on it. From the list, choose "correlation." A drop-down box appears.

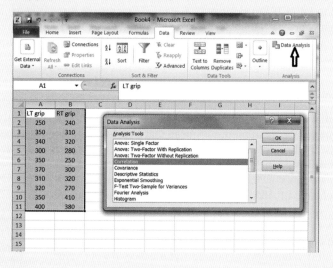

SPECIAL INTEREST BOX 11.2 (*Continued*)

3. From the drop-down box, pick "correlation." Another drop-down box appears. First, select your input range by dragging over your two columns of data. If your labels are in the first row, be sure to click on "Labels in first row."

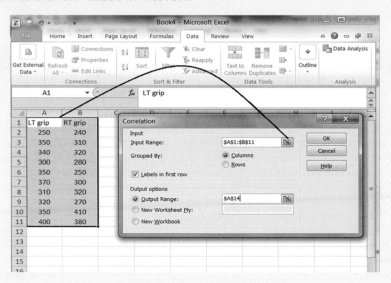

4. Finally, pick where you want your data to go by selecting from the output options list. In our example, the correlation analysis will go just below the data. Click "ok". Your correlation coefficient will appear in your output block.

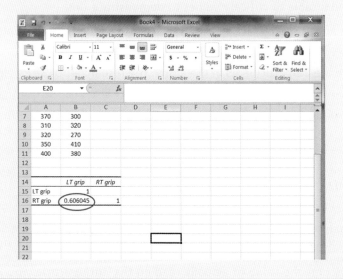

If r_{actual} is greater than $r_{critical}$, then the Pearson's r is significant.

p value (i.e., the real probability of a type I error) without having to consult a table. If the p value is less that the alpha level (generally set at 0.05), then the results are significant. However, it is important to understand how participant number and alpha interact to change $r_{critical}$ (see Special Interest Box 11.3).

SPECIAL INTEREST BOX 11.3

When Is r = 0.70 Significant? You Can't Judge an r by Its Value!

The number of participants within a study, along with the alpha level selected by a researcher, can impact the determination of significance in a big way. In other words, just an r value by itself does not provide enough information to judge significance. The following example should illustrate this point. Imagine that you want to write a paper about different types of knee rehabilitation for ACL injuries. You uncover an abstract on a new protocol that looks promising. The researcher examined the relationship between number of times per week participants received the new protocol and score on a balance test. The researcher found r = 0.70 and was excited to report that with more sessions of training using his new protocol each week, the ACL patients improved their balance! You dig deeper and discover that all rs of 0.70 are not created equal. In fact, the researcher's findings were not even significant. How could that be?

Remember that statistical significance is not determined simply by how far an r is away from 0.0. Researchers must also consider the sample size and the alpha level that the researcher set before starting the study. Without these two values, you have no means by which to assess statistical significance. Furthermore, as these numbers change, so does the interpretation of the r value calculated by the researcher, because these change the $r_{critical}$ value (see Table 11.3). We have included a table of critical r values to demonstrate this.

Scenario I. There are 12 participants in the study. The researcher picks an alpha level of 0.05:

   $r_{critical}$ = 0.576 → Decision: 0.576 < 0.70; reject the null, r is significant.

Scenario II. There are 12 participants in the study. The researcher picks an alpha level of 0.01:

   $r_{critical}$ = 0.708 → Decision: 0.708 > 0.70; Do NOT reject the null; r is not significant.

Scenario III. There are 12 participants in the study (N = 12; df = 10). The researcher picks an alpha level of:

   $r_{critical}$ = 0.658 → Decision: 0.658 < 0.70; Reject the null; r is significant.

Scenario IV. There are 10 participants in the study (N = 10; df = 8). The researcher picks an alpha level of 0.02:

   $r_{critical}$ = 0.716 → Decision: 0.716 > 0.70; Do NOT reject the null; r is not significant.

In the research paper's abstract, the researcher indicated that there were 10 participants in the study, but failed to mention the alpha level set for the study and did not indicate if the test was significant or not. Therefore, you cannot conclude that the r value of 0.70 is significant! This underscores the value of actually reading the entire article. You may believe that researchers may not make such mistakes, but as reviewers and editors, we have both seen manuscripts where the researcher provides only an r value without other, important information; these manuscripts tend to get rejected.

TABLE 11.3   Critical Values of *r* for Different Sample Sizes and Alpha Levels

# of Participants	Level of Significance (Alpha)			
	0.10	0.05	0.02	0.01
...				
8	0.622	0.707	0.789	0.834
9	0.582	0.666	0.750	0.798
10	0.549	0.632	716 IV	0.765
11	0.521	0.602	0.685	0.735
12	0.497	.576 I	.658 III	.708 II

✓ Check Your Understanding

1. What is $r_{critical}$ if df = 15 and alpha = 0.01?
2. What does it mean if a researcher determines that *r* is significant?

HOW MEANINGFUL IS THE RELATIONSHIP?

As you looked over the critical values in Table 11.3, you might have noticed that with more than 10 degrees of freedom (or 12 participants), and the values seem to drop off rather quickly. In fact, if you have 22 participants in your study, even with the smallest alpha level (0.005), you would need an *r* value of only 0.55 to be significant. Furthermore, if you used an *r* value of 0.05, which is a far more commonly accepted value, you would only need an *r* value of 0.361 to reach significance. Surely, all significant *r*s are not the same. The *r* value, in and of itself, tells us that an association exists between the variables; it doesn't indicate how strong that relationship is. This is why we also examine the strength of the association.

The critical value of r can change based on the sample size as well as the alpha level.

Coefficient of Determination r^2, which measures the strength of a significant relationship

Fortunately, there is an easily calculated statistic that allows us to interpret the strength of a significant relationship, called the **coefficient of determination**. The symbol for the coefficient of determination is r^2, and that is exactly how you calculate it—by squaring the *r* value. So, if you have an $r = 0.70$, then $r^2 = 0.49$. This measures the amount of shared or common variance by the two variables. You can also report it as a percentage of shared variance by multiplying r^2 by 100. The notion of shared or common variance is an indication of how much of the change in one variable can be explained by a change in the other. If two variables are tightly related, they tend to change together. Think back to our hand grip example: With an *r* of 0.97, r^2 will equal 0.94. This means the shared or common variance is 94%; in other words, right and left grip force vary together 94% of the time. This should not be too surprising, since most people are more similar than different between left and right hands.

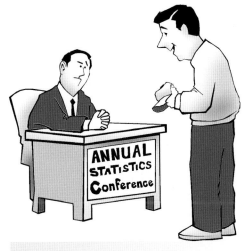

"I'm looking for a meaningful relationship!"

There are no hard and fast rules for interpreting the meaning of r^2; just keep in mind that the larger the value is, the more variance the variables have in common.

If there is 94% common variance between the left and right grip force, what does the remaining 6% mean? This is called unexplained or error variance. The statistical terms "unexplained" and "error" may be a little misleading. In this context, unexplained means that it is the variance unaccounted for by the two variables. In fact, researchers often try to explain that variance, looking for other variables that account for the differences in one variable or the other. In our example, hand dominance or handedness may account for some of unexplained variance.

RULES OF THUMB FOR INTERPRETATION OF r and r^2

In the earlier chapters, we talked about reviewing previous research as a way to understand what is known and unknown within a particular area. If there is a lot of research published within an area, you may be looking for quicker ways to read and summarize the information you obtain from a given paper. To this end, we wanted to provide you with general rules of thumb for evaluating r and r^2. In all cases, you must carefully read the entire journal article first; nothing replaces this! However, if there is no indication of the significance of r, or the authors don't interpret their r^2 values, you can still generally interpret their results using Table 11.4.

As we said, this rule of thumb chart doesn't take the place of thoughtful reading of a paper, nor should it be used alone to judge the merit of an article. At the same time, it gives you a quick look at what these values mean in general, so that if you see an r value of 0.4, you suspect the relationship is only moderate, and if the author of that paper makes magnificent claims of relationship based on $r = 0.40$, you might question the interpretation of those results!

One last reminder about interpreting r values, and that is that the sign (positive or negative) just signifies the direction of change between the two variables. Many students often misinterpret a negative value to mean less of a correlation. However, a -0.50 and a $+0.50$ signify the exact same strength of relationship.

TABLE 11.4 Rules of Thumb for Interpreting r and r^2		
r	r^2	Interpretation
0.8 and above	0.64 and above	Very strong
0.6–0.8	0.36–0.64	Strong
0.4–0.6	0.16–0.36	Moderate
0.2–0.4	0.04–0.16	Weak
0.0–0.2	Below 0.04	Very weak

✔ Check Your Understanding

1. How is r^2 interpreted differently from r?
2. What does the coefficient of determination mean?
3. Can a relationship between two variables be significant but not meaningful?

CORRELATION MATRICES

Unexplained or error variance is the variance unaccounted for by the two correlated variables.

More often than not, researchers measure several variables and perform more than one correlation within their study. Performing such analyses is relatively simple using current software programs such as Microsoft Excel

TABLE 11.5 Correlation Matrix for Data in Table 11.1

	GPA	Mass (kg)	L Grip Force	R Grip Force
GPA	1			
Mass (kg)	−0.09	1		
L grip force	0.03	0.71[a]	1	
R grip force	0.07	0.61[a]	0.97[a]	1

[a]Indicates significance at the 0.05 level.

and IBM SPSS and their output is placed into a **correlation matrix**. This matrix organizes the correlations in an orderly way so you can easily read and interpret the information. Each number within the matrix is a distinct r value derived through the formulas we have already presented. We will use our previous example from Figure 11.1 and place this information into a correlation matrix for an example (Table 11.5). Where each column and row intersect, there is a value for that specific correlation. So, if you read across row 1 (left grip strength) to column 2 (right grip strength), you will see the r value of 0.97. The next value in that row is r = 0.71, which is the correlation between left grip strength and mass. Generally, you will see the significant values labeled with an asterisk or star, with p value listed below the matrix. Notice that no values are provided when a variable is plotted against itself (since this is always 1.0 and, really, that doesn't tell us anything). Further, only one set of values are given, and only ½ of the matrix is filled. Note that a star next to a value indicates that it is significant.

Correlation Matrix An efficient manner of reporting Pearson's *r* when three or more variables are being compared

Check Your Understanding

1. Is as r in a correlation matrix interpreted differently from an r between two variables?
2. What does the "1" in a correlation matrix represent?

REGRESSION

When there is a significant, strong correlation, you know that as one variable changes, so does the other variable. That provides a powerful tool for predicting the value of one variable from the corresponding value of the other variable. The statistical tool used for this is called linear **regression**.[2] If you have taken exercise physiology, you may have encountered regression when calculating percentage of body fat using skin fold calipers to measure three or four skinfold sites around the body (e.g., triceps or superior iliac crest). These values are placed into a regression equation to predict overall percentage of body fat. The most basic form of regression is simple, linear regression, where one variable is predicted from another variable to which it is correlated. This is represented by a straight line on the scatter plot (see Fig. 11.2A–C). The equation used for simple linear regression is

Regression A statistical method for predicting one variable based on the value of another variable

When interpreting r, a positive or negative sign refers to the direction of the correlation, not its value

$$Y = a + bX \qquad \text{Equation 11.2}$$

where Y is the value of the variable to be predicted; a is the y intercept; b is the slope of the regression line, which represents the rate of change of Y for each unit change of X; and X is the value of variable that has already been measured. Below, we have the regression line for the relationship between left and right grip strength. The equation is

$$\text{Left grip force} = -53 + 1.06\left(\text{Right grip force}\right)$$

What is a regression line, exactly? This line represents line of best fit for all the X–Y coordinates on the graph (a straight line that most closely represents the correlation between the variables), which is where the X and Y means intersect. The closer the correlation is to ± 1.0, the tighter the fit of the line is to the points on the scatter plot. So, the regression line is generated from the means of the X and Y values, and it is this line from which the regression equation comes.

Regression equations allow you to predict the value of one variable from the corresponding value of another variable, based on an analysis of how these variables correlate in prior research. Such equations can be useful when exact values are difficult (predicting percentage body fat from skinfold sites) or impossible to obtain (e.g., predicting future performance in academics based on scores on placement tests). At the same time, it is always important to remember that the regression equation is only as good as the correlation from which it comes. If a weak correlation exists between two variables, then predicting one based on the other will not yield meaningful results. Unless a perfect relationship exists, then the actual Y values differ from the estimated Y values, and the differences between estimated and actual Y values are called residuals. Residuals represent the error in the prediction equation. One way to determine the accuracy of a regression line is to calculate the standard error of estimate, which provides a measure of the amount of error in a regression equation and is the standard deviation of the residual scores. The smaller the standard error of estimate is, the more accurate the regression equation is at predicting Y values.

Multiple Regression

Although some estimated variables may be predicted well through the use of one predictor variable, more often, the prediction can improve through the use of two or more predictor variables. For example, a researcher may be interested in predicting how far a young child can throw a baseball and has previously determined that a positive correlation of 0.60 exists between distance thrown and strength. With an r^2 of 0.36, this means 67% of the change in throwing distance is not accounted for by change in strength. If the researcher used "strength" as the only predictor, the resultant equation would have large error variance. However, if the researcher added other predictors such arm velocity, pelvic rotation, and step length, the resultant equation could more accurately predict throwing distance. Not only does this make statistical sense (use more predictor variables to explain the "error"), it makes intuitive sense—proficient throwers are more than athletes with strong arms; they have to have proper technique as well.

If a correlation is weak, a regression equation will not provide accurate predictions.

The type of equation that you might see for a multiple regression equation would look similar to that of a simple regression, except more predictor variables would be included. A multiple regression equation with three predictors would look like this:

$$Y = a + b_1 X_1 + b_2 X_2 + b_3 X_3 \qquad \text{Equation 11.3}$$

where Y is the dependent variable to be predicted, X_{1-3} are the predictor variables, and a and b are constants. More bX components are added for each additional predictor variable. It may be tempting to add many different predictors in order to get the best possible fit; however, there are often only several primary predictors after which variables add little to the equation. Through a multiple correlation analysis, the resultant correlation coefficient of all the variables, R, can be calculated.

Check Your Understanding

1. How is correlation used within regression?
2. What does a regression equation based on a nonsignificant correlation tell us?
3. What is a multiple correlation coefficient, R, and how does it relate to multiple regression analysis?

CHAPTER SUMMARY

- Correlation refers to relationships in variables.
- In simple correlation, the relationship exists between two variables. This is represented by an r value ranging from -1.0 to $+1.0$.
- If small values of one variable are associated with small values of the other variable, and large values in one are associated with large values in the other, the relationship is positive.
- If small values in one variable are associated with large values in the other and large values in the first are associated with small values in the second, the relationship is negative.
- The fact that a relationship is either positive or negative is not related to the strength of the relationship.
- You can estimate the strength of the relationship based on the distance between the r value and 0.0. The farther the number is from 0.0 (which signifies no relationship), the stronger the correlation is.
- The most common correlation statistic used is Pearson's r.
- The significance of Pearson's r is by comparing $r_{critical}$ (determined using degrees of freedom, and level of significance.) to the calculated r. If r calculated is greater than $r_{critical}$, it is significant. This means there is a real relationship between the variables.
- The strength of the relationship is determined by calculation the coefficient of determination (r^2).
- Simple linear regression uses correlation to predict the value of one variable from the corresponding value of another, measured variable.

REFERENCES

1. Vincent WJ, Weir JP. *Statistics in Kinesiology*, 4th ed. Champaign, IL: Human Kinetics, 2012:106–111.
2. Field AP. *Discovering Statistics using SPSS*, 4th ed. Washington, DC: Sage, 2013:12.
3. Porter TM. *Karl Pearson: the Scientific Life in a Statistical Age*. Princeton, NJ: Princeton University Press, 2004.
4. Norton BJ. Karl Pearson and statistics: The social origins of scientific innovation. *Soc Stud Sci* 1978;8(3):3–34.
5. Chung, MK. Correlation Coefficient. In Salkind NJ, Rasmussen K, eds. *The Encyclopedia of Measurement & Statistics*, 2nd ed. Thousand Oaks, CA: Sage Publications, 2007.

RELATED ASSIGNMENTS

1. **You want to determine if there is a relationship between mental status after concussion (as assessed by the Standardized Assessment of Concussion [SAC]) and balance (as measured by the Balance Error Scoring System [BESS]).**

   Is balance related to postconcussion mental status? Draw scatter plot.

Athlete	SAC	BESS
John	27	12
Sarah	29	15

Thomas	21	19
Janet	23	16
Jim	26	18
Phillip	25	12
Jen	22	17
Allan	23	14

a. What are the important variables that you need to know in order to establish SIGNIFICANCE?

$N =$		$r_{critical} =$	
$df =$		$r_{actual} =$	
$\alpha =$			

b. What is your decision? How do you interpret the data?
c. What is the MEANINGFULNESS? Calculate and *discuss* the coefficient of determination.
d. Can you predict BESS from SAC? Why or why not?

2. A researcher noted that older women have a tendency to fall frequently and wanted to study why this might be. He wanted to look at the relationships among two psychological factors and two physical parameters and the number of falls experienced by these women. He tested 18 women over the age of 65 who had experienced falls in the past 6 months on two psychological variables and two physical parameters and counted the number of times they fell down. Psychological: *perceived physical competence* (PPC), *fear of falling* (FOF; 1 = low, 10 = high). Physical: *balance, quadriceps strength* (1 = low, 10 = high). He got the following results:

# Falls	PPC	FOF	Balance	Strength
4	3	4	9	3
6	8	6	5	6
2	5	4	8	7
12	9	10	1	2
8	6	10	3	9
2	2	4	2	3
1	6	3	7	4
5	7	9	6	8
6	6	6	7	7
2	4	3	9	9
3	1	2	7	3
7	10	8	3	4
4	2	5	4	1
3	5	4	2	9
2	3	1	4	2
4	4	5	10	4
13	9	10	2	6
2	1	3	5	8

a. Using Excel, create a correlation matrix. Next, determine your $r_{critical}$. What are your decisions about the actual r values? Star the significant r values.

b. Interpret the meaningfulness of the significant results.

c. What variable appears to be most highly related to number of falls? Describe the relationship in words.

IN-CLASS GROUP EXERCISES

1. **For this exercise, you will need a scale and a tape measure. Randomly divide the class into groups of no more than 10 students. In all groups, you will measure each person's mass, height, and maximum vertical jump height. Also, for each student, determine the total number of hours each week spent in physical activity (each group should agree on an operational definition).**

    a. Create a spreadsheet in Excel with 4 columns of data. Calculate a correlation matrix for your data. For the two values that are most highly correlated, create a regression equation (your instructor can help you with this), so that you predict one variable (Y) from one other (X).

    b. Join with 1 other group. Calculate their predicted Y variables using their X variables and your regression equation.

    c. Write a brief report answering the following questions:
       - What (if any) were the significant correlations? Why do you think they are significant?
       - How meaningful were the significant correlations?
       - How well did your regression equation predict their Y variable?
       - Explain why your predictions were close (or not) to the actual values.

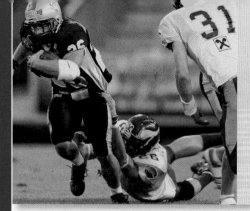

12

Finding Differences among Groups

"There are basically two types of people. People who accomplish things, and people who claim to have accomplished things. The first group is less crowded."—Mark Twain

CHAPTER OBJECTIVES

After studying this chapter, you will be able to:

1. Explain the steps in the process of hypothesis testing.
2. Select appropriate alpha levels and explain your selection.
3. Describe and perform a Student's *t* test.
4. Interpret significance and meaningfulness of an independent *t* test.
5. Compare and contrast different *t* tests.
6. Explain when to use a one-way, two-way, or repeated measures ANOVA.
7. Discuss the purpose of post hoc testing.
8. Describe situations when researchers use ANCOVA.

■ To this point in the book, you've learned to use statistics to describe data as well as to uncover relationships among variables. However, researchers often experiment to see if they can cause some sort of change and, therefore, use a different type of statistics to uncover differences among groups. We have alluded to the fact that different types of statistics can actually help evaluate cause and effect relationships, and in this chapter, we will discuss inferential statistics, which we introduced in Chapter 10. The word *inferential* is used because researchers sample from the population of interest (i.e., test a randomly selected 15 children with cerebral palsy (CP) and then infer that the results of the study hold for the population of interest (all children with CP). Researchers use true experimental designs (see Chapter 6) and pair them with appropriate inferential statistics as part of the process of establishing cause–effect relationships. This is an important part of the process of developing evidence-based practice, as researchers can show statistically that treatments affect patients' outcomes.

HYPOTHESIS TESTING

Hypothesis testing is a process by which investigators move from hypothesis to inference. Most researchers who use inferential statistics follow a specific procedure of hypothesis testing as an objective way to show differences among groups. The process involves creating hypotheses, setting probability levels, calculating critical statistical levels, performing the statistical analysis, and then making a decision about group differences by comparing critical to calculated statistical values.[1] Researchers often perform experiments in order to test or confirm whether a treatment has an effect on the population under study. In other words, researchers want to see if specific dexterity training helps improve hand function in stroke patients, if the drug REGN727 decreases serum cholesterol for individuals with atherosclerosis, or if a group of athletes receiving specialized cognitive treatment after concussions improves more quickly than a group that does not. They will use hypothesis testing as a way to confirm their hypothesis that a treatment works or clarify that a treatment has no effect.

Imagine that a researcher has developed a novel rehabilitation training protocol for stroke patients to use at home in between physical therapy visits. Patients take home a 45-minute instructional DVD that takes them through exercises that help with balance and gait control. Before the study began, the researcher conducted pilot testing to look at the relationship between hours spent in the novel training with scores on a balance test for 20 patients and found a positive correlation of 0.68. Encouraged by early results, the researcher wanted some solid evidence that the protocol improves balance over a 10-week period and followed up with an experiment that compares a treatment group that receives the novel protocol with a control group that does not receive any special training. What must the researcher do next to statistically test for differences in these groups? Below, we outline a general procedure for hypothesis testing that can be used with a variety of inferential statistics.

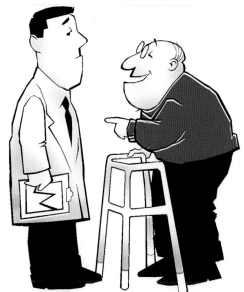

Creating a Null and Directional Hypothesis

One of the most important parts of any research study is the development of an appropriate statistical hypothesis.[2]

Researcher: Do you feel like your walking speed has improved? Old geezer: Only when there is a line at the buffet table!

In Chapter 10, directional and null hypotheses were introduced. Recall that researchers must translate their research hypothesis—a statement of the anticipated outcomes—into a pair of hypotheses that are statistically testable and opposite of each other. In the case of inferential statistics, these hypotheses relate to group differences. The **null hypothesis** states that groups do not differ from each other. Examples of general null hypotheses in testing group differences are as follows:

> **Null Hypothesis** Statistical hypothesis stating no differences exist between or among groups.

- The treatment group will not differ from the control group.
- There will be no differences from pretest to posttest.

> *Statistical hypotheses must be testable through experimentation, so should include variables that are measurable.*

So, for example, if our researcher wanted to examine the impact of his novel rehabilitation protocol on balance in stroke patients, the null hypothesis might be the following:

- After 10 weeks of training, the group receiving novel rehabilitation will not differ from the control group on a standardized balance test.
- There will be no differences in balance test scores before and after 10 weeks of a novel rehabilitation training.

> **Directional Hypothesis** Statistical hypothesis stating differences exist between or among groups.

In contrast, the **directional hypothesis** indicates that one group differs from another as a function of the independent variable. The following examples are directional hypotheses replacing the above null hypotheses:

- The group receiving novel rehabilitation will score significantly higher on a standardized balance test than the control group.
- Standardized balance test scores will be significantly higher after 10 weeks of novel rehabilitation training than before training.

When researchers are unsure about the direction of change, they can use a bidirectional hypothesis and then use a two-tailed test to evaluate (more on that later):

- Standardized balance test scores will be significantly *different* after 10 weeks of novel rehabilitation training than before training.

Select an Appropriate Alpha Level

> *In experiments with human participants, researchers generally use 0.05 or 0.01 as their alpha levels.*

After creating null and directional hypotheses, researchers must set the type I error probability, or alpha level (α).[2] Remember, because researchers cannot test every person within a population, they randomly sample from that population in order to get a group of participants who appropriately represent the population. In our example, the researcher randomly selects a group of stroke patients representative of all stroke patients. The purpose of inferential statistics is to objectively indicate whether sampled groups differ from each other, and then we infer that result to the population as a whole. However, a chance of an erroneous result always exists. In reality, two possibilities exist:

- Within the population, the treatment actually causes balance differences, which are reflected in sample differences.
- Within the population, the treatment *does not* cause balance differences, so the sample differences are based on random error.

By selecting an alpha level, researchers limit the chance that they will incorrectly reject the null hypothesis (i.e., there are group differences) when, in fact, the null hypothesis should not be rejected (i.e., there are no group differences) to that probability. Researchers commonly use the values of either 0.05 (which is most commonly used in research with human participants) or, for a more stringent comparison, 0.01.[3] Occasionally, a researcher whose investigation is pilot work, exploratory, or proof of concept may use an alpha level of 0.10 or even 0.15; however, such studies may prove difficult to publish because these alpha values are not considered very stringent.

In our example, the researcher considers using alpha levels of both 0.01 and 0.05. On the one hand, if the researcher selects 0.01, that means that if the group receiving novel rehabilitation has a higher average score on the balance test than the control group, there is only a 1% chance that this is due to error rather than a real effect of the treatment. That sounds pretty good! On the other hand, using an alpha level of 0.05 will make finding statistical differences somewhat easier and is still the most widely accepted value of alpha level when performing research with human participants, so the researcher selects $\alpha = 0.05$.

For novices in statistics, this second step may seem confusing or out of place ("why not wait until you see the results!"). In fact, a proper procedure dictates that you must *always* select your alpha level before you run your statistics rather than after the fact. That is simply a good statistical practice. You cannot select alpha after the data are collected. Computer programs cannot evaluate hypotheses or make decisions—they just run through equations very quickly and spit out results. Therefore, researchers must be the brains behind the operation, making decisions prior to testing (termed a 'priori') on alpha levels that will guide their decisions to reject the null hypothesis or not.

Researchers can assign their alpha value as either a one- or a two-tailed test. A two-tailed test means you split your alpha in half and test for statistical significance in both sides of the normal curve. Two-tailed tests are frequently used, particularly if a researcher does not specify a direction within the hypothesis. For example, if a researcher is examining running velocity in two groups of third graders, one of which received special training, the hypothesis states "the experimental group will differ in velocity from the control group," and the researcher would use a two-tailed test. A one-tailed test tests for statistical significance on only one side of the normal curve. In this case, the researcher compares a third and sixth grade group on running velocity and is sure that the sixth grade group is faster. The researcher would hypothesize "the sixth grade group will have faster velocity than the third grade group." Using a one-tailed test provides more statistical power to detect differences, but should only be used when the direction of the difference is known.

Collecting Data and Running a Statistical Analysis Using Computer Programs

Back in the first three quarters of the 20th century, researchers had to conduct statistical tests using a pencil, paper, and, if they were lucky, a calculator. Researchers calculating statistics this way needed to consult a table of critical values (serving as benchmarks) to determine whether the result of a statistical test was significant (very similar to the process described in Chapter 11 with regression). If the calculated value equaled or exceeded the critical value, then the null hypothesis was rejected. What a long, arduous process that was! Thankfully, we have computers and computer programs that make calculating statistics and determining significance much quicker and easier.

Statistical programs often provide the actual/critical values of the statistic of interest as well as the p value. Both can be used to make a statistical decision.

Modern-day statistical programs, such as SAS (Statistical Analysis System, from SAS Institute, Inc.), Statistica from StatSoft, or IBM SPSS store critical values for statistical tests within the software, so researchers do not need to look these up in tables. They simply input the alpha level, and the statistical program presents the result along with the *p* value, typically starring the *p* value when it is significant.

Making a Decision Regarding the Null Hypothesis

At this point, researchers must make the decision to either reject the null hypothesis or not. The statistical software provides the results of the statistical test in the form of a *p* value, and researchers must evaluate these based on the alpha level provided before the test was run. The *p* value is the probability of committing a type I error. In other words, the *p* value indicates the probability that random error (rather than treatment effects) caused the sample differences that are seen. If the *p* value is equal to or less than the alpha level, then researchers can reject the null hypothesis and conclude that there are significant differences between or among groups.[3] For example, with alpha level set at 0.05, we would decide the following with these *p* values:

- *p* value = 0.049—reject the null hypothesis; there are real differences between the groups.
- *p* value = 0.055—do not reject the null; there are no differences between the groups.

This procedure for hypothesis testing is used for many different inferential statistical tests that researchers commonly use within the field of kinesiology and the health sciences. As we move on to discuss each individual test, we will describe the procedure in more detail. We will start by discussing the simplest tests, *t* tests, and move on to analysis of variance (ANOVA), as well as some other tests.

INTERPRETING RESULTS FOR MEANINGFULNESS

Before moving on, recall that in correlation analysis, researchers had to make a decision not only about significance but also about meaningfulness of the results. This is also true with inferential statistics. When interpreting statistical results, it is insufficient to state that significant differences exist among groups. Researchers must follow that with an assessment of how meaningful those differences are. We touched on this briefly in Chapter 10 with a discussion of effect size. The process of determining effect size requires separate calculations than those used for calculating significance, as you might expect.

✔ Check Your Understanding

1. Describe the procedure used in hypotheses testing, specifying each step.
2. What is the difference between a null and directional hypothesis?
3. Why do researchers need to select appropriate alpha values prior to statistical testing?

TYPES OF *T* TESTS

_t_ Test A statistical test used when comparing two groups on one dependent measure.

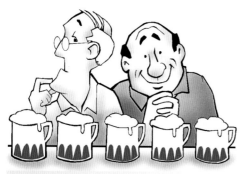

"Do you suppose we need a larger sample size?"

A *t* **test** is a statistical test used when comparing two groups on one dependent measure. A history lesson may make the study of *t* tests go down a little easier.... Student's *t* test was developed around 1908 by a chemist named W. Steven Gosset.[4] Administrators at the Irish stout company, Guinness, had hired Gosset (whose nickname was Student) to help them brew better beer. They wanted to develop a statistical method to determine optimal types of hops, barley, etc. rather than relying on less formal information handed down from brewer to brewer. Gosset went on to develop the one-sample *t* test, revolutionizing both the statistical world and the beer industry.[4]

Student's *t* Test: Comparing a Sample to a Population Mean

The previous example is a great segue into a description of the one-sample *t* test, called a **Student's *t* test**. Researchers use this test to determine if a sample differs from the larger population. Population data exist on many different measures, which can provide normative information about the population. For example, a researcher may be interested to see how a group of senior citizens that have gone through a walking regime compare to age norms for the 6-minute walk. In this case, the t test is used to determine if this group of seniors differs from age normative data.[5] The statistical formula used is the following:

Student's t Test Used to compare a sample mean to the population.

$$t = \frac{M - \mu}{s / \sqrt{n}}$$

Equation 12.1

where M is the population mean, μ is the sample mean, s is the standard deviation for the sample mean, and n is the number of observations in the sample.

Let's follow the procedure we provided in the previous section to walk through an example of the use of Student's t. Imagine a local senior center Director wants to determine if the older adults at his center, who have started a walking group within the past 6 months, differ from the general population of seniors in their walking ability (he wants to tout his center as one that helps keep seniors in shape). He calls a researcher to help. The researcher decides to test the 30 older males aged 70 to 74 years ($n = 30$) on the 6-minute walk test, in which the participants walk as far as they can for 6 minutes; the population mean (M) is 612 yards:[5]

- First, the researcher creates null and alternative hypotheses. The null hypothesis states that sample mean (μ) is not different from the population mean ($M = 612$). The directional hypothesis is that the sample mean exceeds the population mean.
- Next, the researcher selects an alpha value of 0.05.
- The researcher places the data into a spreadsheet and calculates Student's t. For demonstration purposes, we will calculate it here by hand using Equation 12.1:

$M = 612$ yards

$\mu = 654$ yards

$s = 74$

$n = 30$

$$t = \frac{612 - 654}{74 \sqrt{5.477}}$$

$$t = 3.108$$

- The $t_{critical}$ for a two-tailed test is 2.048, compared to the calculated t value of 3.108. Since 3.108 > 2.048, the researcher rejects the null that the population and sample means are the same and concludes that the sample groups walked farther than the population mean on the 6-minute walk test.

The Independent t Test for Two Groups

More frequently, researchers wish to compare two groups of participants to each other rather than to a population mean. The one-sample t test is not appropriate for this sort of statistical comparison; therefore, other types of t tests must be used, most commonly the **independent t test**. In order to use this test, researchers must sample either two independent groups from the same population (e.g., two samples of older adults

Independent t Test Used to compare two independent groups.

TABLE 12.1 Independent *t* Test			
Group	**Mean**	**Standard Deviations**	**Participant Numbers**
1	$\bar{x}_1$	S_1	n_1
2	$\bar{x}_2$	S_2	n_2

from different senior centers) or a single sample from two different populations (e.g., a sample of older adults and a sample of younger adults). In both cases, the samples are independent from each other, which is one of the assumptions of this test (see Table 12.1). With this test, researchers attempt to determine if differences exist between the groups, in which case, they will infer that differences exist in the population from which they sample.[6]

Mathematically, the equation for the independent *t* test is quite similar to that previously presented:

$$t = \frac{\bar{x}_1 - \bar{x}_2}{\sqrt{\dfrac{s_1^2}{n_1} + \dfrac{s_2^2}{n_2}}} \qquad \text{Equation 12.2}$$

To continue with our example, the senior center Director continued his quest to improve the health and physical fitness of his clients at the center and hired a certified personal trainer to work on a more sound walking program, along with armchair exercises and weekly goal setting. He called the researcher back after an additional 8 weeks of training, and the researcher compared this group of seniors on the 6-minute walk to a group of 15 seniors at another center in the next town who have had no training at all. After testing these groups, the researcher got the following values (Table 12.2):

Let's go through the steps to determine if significant differences exist between these groups:

- First, the researcher creates null and alternative hypotheses. The null hypothesis states that the walking group $\bar{x}_1$ is not different from the control group $\bar{x}_2$. The directional hypothesis is that the walking group travels farther than the control group during the 6-minute walk test.
- Next, the researcher selects an alpha value of 0.05.
- The researcher places the data into a spreadsheet (see Special Box 12.1 for step by step instruction on independent *t* test with Excel) and calculates an independent *t* value. For demonstration purposes, we will also calculate this by hand using Equation 12.2:

$$t = \frac{507 - 351}{\sqrt{\left(77^2/15 + 73^2/15\right)}} = 5.68$$

- The t_{critical} for a one-tailed test is 1.701. The calculated *t* is 5.68. Because t 5.68 > t_{critical} 1.701, the researcher rejects the null hypothesis and concludes that the walking group walked significantly farther than the control group on the 6-minute walk test.

TABLE 12.2 Data from the 6-Minute Walk Test from the Two Senior Center Groups			
Group	**Mean**	**Standard Deviation**	**Participant Numbers**
1	507 min	77 min	15
2	351 min	73 min	15

SPECIAL INTEREST BOX 12.1

Using Excel to Calculate an Independent t Test

As mentioned in Chapter 11, Excel spreadsheets provide a simple way in which to do basic statistics. Here, we will walk you through the steps necessary to perform an independent *t* test. We will use the senior center walking data discussed above. Once you have opened Excel, take the following steps:

1. Input all of data into two columns, one for each independent sample. Each cell represents the data from one participant in that column's group. Along the task bar, click on "Data," and then, click on "Data Analysis" on the far right of the Data task bar.

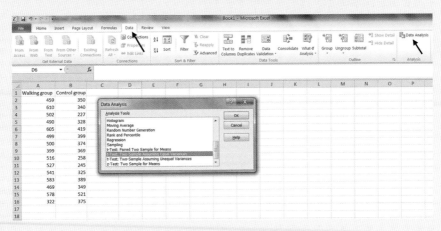

2. A text box pops up with different statistical choices. Select "t Test": Two Sample for Equal Variances. This will open another text box, one that allows you to set up your analysis. Under "Input," select the first group data by clicking on the box at the end of the Variable 1 range row. Click on the label for the first group, and then drag down over the entire column of data. Repeat this for the second group in the Variable 2 range row.

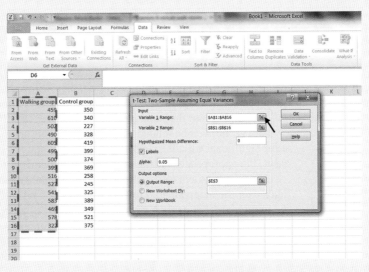

SPECIAL INTEREST BOX 12.1 (*Continued*)

Select hypothesized mean difference as 0 (this is the null hypothesis), check Labels for labels in the first row, and select alpha level and output range. Then, click "Ok."

3. The *t* test results will quickly appear in your output range. That's it! The statistical analysis is finished. Results will look like this:

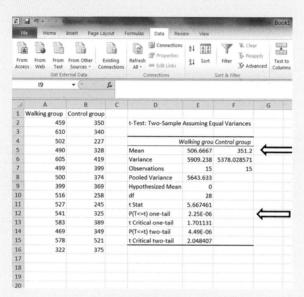

Reading down the columns, you can see the means of the two groups, the *t* statistic, the *p* value, and $t_{critical}$ for a one-tailed test and the *p* value and $t_{critical}$ for a two-tailed test. Evaluate significance for a one-tailed test by comparing *t* stat to $t_{critical}$ (5.66 > 1.70) or alpha to *p* value (0.000002 > 0.05). In both cases, significance is reached, and the null is rejected—significant differences exist between the groups.

The Dependent *t* Test for Two Groups

In many cases, researchers may want to examine two groups that are related to each other in some way. For example, if researchers investigate the effects of an intervention, they will want to compare the outcome or posttest to how the group performed before the intervention, or pretest. This type of experiment is called a "repeated measures" design, because the same measure is taken repeatedly on the same group of participants. Another case where groups can be related is if the participants are matched according to some significant variable, such as strength, age, and physical fitness. In these cases, the appropriate statistic to use is the **dependent *t* test.**[6]

Dependent *t* Test Used to compare two related data sets, such as pre-/posttest, or matched pairs.

Using a dependent (also called "paired sample") *t* test has several advantages over the independent *t* test. In the case of a repeated measures design, the participants act as their own controls, and they all receive the treatment provided. With independent groups, the assumption is that the control group is the same as (or quite similar to) the treatment group, but in a repeated measures design, the control group is the treatment group, which may improve the accuracy of the outcome. The same is true for the matched pairs design. With independent samples, researchers assume that the control group is equivalent to the treatment group due to random selection or assignment. In comparison, researchers create two equivalent groups by matching each participant on some important variable of interest. Again, this should help to improve accuracy of results.

We can continue with our senior center example to illustrate the procedure of going through the dependent *t* test. In this case, rather than randomly selecting a group of seniors from a different senior center, the researcher decides to match the participants from the senior center with the walking program for age and gender. After selecting 15 age- and gender-matched seniors from the new center, the researcher tests them on the 6-minute walk test:

- The researcher's null hypothesis is that no differences exist between the groups on the 6-minute walk test. The researcher's directional hypothesis is that the walking group walks farther on the 6-minute walk test than the control group.
- The researcher selects an alpha level of 0.05.
- Using statistical software, the researcher compares the two groups by placing the information in two columns and running the appropriate statistical program. Because of the complexity of the formula, we will report the values obtained from the statistical program.
- Based on a *p* value of 0.021, which is less than alpha = 0.05, the researcher rejects the null hypothesis and claims that significant differences exist between the walking and control groups.

INTERPRETING THE SIGNIFICANT *T* STATISTIC: MEANINGFULNESS

As we discussed in Chapter 10, the process of interpreting statistics requires more than just identifying the presence or absence of statistical differences. Just because researchers determine that significant differences exist doesn't necessarily mean that they have found large, consequential differences. In fact, researchers need to determine how statistically meaningful those differences are. The easiest way to do this with *t* tests is to examine the **effect size** of the differences, which was mentioned briefly in Chapter 10. As you may recall, effect size provides an estimate of the strength of group differences.[7] In other words, significance testing tells us that the groups are different, and effect size tells us how different they are. In the case of *t* tests, we will calculate Cohen's *d* for an estimate of effect size:

Effect Size An estimate of the strength of group differences, which represents the meaningfulness of the results.

$$d = X_t - X_c / s_{pooled} \qquad \text{Equation 12.3}$$

where X_t is the treatment mean, X_c is the control mean, and S_{pooled} is the pooled standard deviation. In order to pool the standard deviations of the two group, all that is necessary is the individual standard deviations and the number of participants per group.

If researchers don't report effect size, you can calculate it on your own and interpret it using the rules of thumb provided in Table 12.3.

$$s = \sqrt{\frac{(n_1 - 1)s_1^2 + (n_2 - 1)s_2^2}{n_1 + n_2}},$$

The resultant value of Cohen's *d* will range between the values of 0 and 2.0. Use Table 12.3 below as a rule of thumb for interpreting Cohen's *d*.

TABLE 12.3 Rules of Thumb for Interpreting the Cohen's d Effect Size	
Cohen's d Value	**Interpretation**
0.20 and below	Small
0.50	Medium
0.80 and above	Large

✔ Check Your Understanding

1. Differentiate among the three types of *t* tests.
2. What are the two ways to determine the significance of *t* tests?
3. What measure is used to assess meaningfulness of significant differences?

ANALYSIS OF VARIANCE

Researchers looking for quick ways to distinguish differences between two groups can perform a *t* test and be satisfied with the statistical results. Often, however, researchers want to investigate differences among more than two groups or between two groups at multiple points in time. One way to address this would be to perform a series of *t* tests, which can get complicated with more than three comparisons, and also compounds type I error. Alternatively, researchers can perform another type of test, called **analysis of variance** (ANOVA), which allows for multiple comparisons.[6] The symbol for the result of an ANOVA is *F*, also known as an *F* ratio. Various types of ANOVAs exist, including a one-way, repeated measures, and two-way, among others.

ANOVA Analysis of variance, which is a statistical test used to compare two or more data set means.

One-Way ANOVA

One-Way ANOVA An ANOVA comparing two or more groups of one independent measure on one dependent measure.

*When testing more than two groups on one independent variable, use a one-way ANOVA rather than a series of **t** tests in order to maintain the type I error rate.*

The **one-way ANOVA** is the most basic form of ANOVA, essentially an extension of the *t* test to include three or more groups, all of which represent different levels of the same independent variable or factor. For example, if a researcher wanted to compare the effect of 0 (control), 20, 40, and 60 minutes of rehabilitation training (the factor), then each time value represents a distinct level of that factor. A one-way ANOVA evaluates the null hypothesis that no differences exist among the groups.

As the name implies, the one-way ANOVA partitions out variability of scores into either variance between two or more groups (this represents how the groups differ from the population mean) and the variance within groups, or error (this represents how individuals differ from the group means). If the variance between groups is similar to the variance within groups, then this suggests that the treatment does not have an effect. This makes intuitive sense, since the within groups variance represents error or how much the individuals differ from the population mean—if the variance among the groups isn't different from the variance of individuals from the population, then the impact of the treatment is negligible. However, if the variance between groups exceeds that within groups, then the null hypothesis can be rejected.

From the data, several measures are calculated. First, the "sum of squares between (or explained)" calculates the variability between groups. If this equals 0, then there are no differences between the groups. The "sum of squares within (or error)" is calculated. Finally, the mean squares (MS) for between and within are calculated by dividing each of the sums of squares (SS) values by their respective degrees of freedom. (The degrees of freedom for between are calculated as the number of groups—1. The degrees of freedom for within are calculated as the number of participants—the number of groups.) The ratio of these MS represents the *F* ratio or statistic. All of these measures are provided in the computer output of the ANOVA table that we show below.

For an example, let's look to the researcher exploring the walking program at the senior center again. The researcher wants to compare the impact of walking for 45 minutes at a target heart rate zone for 2 versus 4 days a week (with 0 day a week as a control) over a 10-week period. There are 10 participants in each group, and the following data are generated (Table 12.4).

TABLE 12.4	Data from the 6-Minute Walk Test for Three Senior Center Groups	
Control	**2 ×/Week**	**4 ×/Week**
352	462	524
299	589	576
251	499	482
327	432	578
420	521	322
366	482	621
325	511	255
399	259	378
247	352	499
245	521	510

The procedure remains the same as for t tests:

- The researcher's null hypothesis is that no differences exist among the groups in the 6-minute walk test. The researcher's directional hypothesis is that the two and four times per week walking groups will travel a greater distance on the 6-minute walk test than the control group.
- The researcher selects an alpha level of 0.05.
- Using statistical software (see Special Interest Box 12.2 for an example), the researcher compares the three groups by placing the information in three columns and running the appropriate statistical program (see Table 12.5).
- Significance is evaluated by comparing the F_{actual} to $F_{critical}$, in which case 7.833 > 3.354, so the null hypothesis is rejected indicating there are differences among walking 0, 2, and 4 days each week.

Note that all the important components of the equation are clearly labeled within the ANOVA table so that you could calculate them yourself if you chose to.

TABLE 12.5	Results from One-Way ANOVA of Table 12.4 Data						
ANOVA: Single Factor							
Summary							
Groups	**Count**	**Sum**	**Average**	**Variance**			
Control	10	3231	323.1	3946.1			
2×/week	10	4628	462.8	9051.511			
4×/week	10	4745	474.5	14176.94			
ANOVA							
Source of Variation	**SS**	**df**	**MS**	**F**	**p-value**	**F crit**	
Between Groups	141916.5	2	70958.23	7.833604	0.002076	3.354131	
Within Groups	244571	27	9058.185				
Total	386487.5	29					

SPECIAL INTEREST BOX 12.2

Calculating a One-Way ANOVA Using Excel

Just like *t* tests, ANOVAs are relatively simple to perform using Excel.

A. Place data in columns with appropriate labels. Click "Data" tab and then "Data Analysis" on the far left in the task bar that pops up. Select "ANOVA: Single factor," and then click "Ok."

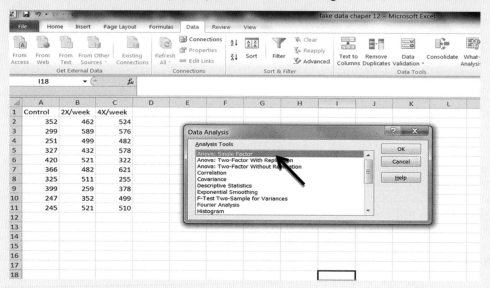

B. In the pop up box, select the input range by clicking on the button and then by dragging the cursor over the appropriate three columns of data. Click "Columns" and "Labels in First Row," and select appropriate alpha level. Select where you would like the output to go, and then click "Ok."

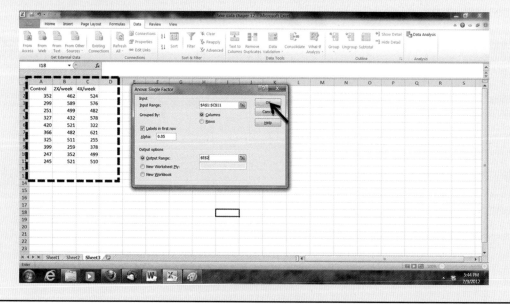

C. The one-way ANOVA will be written to your output location and will look like this:

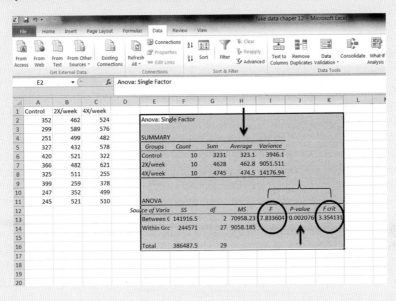

The output provides the average values, SS and MS between and within groups, F_{actual} (7.83), p value (0.002), and $F_{critical}$ (3.35)—everything you need to evaluate for significance!

After looking at the results, you may have noticed that several questions still remain. Most prominently, the ANOVA indicated that there were significant differences among the three groups. However, it did not indicate which groups differ from each other. That is, if only the one-way ANOVA was performed, the researcher could only say that the groups differed, but would not be able to indicate if the walking groups differed from each other (e.g., which walking protocol might be better) or if they truly differed from the control group. More work needs to be done, and this comes in the form of post hoc testing. We will cover this topic following our discussion of repeated measures and two-way ANOVAs.

Check Your Understanding

1. How is a *t* test different from an ANOVA?
2. What are the sources of error in an ANOVA?
3. What does a significant F mean when comparing four groups (three treatment, one control)?

Repeated Measures ANOVA

In many studies that are designed to produce evidence-based practice, researchers want to show that some sort of change over time occurs. In order to show that an intervention works, participants need to take a pretest before the intervention and then one or more follow-up tests after the intervention. If the intervention worked as planned, then the test results should be significantly different from each other. This gives researchers a powerful tool to track the course of change in a dependent measure.

In the most simple repeated measures ANOVA, a single group of participants is measured at least two times on a single dependent measure. Participants act as their own controls, with the pretest indicating preintervention measures. This controls for individual differences in participants, which is a substantial source of variation or error within studies. Another type of repeated measures ANOVA includes two or more groups.

Two-Way ANOVA

Often, researchers may want to examine the effect of more than one independent variable on a dependent measure, because more than one variable can impact the outcome of the research. For example, researchers know that intensity of exercise is one variable that can impact VO_2max, but so can frequency of exercise. It would be convenient to design an experiment that manipulates both intensity and frequency and then compares their effects—both independently and together—in one statistical test. A **two-way ANOVA** is the type of statistical test to use in this case, because it allows the researcher to examine two independent variables at the same time. Unlike a one-way ANOVA, a two-way ANOVA also allows for the evaluation of **interactions** between the independent measures. Thus, in our example above, we could look at the impact of frequency alone and intensity alone (called **main effects**) and interaction of frequency and intensity together (called **interaction effects**). With the main effects, all data are compared on one independent variable and pooled on the other independent variable. We will use this example to illustrate the use of a two-way ANOVA.

Two-Way ANOVA An ANOVA comparing two independent measures with two levels of each factor on one dependent measure.

Interactions The effect of two independent measures acting together on a dependent measure.

Main Effects The effect of an independent variable when all other independent variables are held constant.

Imagine that a high school football coach is looking for a more efficient way to improve the cardiovascular fitness of the players on his team. The coach has the athletes run 1 mile each day at the beginning of practice, at a self-determined pace that is supposed to be "as fast as possible" (although some players look suspiciously slow) to try to improve basic levels of fitness during the first month of football practice. However, the coach wants to spend as much time as possible in practice working on teamwork and skills and so wants to find the optimal combination of frequency and intensity for these running workouts. The coach consults with an exercise physiologist from the local university Kinesiology department, who designs an experiment. The researcher selects two levels of frequency (3 and 5 days per week) and two levels of intensity (65% and 85% of maximum heart rate during a 1-mile run). The researcher selects VO_2max as the dependent variable. With this experiment, the researcher will answer the following questions. First, does a group that runs 3 days a week differ in their VO_2max from group that runs 5 days a week? Second, does a group that runs at 65% intensity differ from a group that runs at 85% intensity? Finally, does intensity interact with frequency? The answer to this final question would indicate if there is a best combination of frequency and intensity for this sample of football players.

The researcher recruits 80 football players from area high schools during the summer and randomly assigns the players into one of four groups: (a) 3 days per week at 65% intensity, (b) 3 days per week at 85% intensity, (c) 5 days per week at 65% intensity, and (d) 5 days per week at 85% intensity. The researcher pretests the players for their VO_2max and then has them follow their running regime for a

TABLE 12.6   Intensity and Frequency Data for the 2 × 2 ANOVA

		Frequency	
		3 Days/Week	5 Days/Week
Intensity (mL/kg/min)	65	57	60
	85	71	65

TABLE 12.7 ANOVA Table for Table 12.6 Data

Effects	F Statistic	p Value
Main effect for frequency	1.40	0.136
Main effect for intensity	10.0	0.001[a]
Interaction effect for frequency × intensity	5.0	0.045[a]

[a]Indicates significance at 0.05 level.

month, using heart rate monitors to provide measures of exercise intensity. Finally, the researcher collects posttest data and is ready to calculate a two-way ANOVA. Table 12.6 depicts these groups below:

- The researcher develops a null and directional hypothesis. The null hypothesis states that no differences exist among any of the four groups in their VO_2max. The directional hypothesis states that the groups will differ in their VO_2max.
- The researcher selects alpha = 0.05.
- The researcher collects the data.
- The researcher places the data into a spreadsheet and uses statistical software to calculate the F statistic. Just as with one-way ANOVA, SS and MS are calculated, and an F ratio is derived (we will not go through the equation here). From the software, the following results are derived (Table 12.7).

Graphically, the results look like this (Figure 12.1):

- The researcher uses the p values to interpret the main effects first. Because the p value for frequency is > 0.05, the researcher does not reject the null hypothesis and concludes that groups running 3 days and 5 days a week do not differ across all levels of intensity. Because the p value for intensity is < 0.05, the researcher rejects the null hypothesis and concludes that the groups differ at 65% and 85% intensity levels.
- The researcher then examines the p value of the interaction. Because the p value for frequency by intensity is < 0.05, the researcher rejects the null and concludes that the groups differ based on frequency and intensity together.

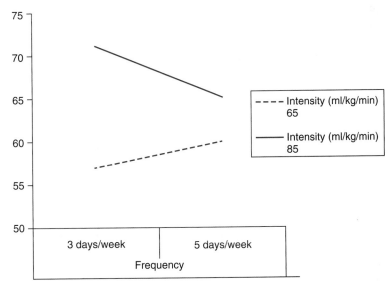

■ **FIGURE 12.1** VO_2max after a 1-month training period based on two exercise intensities (65% or 85% max) and two exercise frequencies (three or five times per week).

INTERPRETING A TWO-WAY ANOVA

We will use the example above to illustrate how to interpret a two-way ANOVA. Because there are just two levels of each independent variable, the researcher can make specific inferences about the effectiveness of frequency and intensity. In terms of the main effects, the researcher can tell the coach that both 3 and 5 days a week don't provide different VO_2max values when pooling across the different intensity levels. For the coach, this means that if intensity is not monitored (some players go as fast as possible and some slack off), then running 3 days a week will be just fine. On the other hand, those players who train at 85% of their maximum intensity significantly outperform their peers who train at 65% max. The results from the interaction suggest that training at 85% max for 3 days a week results in the highest levels of VO_2max. The coach then modifies his practice schedule so that the players run Monday/Wednesday/Friday at the beginning of practice and they use heart rate monitors to ensure that they work at 85% of their maximum heart rate.

In this example, there were both a significant main effect and a significant interaction effect. Occasionally, a significant interaction will occur without any significant main effects. Results of this nature indicate that the effect of the independent variables alone is not strong enough to result in group differences, but together, they do make a difference. Alternatively, significant main effects may exist in the absence of interaction effects. When completing statistical analyses, it is important to always check on both main and interaction effects. Further, when reading published research, be sure the authors interpret these effects correctly.

Factorial ANOVAs

Factorial ANOVA ANOVA with two or more independent variables, each with two or more levels.

The two-way is actually the most basic case of a **factorial ANOVA**. A factorial ANOVA allows for simultaneous evaluation of two or more levels of independent variables. Factorial designs are referred to by the number of levels of each of the independent variables. Therefore, researchers will refer to a two-way ANOVA as a 2 × 2 ANOVA. If, in our example, the researcher had compared three intensity levels (65%, 75%, and 85%), then the resulting statistical analysis would be called a 2 × 3 ANOVA, indicating two levels of one independent variable and three levels of the second independent variable. Factorial analyses can be extended to more than two independent variables as well. If the researcher had included running distance as a third independent variable with two levels (1 and 1.5 miles), this would have resulted in a 2 × 2 × 3 ANOVA. Sometimes, to help provide clarity, a researcher may notate an ANOVA as 2 (frequency) × 2(distance) × 3 (intensity) factorial ANOVA. Once researchers start adding more than three independent variables, the statistical analysis can be challenging to interpret, particularly if many significant interaction effects result.

POST HOC TESTS

In all of the ANOVA statistical tests where there are at least three sets of data being compared, significant results indicate that differences exist, but do not show which groups differ from each other.

When three or more groups are compared using ANOVA, researchers must always use post hoc tests to determine which groups differ from each other.

In a one-way ANOVA with two groups, or a 2 × 2 ANOVA, interpreting significant differences is simple because one group will be higher (or more or faster) than the other group. On the other hand, if an independent variable has more than two levels, then a significant ANOVA indicates only that differences exist somewhere between two or more of the groups. However, the results of the ANOVA do not indicate which groups differ from each other.

Let's go back to our example from page 12. The researcher compared older adult groups on walking 0, 2, and 4 days a week. $F = 7.833 > F_{critical} = 3.354$, so the null hypothesis was rejected, indicating differences exist among walking groups. A novice researcher may then follow this with an incorrect interpretation that walking 4 days a week results in the best 6-minute walk times. However, the results of the ANOVA do not allow for that interpretation. All we can say is that at least one of the groups differs from at least one other group. This could mean that the group walking 0 days differs from the groups walking 2 and 4 days—or it could mean that the group walking 2 days differs from the 0 day group, but not the 4-day group. In order to figure out which groups are significantly different, researchers must use **post hoc tests**. These tests are used to follow up a significant ANOVA and so have also been called follow-up tests.

Post Hoc Tests Tests that follow up ANOVA to show where significant differences between specific groups exist.

Basically, post hoc tests compare each group to every other group, similar to performing a set of *t* tests on all of the groups. You may wonder why the researcher chose an ANOVA with post hoc tests rather than just performing a set of t tests from the start. Although that sounds reasonable, problems exist with performing more than one *t* test on a data set. The biggest problem is that *t* tests are designed to compare two, and only two, groups. Therefore, each additional analysis compounds type I error, which is concluding that differences exist when in fact there are no differences between groups. If alpha is set at 0.05, then each subsequent *t* test increases the overall type I error by 0.05, resulting in an ever-increasing probability of falsely concluding that differences exist (called experiment-wide alpha). In our example above, if the researcher chose to perform three independent *t* tests, the experiment-wide alpha would be 0.05 + 0.05 + 0.05 = 0.15—that means the researcher would have a 15% chance of concluding differences between groups existed when in fact all groups were not different. Alternatively, post hoc tests retain alpha at its original level while providing the comparisons of each individual group to every other one. By retaining the original alpha level, post hoc tests provide a much better way to determine where the significant difference or differences appear between groups.

Several different post hoc tests exist. In cases where the groups or data sets being compared are of equal size, post hoc tests include Fisher's least significant difference (LSD), Tukey's honestly significant difference (HSD), Duncan's multiple range, and Newman–Keuls. Tests that can be used whether the data sets being compared are of equal or unequal sizes include Scheffé, Tukey–Kramer, and Bonferroni–Dunn. Each post hoc test differs in the amount of adjustment to alpha; in other words, some post hoc tests are more conservative and less likely to lead to rejecting the null hypothesis, whereas others are more liberal and more likely to lead to rejecting the null hypothesis (see Fig. 12.2 for an example).

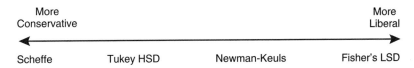

■ **FIGURE 12.2** The relative strength of post hoc tests to detect differences. The more conservative the test, the more difficult it is to detect differences.

ANALYSIS OF COVARIANCE

The final type of ANOVA we will discuss is used in cases where group means are known to be different at the beginning of an experiment. In order to statistically adjust for these differences, an **analysis of covariance**, or ANCOVA, is used.[6] In certain situations, a variable termed a covariate has an impact on the values of a dependent measure

ANCOVA Analysis of covariance, used to adjust for a variable that covaries with the independent variable and may impact the outcome of the test.

Use ANCOVA on repeated measures designs in order to account for differences in pretest scores among the different groups.

and will impact the results of the statistical analysis. In a way, ANCOVA allows for the statistical control of confounding variable just as inclusion and exclusion criteria allow for manual control of confounding variables.

For example, researchers may be interested in the impact of a new weight loss drug over an 8-week period. They may use percentage body fat as inclusion/exclusion criteria, so that only individuals with a percentage body fat between 30% and 40% may be included in the study. An important variable to consider in any weight loss experiment is the amount of physical activity each participant gets each day. The researchers may determine that daily physical activity covaries with the percentage of body fat and want to remove physical activity as a potential confound. Therefore, this range of body fat measures can be statistically adjusted using ANCOVA to account for differences in daily physical activity.

Another way in which ANCOVA can be used is to adjust for initial group differences. In certain situations, random sampling may be impossible, and group differences in pretest scores need to be accounted for. For example, researchers may want to determine the impact of a 10-week movement education program on preschoolers. Ideally, the researchers could randomly assign preschoolers to either a treatment group or a control group. However, within a preschool setting, this is not feasible over a long time period; for a variety of reasons, each class needs to stay together as a cohort. As a result, initial group scores on a motor skills test differ due to different teachers' uses of movement education within their teaching plans. To adjust for these differences, ANCOVA can be used.

CHAPTER SUMMARY

- A systematic procedure can be used in which to test hypotheses in experiments examining group differences.
- The first step of this process involves the development of testable null and alternative hypotheses.
- Alpha levels of 0.01 or 0.05 are frequently used in research with human participants. The alpha level must be selected before the study begins.
- Many computer programs such as Excel or SPSS are available for statistical computations, although statistics can also be compiled using a calculator.
- Researchers can compare the calculated statistic to a critical value or use the p value to determine if they reject or do not reject the null hypothesis.
- Two groups can be compared using a t test.
- Student's t test compares a sample mean to a population mean.
- An independent t test compares means of two independent groups.
- A dependent t test compares means of dependent groups. These can be groups that are matched on some characteristic or two repeated measures (pre/post) in one group.
- ANOVA compares two or more data sets on one dependent variable.
- One-way ANOVA compares two or more groups on one dependent variable.
- Repeated measures ANOVA compares one dependent variable two or more times for a single group. Two-way ANOVA compares two groups on two independent variables.
- Factorial ANOVA compares two or more independent variables simultaneously. Post hoc tests are necessary to determine where significant differences occur when more than two groups are compared in an ANOVA.
- Analysis of covariance (ANCOVA) adjusts for a covariate that may impact the dependent measure.

REFERENCES

1. Kaye DH, Freedman DA. Reference guide on statistics. In: *Reference Manual on Scientific Evidence*, 3rd ed. Washington, DC: West National Academies Press, 2011:249–247.

2. Marczyk G, DeMatteo D, Festinger D. *Essentials of Research Design and Methodology*. Hoboken, NJ: John Wiley & Sons, 2005:9–12.

3. Gravetter FJ, Wallnau LB. *Statistics for the Behavioral Sciences*, 8th ed. Pacific Grove, CA: Wadsworth-Thompson Learning, 2009.

4. Fisher Box J. Guinness, gosset, fisher, and small samples. *Stat Sci* 1987;2(1):45–52.

5. Rikli R, Jones J. Functional fitness normative scores for community-residing older adults, ages 60–94. *J Aging Phys Act* 1999;7:162–181.

6. Field AP. *Discovering Statistics Using SPSS*, 4th ed. Washington, DC: Sage, 2013.

7. Kelley K, Preacher KJ. On effect size. *Psychol Methods* 2012;17:137–152.

RELATED ASSIGNMENTS

1. A renowned researcher at Drugtopia University wants to investigate the effect of a secret supplement that she developed on weight loss. She believes that the supplement, Drug X, leads to rapid loss of body fat. She uses a pretest/posttest design and examines 20 participants who take Drug X over a 10-week period. Her dependent measure is percentage body fat. She sets alpha at 0.05 and finds $t_{critical}$ at 2.101. Statistical analysis of the data leads to a t_{actual} of 2.75, $p = 0.032$. Interpret the significance and meaningfulness of these results.

2. Encouraged by the results of her previous research, the researcher plans more extensive tests on Drug X. She decides to vary the amount of the drug that different groups get, so examines three groups: a control group, a group that gets a "moderate" amount of Drug X, and a group that gets a "large" amount of Drug X. Prior to starting, she sets alpha at 0.05. Next, she randomly assigns 15 participants in each group, pretests them, gives them 10 weeks of treatment, and then posttests them. She reports her results as "$F(2, 42) = 4.31, p = 0.027$." Interpret these results.

IN-CLASS GROUP EXERCISES

1. In this exercise, your class will investigate the impact of starting body position on long jump distance. You will need tape measures and an area suitable for jumping, such as a long hallway or field. First, randomly assign classmates into one of three groups. Group one has no restrictions on their long jump. Group two must keep their arms on their waist throughout the long jump. Group three must keep their hands on their head throughout the long jump. Divide into each group, and generate data for the long jumps. Collate the data into one spreadsheet, and each group should perform a one-way ANOVA on the entire data set. As a group, discuss the results in terms of statistical significance and meaningfulness. What have you determined regarding body positions and long jumping?

2. Within a small group, discuss the covariates that may exist in the following research questions:
   - Does dynamic balance training improve balance in TBI patients?
   - Which of the three strength training protocols leads to the greatest amount of improvement in quadriceps power?

Next, design experiments that would test for group differences for these questions. Start by developing hypotheses. Discuss statistical and nonstatistical ways to account for the covariates.

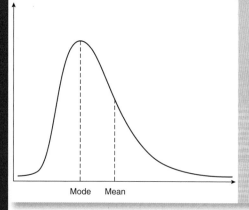

Mode   Mean

13

Nonparametric Statistical Tests

"To study the abnormal is the best way of understanding the normal"—William James

CHAPTER OUTLINE

Chi-Square
  One-Way Chi-Square
  Two-Way Chi-Square

Correlation: Spearman's Rho
  Interpreting Spearman's Rho

Differences Among Groups
  Two-Group Comparison:
    Mann–Whitney U
  More than Two-Group Comparison:
    Kruskal–Wallis One-Way ANOVA

CHAPTER OBJECTIVES

After studying this chapter, you will be able to:

1. Understand when researchers should use nonparametric statistical tests.
2. List nonparametric equivalents for common parametric statistical tests.
3. Describe two different types of chi-square tests.
4. Compare and contrast a Spearman's *rho* with a Pearson's *r* test for correlation.
5. Describe the basic elements of the Mann–Whitney U test and Kruskal–Wallis ANOVA.

■ THE statistical tests described to this point have been parametric. As we discussed in Chapter 10, in order to use parametric statistics, researchers must use data that meet three assumptions:

- The variable of interest must be normally distributed within the population.
- The variable of interest must have the same variance within samples drawn from the population.
- Scores or measures for the variable of interest must be independent.

In addition, parametric statistical tests use means and standard deviations to calculate either relationships or differences and use data that are interval or ratio. If researchers cannot meet these assumptions with their data, or if they want to collect nominal or ordinal data, do they have to rely on descriptive techniques? Fortunately, there are alternative types of statistics called **nonparametric statistics**. These statistics are distribution free, which means the data do not need to fit to a normal distribution.[1]

> **Nonparametric Statistics**
> Statistical tests that do not require the assumption of a normal distribution of the sample

Clearly, nonparametric statistics offer an alternative when one or more of the parametric assumptions cannot be met. In fact, it is tempting to consider using nonparametric tests all the time, given the diversity of data with which they can be used. However, there are some disadvantages associated with nonparametric statistics, as well. First, nonparametric tests have less statistical power, which increases the chances of deciding not to reject the null hypothesis when differences do exist. Second, fewer options exist for accessing nonparametric statistical tests with contemporary software such as IBM SPSS or SAS, which focus primarily on parametric statistics. In fact, the basic data analysis package for Excel does not include a nonparametric test (Although nonparametric statistics can be done with Excel, the process is more complicated than the Excel procedures we have presented to this point.).

If you are not sure if your sample comes from a population with a normal distribution, you should use a nonparametric test.

It is important to note that for each parametric test, a nonparametric equivalent exists (see Special Interest Box 13.1 for ways to choose between tests, and Table 13.2 for some examples of equivalent tests). We will discuss several of the more commonly used nonparametric tests, including chi-square, Spearman's rank, and Kruskal–Wallis.

✔ Check Your Understanding

1. With what types of data should someone use nonparametric statistical tests? Provide examples of each type of data.
2. What does it mean to violate the assumption of a normal distribution? How would you know if your data had violated this assumption?

SPECIAL INTEREST BOX 13.1

Choosing Between Parametric and Nonparametric Tests

The process by which researchers choose parametric versus nonparametric tests is not always straightforward. At the same time, understanding basic guidelines to help make such a choice can help with both selecting as well as critiquing other researcher's uses of specific statistics (see Table 13.1).

Here are a series of questions to ask; if answered "yes," then a nonparametric test should be used:

- Is the sample size small ($n < 10$ per group)?
- Are the data ordinal or nominal?
- Are the data presented in ranks?
- Are the data presented as a scale (such as a 5-point Likert scale)?
- Are the data presented as frequencies or percentages?
- Is the population distribution unknown?
- Is the population distribution known and not normal?

TABLE 13.1 Guidelines for Selecting Parametric or Nonparametric Statistical Tests

Assumption	Parametric	Nonparametric
Population distribution	Normal	Skewed, kurtosis, other
Variance	Equivalent per group	Any
Observation relationships	Independent	Any
Data type	Ratio, interval	Nominal, ordinal, ratio, interval

CHI-SQUARE

One of the situations for which researchers must choose a nonparametric statistic is comparison of frequencies or percentages among different categories of participants. Are the percentages observed the same or different than what we expected to observe? Chi-square offers a way in which to answer this question. Chi-square compares the expected frequency or distribution of values in the population based on chance to the observed frequency or distribution.[2]

Chi-Square Statistic used to compare frequencies

One-Way Chi-Square

Researchers use one way or goodness of fit chi-square tests when they want to determine if two or more groups differ on one variable category.

The formula for a one-way chi-square is

$$X^2 = \sum \frac{(Observed - expected)^2}{Expected}$$

Equation 13.1

For example, imagine that an athletic director (AD) at Jock University is concerned that a seemingly large number of athletes sprain their ankles on the new AstroTurf practice field, more so than on the grass practice field that had been replaced. The AD asks a researcher in the Kinesiology Department to investigate. The researcher accesses data on the numbers of sprains of all the athletes over the past 2 years (1 year on grass, 1 year on turf). The actual number of sprains is the *observed frequency* on each field. For the *expected frequency*, consider what the researcher would anticipate if there were no differences between the fields—in this case, the researcher would expect that half the sprains occurred on the grass field and half occurred on the turf field. Therefore, the researcher

TABLE 13.2 Parametric and Nonparametric Test Equivalents

Type of Comparison	Parametric Test	Nonparametric Test
Relationships among variables	Pearson Product Moment Correlation	Spearman's rho (ρ)
Differences between two independent groups	*t* test	Mann–Whitney U, chi-square
Differences between two dependent groups	Matched-pair *t* test	Wilcoxon
Differences in + 2 groups	One-way ANOVA	Kruskal–Wallis, chi-square
Repeated measures in + 2 groups	Repeated measures ANOVA	Friedman

TABLE 13.3   Data and Chi-Square Calculations for Frequency of Ankle Sprains on Grass Versus AstroTurf Fields at Jock University

	Grass	Turf	Total
Observed number of sprains	24	36	60
Expected number of sprains	30	30	60
O – E	– 6	6	
$(O - E)^2$	36	36	
$(O - E)^2/E$	1.2	1.2	2.4

divides the total number of sprains over the course of the 2 years (60) by half to get the expected number for each field (see Table 13.3). We can follow along with the procedure for hypothesis testing procedure as we did with parametric statistics:

- The null hypothesis is that ankle sprains occur at the same frequency on both of the fields—this relates to the expected results (30 on turf, 30 on grass). The researcher's directional hypothesis is that athletes sprain their ankles more frequently on AstroTurf fields than on grass fields.
- The researcher selects an alpha level = 0.05.
- Using statistical software, the researcher places the data in a spreadsheet and calculates $X^2 = 2.4$. For demonstration purposes, we will use the equation here (see Table 13.3).
- The critical X^2 is 3.84. Since 3.84 > 2.4, the researcher does not reject the null hypothesis and concludes that the fields have yielded the same frequency of ankle sprains and that any differences are due to chance.

Two-Way Chi-Square

Two-way or contingency table chi-square tests are used when two or more groups are compared on more than one category of occurrence. The **two-way chi-square** determines if some interaction exists between group and category.

Expanding on the investigation of ankle sprains on different field types offers a good example of a contingency table. The results indicated that no differences exist in the frequency of ankle sprains from one field to the next. However, the researcher suspects that the differences may occur in the frequency of more severe sprains rather than just the overall number of sprains. Therefore, the researcher breaks down the data even further, to first-, second-, and third-degree sprains. Table 13.4 shows the observed data for degrees of ankle sprains on each field:

Two-Way Chi-Square A Chi-Square where two or more groups are compared on more than one category of occurrence. Also called a contingency table

- The null hypothesis is that degrees of ankle sprain and field type are independent of each other. The researcher's directional hypothesis is that degree of ankle sprain depends on field type; AstroTurf has yielded a higher frequency of second- and third-degree sprains compared to the grass field.
- The researcher selects an alpha level = 0.05.

TABLE 13.4   Observed Data for Severity of Ankle Sprain on Each Field Type

Observed Sprain Severity	Grass Field	AstroTurf Field	Total
First degree	20	7	27
Second degree	6	13	19
Third degree	4	10	14
Total	30	30	60

TABLE 13.5   Expected Frequency of Severity of Ankle Sprain on Each Field Type

Expected Sprain Severity	Grass Field	AstroTurf Field	Total
First degree	30 × 27/60 = 13.5	30 × 27/60 = 13.5	27
Second degree	30 × 19/60 = 9.5	30 × 19/60 = 9.5	19
Third degree	30 × 14/60 = 7	30 × 14/60 = 7	14
Total	30	30	60

- Using statistical software, the researcher places the data in a spreadsheet and calculates X^2. For demonstration purposes, we will use the equation here. Table 13.5 shows the expected frequencies, which are calculated by multiplying the column total by the row total and dividing by n.

  The researcher now needs to calculate the X^2 (Table 13.6). The sum of these values results in an X^2 of 9.24:

- The critical X^2 is 5.99. Since $5.99 < 9.24$, the researcher rejects the null hypothesis and concludes that the observed degree of sprain differs between grass and AstroTurf.

✔ Check Your Understanding

1. What sort of comparisons are made when using a chi-square?
2. What is the difference between a one-way and two-way chi-square?

CORRELATION: SPEARMAN'S RHO

Spearman's Rho The nonparametric test for correlation, analogous to Pearson Product Moment correlation

To test for correlation with ordinal or nominal data, use Spearman's rho.

The nonparametric equivalent for the Pearson Product Moment correlation, r, for determining relationships between variables is called the Spearman's rank correlation or **Spearman's rho**. Spearman's rho is used when the two variables are ordinal, when one variable is ordinal and one is continuous, when both are continuous, or when the sample size is small.[1] To calculate Spearman's rho, variables need to be assigned ranks. Ranking is a simple process—simply assign "1" to the highest score, "2" to the next highest score, and so on. When two variables have the same value, the ranks are averaged. For example, if two variables are tied for the top rank, each is assigned a 1.5 $(1 + 2)/2$. If three variables tie for the third highest rank, then take the average of the ranks 3, 4, and 5, which is $(3 + 4 + 5)/3 = 4$, and assign all of them a 4 ranking.

TABLE 13.6   Two-Way Chi-Square Calculation from Data in Tables 13.4 and 13.5

Sprain Frequencies	O – E	(O – E)²	(O – E)²/E
Grass, first degree	20 – 13.5 = 6.5	42.25	3.14
Grass, second degree	6 – 9.5 = – 3.5	12.25	1.29
Grass, third degree	4 – 7 = – 3	9	0.14
AstroTurf, first degree	7 – 13.5 = – 6.5	42.25	3.14
AstroTurf, second degree	13 – 9.5 = 3.5	12.25	1.29
AstroTurf, third degree	10 – 7 = 3	9	0.14

TABLE 13.7	Hundred Meter–Sprint Data from Quad Rugby Players	
Athlete	Heart Rate	Perceived Exertion Rating
1	153	7
2	192	8
3	142	4
4	157	10
5	154	5
6	138	6
7	169	8
8	193	9
9	176	10
10	180	8

The formula for calculating Spearman's rho is

$$\rho = 1 - \frac{6\sum d_i^2}{n\left(n^2 - 1\right)}$$
Equation 13.2

where d is the difference in ranks between two paired scores and n is the number of observations.

Here is an example of the use of Spearman's rho. With a growing interest in the Paralympics and adaptive sports, a researcher became intrigued with quad rugby after watching the documentary "Murderball." The researcher was particularly interested in the intensity of effort among the quadriplegic athletes and wanted to better understand the relationship between their perceived physical exertion and their heart rates during activity. To determine perceived physical exertion, the researcher used a 10-point Likert scale, with 0 = no effort and 10 = maximum effort. Since this is an ordinal scale, Spearman's rho is the appropriate test for evaluating the association. The researcher recruited 10 players from the U.S. National Quad Rugby team to participate and had them complete a 400-m sprint around a track as fast as possible. Heart rates were monitored using Actiheart monitors. At the finish line, participants rated their exertion levels, and the researcher collected heart rate information. The following data were collected (Table 13.7):

Here is the process by which the researcher calculated Spearman's rho correlation:

- The null hypothesis was that no relationship exists between perceived physical exertion and heart rate. The directional hypothesis was that there is a positive relationship between these two variables.
- The researcher set alpha at 0.05.
- Using statistical software, the researcher calculated Spearman's rho $\rho = 0.66$. For demonstration purposes, we will calculate it here by hand. This involves taking the data from Table 13.8, ranking both columns of data, squaring the ranks, and then totaling the squared ranks using Equation 13.2:

$$\rho = 1 - 6\left(55\right)/10\left(100 - 1\right) = 0.66$$

- The critical value of ρ was 0.450. Since $0.66 > 0.450$, the researcher rejected the null hypothesis and concluded that there was a significant correlation between perceived exertion and heart rate during a 400-m sprint in quad rugby athletes.

TABLE 13.8   Ranks, Differences, and Differences Squared for Spearman's Rho Calculation of Data from Table 13.7

Athlete	Heart Rate	HR Rank	Perceived Exertion Rating	PE Rank	HR Rank— PE Rank (Difference)	Difference Squared
6	138	10	6	8	2	4
3	142	9	4	10	− 1	1
1	153	8	7	7	1	1
5	154	7	5	9	− 2	4
4	157	6	10	1.5	4.5	20.25
7	169	5	8	5	0	0
9	176	4	10	1.5	2.5	6.25
10	180	3	8	5	− 2	4
2	192	1.5	8	5	− 3.5	12.25
8	192	1.5	9	3	− 1.5	2.25
Σ = 55						

Interpreting Spearman's Rho

Fortunately for us, the interpretation of Spearman's rho is the same as for Pearson's r. If the value is positive, then we expect small values of one variable to go with small values of the other, large values of one to go with large values of the other, and for the data points on the scatter plot to go from bottom left to top right. Negative relationships are opposite of positive, and points on the scatter plot trend from top left to bottom right. Further, the value of Spearman's rho is also from − 1 to + 1, with 0 indicating no relationship and ± 1 indicating a perfect relationship. After significance is established, you can square rho to get a value of meaningfulness or strength of the association (just as with the coefficient of determination); this is interpreted the same way as r^2 is as well (refer to Table 11.4). So, in the case of the previous researcher's investigation, the $\rho = 0.66$, once squared, becomes 0.44, which indicates a moderately strong relationship. If that value is multiply by 100%, this tells us that 44% of the variance is explained by the relationship between these two variables.

✔ Check Your Understanding

1. When should a researcher use a Spearman's rho instead of a Pearson's r?
2. How would you interpret $\rho = 0.60$ versus $r = 0.60$?
3. What can be interpreted from the value $\rho = -0.90$?

DIFFERENCES AMONG GROUPS

Nonparametric tests for group differences exist that researchers use in place of parametric tests if violations to the assumptions are present or the sample size is small. We will discuss two of these tests, the Mann–Whitney U and the Kruskal–Wallace test.

Two-Group Comparison: Mann–Whitney U

It is interesting to note what ultimately became known as the **Mann–Whitney U** test for independent groups was proposed by neither Henry Mann (a mathematics professor at Ohio State University in the 1940s) or Donald Whitney (his graduate student), but originally by Gustav Deuchler in 1914, and later by Frank Wilcoxon in 1945[3] (Mann and Whitney, however, extended the statistic so that it could be used with unequal sample sizes, which greatly increased its utility[4]).

Mann–Whitney U The nonparametric equivalent of a t test, used to compare two groups

The Mann–Whitney U is a test that uses ranked data, just like Spearman's rho, and then determines if the ranks of one group are different from those of the other. With this test, all the scores are ranked across the entire sample (not just within a group).

The formula for calculating Mann–Whitney U is

$$U_A = n_a n_b + \frac{n_a(n_a + 1)}{2} - T_A$$

Equation 13.3

where T_A = the observed sum of ranks for sample A and

$$n_a n_b + \frac{n_a(n_a + 1)}{2} = \text{the maximum possible value of } T_A$$

Let's go through an example. Imagine the researcher with an interest in quad rugby wants to continue his research. During the previous study, he noted that most players used one of two different types of chairs, either an Eagle Tornado (which cost \$3,500) or a Vesco Metal Craft (VMC) rugby chair (no bargain at \$3,400). The researcher wanted to determine if 100-m sprint times differed in groups using one or the other chair. From the population of quad rugby players, the researcher recruited seven players who use the Eagle Tornado and six who used the VMC. Each player completed a 100-m sprint, which generated the following data (Table 13.9).

Here is the process by which the researcher calculated Mann–Whitney U:
- The null hypothesis was that the 100-m sprint times would not differ between the Eagle Tornado and the VMC groups. The directional hypothesis was that the groups would differ in their 100-m spring scores.
- The researcher set alpha at 0.05.

TABLE 13.9	Times in the 100-m Spring for Quad Rugby Players Using Two Different Types of Wheelchairs	
Participant Number	**Eagle Tornado**	**VMC**
1	16.23	14.98
2	19.84	19.99
3	17.98	21.88
4	21.53	18.61
5	19.48	24.33
6	18.23	17.37
7	17.66	

TABLE 13.10	Rankings of Players from Table 13.9 for Mann–Whitney U Calculation		
Eagle Tornado	**ET Rank**	**VMC**	**VMC Rank**
16.23	2	14.98	1
19.84	9	19.99	10
17.98	5	21.88	12
21.53	11	18.61	7
19.48	8	24.33	13
18.23	6	17.37	3
17.66	4		

- Using statistical software, the researcher calculated U = 25. For demonstration purposes, we will calculate it here by hand. First, we rank the data from 1 to 13, with 1 going to the fastest time across both groups (Table 13.10) using Equation 13.3:

$$U_1 = 7 \times 6 + (7(7+1)/2) - 45 = 25$$

The critical value of U is 36. Because 25 < 36, the researcher does not reject the null hypothesis and concludes that the time in the 100-m sprint is not significantly different for these two types of wheelchairs.

It may be a little hard to understand how Mann–Whitney U works, so we are going to provide another comparison to demonstrate it. The researcher wants to determine how much influence a specialized wheelchair might have on sprint performance and so has the second group use standard hospital wheelchairs instead of VMC chairs to complete the 100-m sprint. Here are the results from the second trial, as compared to the results of the first trial for the first group, followed by the ranking (see Table 13.11).

Clearly, the Eagle Tornado group had faster times than the group using the standard chairs and, therefore, higher rankings. Recalculating the U statistic, the researcher uses Equation 13.3 and finds:

TABLE 13.11	Rankings of Players Using Eagle Tornado Versus Standard Wheelchairs on the 100-m Sprint		
Eagle Tornado	**ET Rank**	**Standard Wheelchair**	**SW Rank**
16.23	1	27.32	9
19.84	6	31.04	11
17.98	3	34.28	12
21.53	7	28.98	10
19.48	5	37.25	13
18.23	4	25.01	8
17.66	2		

$$U_1 = 7 \times 6 + 7(7+1)/2 - 28 = 42$$

In this case, 42 > the critical value of 36. Therefore, the researcher rejected the null hypothesis and concluded that the groups' performance times were different.

More than Two Groups: Kruskal–Wallace One-Way ANOVA

In cases where there are more than two groups to compare, researchers can use the **Kruskal–Wallis ANOVA**, which is a nonparametric equivalent to the one-way ANOVA.[1] Just as with the Mann–Whitney U, researchers rank the data and then compare the sums of the ranks. In fact, the Kruskal–Wallis is an extension of the Mann–Whitney U. The null hypothesis states that the median values of the variable being compared across groups are equal or, in other words, that the groups are sampled from the same population. The directional hypothesis states that differences exist in the group medians, which indicates that the groups are sampled from different populations. Similar to the parametric one-way ANOVA, rejecting the null hypothesis indicates that differences exist between two of the groups, but the results of the test do not indicate where those differences exist. In this case, a multiple comparison test must be performed in order to see where the differences exist.

Kruskal–Wallis ANOVA A nonparametric equivalent to the one-way ANOVA

To this point, the statistical equations we have provided have allowed for a relatively quick computation of the statistics by hand. However, it is unlikely that students will perform a Kruskal–Wallis ANOVA without the use of statistical software or spreadsheet, so we will not include the equation here. For students taking a research methods course, probably the most important point to understand about the Kruskal–Wallis is that researchers use it as they would an ANOVA, except their data do not meet one or more of the parametric assumptions. Should students encounter a journal article where the Kruskal–Wallis is reported, they should interpret the results as they would those of an ANOVA, paying heed to the *p* value for information about significance and strength of the group differences.

✔ Check Your Understanding

1. What is the parametric equivalent to the Mann–Whitney U?
2. A researcher uses a Kruskal–Wallis ANOVA and concludes that significant differences exist among three groups with *p* = 0.045. What has the researcher determined? What remains to be determined?

CHAPTER SUMMARY

- Researchers should use a nonparametric statistical test if the assumption of normal data distribution has been violated.
- When data are ordinal or nominal, nonparametric statistical tests are required.
- Many parametric tests have nonparametric equivalents.
- Chi-square tests are used when examining frequency data.
- With a one-way chi-square test, the observed frequency is compared to the expected frequency.
- A two-way chi-square test involves comparing frequencies in two or more categories of data (e.g., gender and year in college), each of which has two or more levels (male/female and freshman/sophomore/junior/senior).
- Spearman's rho provides a measure of correlation between two groups of ranked data.

- Mann–Whitney U is the nonparametric equivalent to a t test and compares the medians of ranks of two groups.
- Kruskal–Wallis ANOVA is an extension of the Mann–Whitney U and compares more than two groups. Multiple comparisons are necessary after determination of significant differences.

REFERENCES

1. Corder GW, Foreman DI. *Nonparametric Statistics for Non-Statisticians: A Step-by-Step Approach.* Hoboken, NJ: John Wiley & Son, 2009.
2. Field AP. *Discovering Statistics Using SPSS*, 4th ed. Washington, DC: Sage, 2013:764.
3. Kruskal WH. Historical notes on the Wilcoxon unpaired two-sample test. *J Am Stat Assoc* 1957;52(279):356–360.
4. Mann H, Whitney R. On a test of whether one of two random variables is stochastically larger than the other. *Ann Math Stat* 1947;18(1):50–60.

RELATED ASSIGNMENTS

1. Using the data from Table 13.9, perform a t test. Compare and contrast the results to those of the Mann–Whitney U test. Are your conclusions the same or different?

2. Search the Internet for studies that use nonparametric statistics. Find two of each type (chi-square, Mann–Whitney U, Kruskal–Wallace). After reading these studies, determine why the authors chose to use nonparametric statistics. Create an annotated bibliography of the studies that includes this information.

IN-CLASS GROUP EXERCISES

1. Within your group, discuss specific situations where nonparametric statistics should be used. Develop details about hypothetical experiments, such as independent and dependent measures, sample size, and other aspects that would affect your decision of which statistics to use.

2. For this exercise, use chi-square to answer the question "are individuals taking a research methods course in health sciences more likely get the recommended amount of exercise than the typical population?." For this problem, we will use values from the CDC that indicate 20% of the population gets 2.5 hours of moderate to vigorous exercise each week. To get expected values, multiply the number of students in your class by 0.20. Now, survey the class, and see what percentage of students exercise this amount; this is your observed values. Create a chart like the one in Table 13.3, and use the following formula to calculate chi-square:

$$X^2 = \sum \frac{(\text{Observed} - \text{expected})^2}{\text{Expected}}$$

	Do get recommended exercise	Do not get recommended exercise	Total
Observed			
Expected	# in class × 0.02 =	# in class × 0.08 =	
O – E			
(O – E)^2			
(O – E)^2/E			

Given a critical X^2, what is your decision?

4 Measurement of Variables in Research

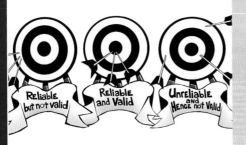

"All science is experiential; but all experience must be related back to and derives its validity from the conditions and context of consciousness in which it arises, that is, the totality of our nature."—Wilhelm Dilthey (1833 – 1911)

CHAPTER OBJECTIVES

After studying this chapter, you will be able to:

1. Define validity and describe why it is important.
2. Differentiate between logical, content, criterion, and construct validity.
3. Compare and contrast validity and reliability.
4. Explain how to determine test–rest and alternate forms reliability.
5. Describe techniques to determine internal consistency of tests.
6. Explain how two researchers can determine if they reliably rate measures the same way.
7. Understand the process of transforming different measures to standard scores.
8. Differentiate between well- and poorly designed rating scales.

■ WE have discussed the many different types of research designs as well as statistical tools to analyze data within those designs. Now, we need to consider characteristics of the variables collected as data. Even the most well-designed study can fail if the researcher does not select the most

Minimizing measurement error will improve the validity of your research findings.

appropriate dependent measures to observe. The number of instruments, tests, and tools available to measure the same phenomena may daunt novice researchers. How does a researcher know what to select? Fortunately, several criteria guide choices of variables that relate to their accuracy and consistency. These include objectivity, validity, and reliability of measures.

At the heart of measurement is error. All measurements have some error associated with them, as do tools, instruments, and equipment. One of the keys to successful research is to maximize true measurements (the actual score or value) while removing as many sources of error as possible, so that results can be attributed to independent variables. For some researchers, this means selecting the most accurate tool available on the market in which to measure dependent variables. For others, this means quantifying how well an instrument measures what it says it is measuring. Others may want to compare how well a new piece of equipment compares to the most accurate measure available. All of these are aspects of measurement of variables in health science research.

Be sure that any equipment you use provides some indication of its validity.

VALIDITY

Part of the challenge of research is matching what you want to study with the best tools to study it. A fundamentally important characteristic of a measurement tool is that it accurately measures the phenomena of interest. This point is easy to illustrate with a simple example. Imagine that a company that produces fitness DVDs has developed a specialized Zumba program that they want to market as "faster fat burning." They have hired you to quantify weight loss from their specialized 20-minute Zumba program. You design an experimental study with a control group using a standard 20-minute exercise DVD and a group following the Zumba program on DVD. You will randomly assign sedentary participants into one of the two groups and have them train three times a week for 3 months. To determine change, you will pre- and posttest them on a dependent variable that measures weight loss. You have several variables available to you. The first and easiest to collect is weight in pounds obtained from a standard scale. As convenient as a scale is, it can only provide a unit of total weight; that number does not necessary reflect what you are actually attempting to measure, which in this case is body composition. If undertaking a new program of physical activity, they may stay at the same overall weight or even gain weight after 3 months! Remaining at the same weight happens, for example, when the amount of adipose tissue lost in pounds (from expended energy) equals the amount of muscle mass gained in pounds. If you used a standard scale and discovered, after all the time put into the research, that the Zumba group actually gained weight (even though participants looked thinner), neither you nor the DVD company would be happy.

Validity The accuracy of a test, instrument, or measure

Validity is the extent to which a test or instrument measures what it is supposed to measure. For the purposes of our hypothetical study, "weight in pounds" as measured by a scale is not a valid variable because the variable of interest is not body weight, but body fat percentage (the weight of fat divided by total body weight). Body fat percentage can be measured using skinfold calipers or a BOD POD. The BOD POD is an egg-shaped chamber that measures body composition by calculating air displacement (similar to the way underwater weighing uses water displacement) to calculate body volume when a participant sits inside it. Either of these tools will allow for the valid assessment of body fat.

In Chapter 4, we discussed the notion of validity as it applied to experiments. As you recall, internal validity relates to how well the researcher has designed the experiment such that differences in dependent variables can be only attributed to manipulation of independent variables (usually improved by controlling for variables that could provide alternative explanations for observed differences). The validity of tests and measurements is an important component of internal validity because this provides evidence that the tools used to measure the dependent variables are, in fact, accurate. There are several different types of validity that can be used to establish measurement accuracy. These include nonstatistical (logical, content) and statistical types (criterion-based, construct).

Check Your Understanding

1. When a test or instrument is described as valid, what does that mean?
2. Are statistical analyses always used to establish validity?

Logical or Face Validity

In terms of establishing validity of measures, logical validity represents the weakest case, because it represents the accuracy of a tool or instrument at its face value. In other words, **logical validity** is stating a tool measures what it is supposed to measure because it seems obvious that it does. Back to our example of using a bathroom scale to measure weight. How do we know if it accurately measures weight? Because that is what a scale is for! That is taking the instrument at its face value.

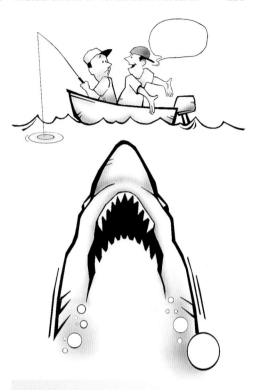

The trouble with face validity is that sometimes it isn't accurate

The issue with logical validity is that no external standard exists by which accuracy is measured. Imagine a professor assigned grades based on the number of questions a student answered in class. The professor might argue that answering questions represents content knowledge on the course subject matter and, therefore, is a valid measure of student ability.

Logical Validity A weak form of validity based on face value

There is logic behind the practice, but that logic doesn't make the measure accurate. At the very least, there would have to be some assurance that the questions posed reflected the content of the course. This is the other type of nonstatistical validity called content validity.

Content Validity

Have you ever taken a test in high school or college and wondered "Did I even attend the right class? This test has nothing to do with what we learned in lecture!" Researchers who study issues of measurement would posit that such a test lacked **content validity**. Content validity is a term that is typically used in relation to questionnaires, surveys, and tests used in educational settings. If a test has content validity, then the questions within the test accurately reflect the content that the student should have learned. All professors strive to make their tests sample accurately from the knowledge base they provide within lecture and textbooks—that is the entire purpose of a test.

Content Validity Validity based on representative sampling of content

When creating questionnaires or surveys, have an expert in that area read through the questions. They can quickly assess if the questions accurately reflect what you are trying to measure.

In order to obtain content validity, researchers must carefully develop their instruments to reflect the content under question. This can be done by creating a list of the contents and then establishing how much of the test or questionnaire should be devoted to each piece of content. These can be expressed as percentages of the test or numbers of questions per content area. Next, the test can be developed around the percentages or numbers so that the whole test reflects the appropriate proportion of content from each of the content areas, or researchers can use experts to agree that content has been correctly sampled.

An example of establishing content validity comes from Resnick and colleagues.[1] They developed the Outcome Expectations for Exercise Scale (OEE), which measured the expectations and benefits that older adults had when participating in exercise. They wanted to establish that their scale sampled the appropriate content, which in this case is the range of expectations that adults can have when exercising. The researchers established content validity of the OEE by initially reviewing the items with a group of four researchers (i.e., this article's authors) who were familiar with the issues related to motivation and exercise adherence in older adults. The four researchers agreed with the items identified and proposed some wording changes so that the measure would be better understood by an older adult. They followed this up by sending the measures to four independent experts within the field, who rated the relevancy of the items on a scale of 1 (not very relevant) to 4 (very relevant). All four reviewers rated the items as either relevant or very relevant.

In the above case, content validity was established through expertise. Although content validity is stronger than logical validity, it still lacks any quantitative standard by which to compare the measure to others. The next section discusses several types of validity exist that use statistics as a quantitative basis of comparison.

✔ Check Your Understanding

1. What is the basis of logical validity?
2. If a test is described as having content validity, what can you say about the test?

Criterion-Based Validity

The most accurate procedure for measuring a given variable is sometimes referred to as a "gold standard." This serves as the standard or criterion for measurement of this variable. For example, we mentioned the use of skinfold calipers to measure percent body fat. The most accurate current tool for measuring body composition, however, is dual-energy x-ray absorptiometry, or DXA scanning, which is the gold standard for measuring body composition (DXA is also frequently used to determine bone mineral density). In order to assess the accuracy of skinfold calipers, researchers can compare values obtained with them to those obtained via DXA scans. In general, the process of establishing criterion validity involves comparing a measure of some variable to the criterion variable. Two forms of **criterion-based validity** exist: concurrent and predictive.

Criterion-Based Validity

Comparing a measure against a "gold standard" criterion

Concurrent Validity

Positively correlating a test or measure to the "gold standard" criterion

Don't assume two pieces of equipment designed to measure the same variable are equivalent.

Concurrent validity involves comparing the new measure to the criterion standard at or close to the same time. The values of each are then statistically compared using a correlation analysis (see Chapter 11). The greater the value of r, the more accurate the new measure is considered to be.

An example of concurrent validity comes from a study where researchers compared body composition in 43 children between the ages of 9 and 11 years.[2] They examined the same children using three different techniques: DXA, skinfold thickness, and bioimpedance analysis (BIA). They performed Spearman's correlations on the data set, which resulted in the following (Table 14.1):

TABLE 14.1 Correlations among DXA, Skinfolds, and BIA	
Comparison	**_r_ Value**
DXA–BIA	0.790
DXA–skinfold	0.898
Skinfold–BIA	0.800

They concluded that the three techniques were highly correlated and therefore had concurrent validity.

Establishing concurrent validity can be very important for a researcher who wants to use a different instrument other than the gold standard. Oftentimes, the most accurate instruments are also the most expensive and time consuming to use and may require a high level of expertise to operate. If cheaper, quicker, and easier alternatives exist that yield measures nearly as accurate as the criterion, then researchers can choose them and still feel confident that their measures are valid.

Another type of criterion validity is called **predictive validity**. As the name suggests, predictive validity involves determining the accuracy of a test, equation, or instrument to predict a criterion or behavior (for an example, see Special Interest Box 12.1). To illustrate, consider the skinfold measurement discussed earlier. To calculate percentage body fat (the criterion), skinfold measurements are taken at several sites, such as the triceps, abdomen, and suprailiac crest. The best predictors were determined using multiple regression techniques, and in order to be useful as an estimate of body composition, the values calculated from resulting regression equation had to be compared to the criterion value, which in 1978 at the time of the study was a value derived from underwater weighing. In 1978, Jackson and Pollock[3] validated a predictive equation for body composition for men based on three sites (chest, abdomen, thigh), and in 1980, Jackson, Pollack, and Ward validated an equation for women[4] (triceps, suprailiac, thigh).

> **Predictive Validity** The extent to which a score, measure, or test can predict a criterion measure

Construct Validity

Within the health sciences, many variables exist that may not be directly measurable, such as motivation, fear, or quickness. These represent constructs that are hypothetical ideas or concepts that have no directly measurable form. At the same time, tests measuring motivation, fear, or quickness are used in the field, so at some point in time, their **construct validity** was established. Construct validity is the accuracy of a test or instrument at measuring a construct.

> **Construct Validity** The extent to which a test or measure correlates to a theoretical construct

Construct validity of a test can be established using the "known group difference" method. In order to use this technique, two groups of participants—one with a high value of the construct and one with a low value—are tested and statistically compared using at test. If significant differences exist, then construct validity is established. An example within the study of physical activity in older adults comes from Jones, Rikki, and Beam.[6] These researchers wanted a valid measure of lower body strength that they could use with older adults. In this case, "lower body strength" is the construct under question, with important functional consequences in an aging population. We all know what lower body strength is as a construct, but how is it measured, particularly in older adults? Jones, Rikki, and Beam developed a 30-second chair stand test as a measure of lower body strength. They established construct validity by comparing scores from a low-active group (who would have lower levels of lower body strength) to those of a high-active

SPECIAL INTEREST BOX 14.1

Predictive Validity: The NFL Scouting Combine

Have you ever noticed that players from the top 10 collegiate football teams are not necessarily the first ones drafted? Also, that many starting players in the National Football League played for lesser known Division 1-A, Division 1-AA, or even Division III schools? This is likely because of the players' performances in the National Football League's Scouting Combine—an invitation-only, 4-day test of physical and mental aptitude that occurs each year in February (http://www.nfl.com/combine). The purpose of the combine is to provide NFL scouts, coaches, and general managers a way to watch players perform in a standard setting rather than in games where their performance depends not only on themselves but on both their teammates and the opposing team. Each player performs a series of tests and receives a score based on the results; the score represents their predicted success in the NFL and is used to help teams draft appropriate players.

The tests included in the NFL Combine include seven general physical tests, such as the 40-yard dash, bench-press, and vertical jump. Players perform drills that are specific to their position as well, conduct interviews, and are screened for injuries and drugs, among other tests.

Players who may have had a sub-par college career or played for a mediocre team have a chance at increasing their odds of being drafted. But, does the NFL Combine actually predict success in the NFL? There are mixed thoughts on this. Research by Lyons, Hoffman, Michaels, and Williams[5] found that a combination of certain scores was not particularly useful in predicting NFL success and that, in fact, playing performance in college acted as a better predictor of success. Yet the NFL establishment goes through a lot of time, money, and effort to put on the NFL Combine, hosting an average of 335 players each year who are observed by about 18 franchises as well as more than 5 million others who watch it on the NFL channel. Clearly, the NFL believes in the predictive validity of the NFL Combine.

If a construct is not well defined, it will be very difficult to establish construct validity.

group (who would have higher values of lower body strength). They performed an ANOVA and determined that test scores were significantly lower for the low-active group as compared to the high-active group (Table 14.2).

Because the high-active group scored significantly higher than the low-active group, the study established construct validity for the 30-second chair stand test for older adults.

✔ Check Your Understanding

1. How do predictive and concurrent validity differ?
2. What is a construct? How does it relate to construct validity?

TABLE 14.2 Comparing High- and Low-Active Older Adults on the 30-Second Chair Stand Test				
Group	***n***	**M**	**F**	***p***
High active	144	13.3	21.9	<0.0001
Low active	46	10.8		

RELIABILITY

Imagine that you have been asked to test BIOFAT, a new, inexpensive instrument designed to measure body composition through bioelectric impedance (resistance to electric current through body tissues). You begin your analysis by trying to establish concurrent validity by correlating BIOFAT values in 40 participants to those obtained from a BOD POD (Life Measurement Instruments, Inc.). For each participant, you take three data samples from the BIOFAT in order to establish an average value of percent body fat. You test your first participant and discover that the scores on BIOFAT vary widely (24.3%, 29.8%, 18.2%). You test your second participant and get a similarly wide dispersion of scores (31.8%, 25.2%, 29.4%). What is this? You question the ability of the instrument to assess body composition in a consistent and repeatable way. That is, the tool does not reliably provide the same or similar values of percent body fat when measuring the same participant. Reliability is the ability of a test or an instrument to consistent yield the same results when measuring the same quantity. In fact, **reliability** is an essential part of validity. In order to be accurate, a tool must provide the same value of a measurement time after time. Of course, an instrument can consistently provide inaccurate scores if it is broken or calibrated incorrectly. Therefore, reliability is a necessary condition for validity, but validity is not a necessary condition for reliability.

Reliability The repeatability of a test or measure

Just because a tool provides reliable measures doesn't mean those measures are valid; the measures could be consistently too high or low.

✓ Check Your Understanding

1. What is reliability?
2. How does it differ from validity?

Stability or Test–Retest Reliability

One of the ways a test can be shown to be reliable is if test scores from 1 day are highly similar to those gotten with the same test on another day. That is, the test score is stable over time. Having stability in measures is critical for practitioners who make health-related decisions based on instrument or test scores. A physician would want to be sure that an individual's blood pressure measures are consistently high on several tests before prescribing medication. It is also important for researchers to be consistent in the measures they take.

Stability, which is also known as test–retest reliability, can be established using correlation techniques described in Chapter 11. The test under question is administered to a group of participants on day 1 and then readministered shortly thereafter on day 2 (sometimes, more retests are taken, depending on the tool). The values are then correlated, and the correlation coefficient can be used to assess test stability over day 1 and 2. One issue with measuring stability is that, if a test is administered that can be learned, test scores on the second administration can be affected. Therefore, stability reliability is generally not used in those situations.

Stability A test that consistently provides the same results on the same individuals one time to the next

As an example, it is easy to understand why practitioners would want stable measures when examining concussions. If a variable was not stable from one test to the next in an individual without a concussion, then it would be impossible to establish the severity of a concussion when it did occur. Therefore, Broglio and colleagues[7] examined stability in three different concussion tests: ImPACT, Concussion Sentinel, and Headminder Concussion Resolution Index tests. They looked at these scores on a baseline day, day 45, and day 50. They calculated interclass correlation coefficients from days 45 and 50 and found these ranged from 0.39 to 0.61 on the ImPACT, 0.39 to 0.66 on the Concussion Sentinel, and 0.03 to 0.66 on the Concussion Resolution Index. Based on these findings, they concluded that these measures had only low to moderate

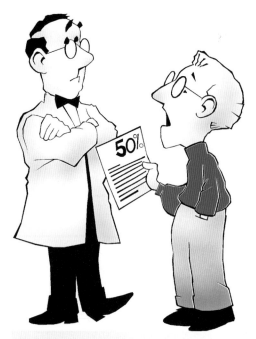

"I suspect that only 50% of the questions accurately reflect my knowledge. Perhaps you should exclude the questions I got wrong."

Equivalence Two forms of a test consistently provide same results on the same individuals

stability and concluded that these tests should be used in conjunction with other types of tests to assess concussions.

Equivalence or Alternate Forms Reliability

Another example of reliability testing relates to comparing two tests designed to measure the same constructs or material. If **equivalence** reliability is determined, the construct can be consistently measured using these two tests (or alternate forms) on two different occasions. In general, this type of reliability is used in educational research, to examine if two tests sample the same constructs.

Equivalence is established much in the same way that stability is. Test one is administered on day 1; then, test two is administered shortly thereafter on day 2. These values are correlated, and the r value is evaluated to determine if the two tests are consistent in their scores.

Imagine how hard it might be to examine the effect of an intervention or practice if the dependent measure were sensitive to that practice. It would be impossible to determine if the intervention had an effect or if the individuals got better on the posttest because of a learning effect from the pretest. Benedict and colleagues[8] acknowledged this dilemma when using the Symbol Digit Modalities Test (SDMT) and, therefore, wanted to identify valid alternate forms of the SDMT. They had 25 healthy individuals take five alternate versions of the test. They found correlations ranging from 0.77 to 0.86 and concluded that at least three of the tests could be considered good alternative forms.

 Check Your Knowledge

1. Under what circumstances would you want to establish stability?
2. If you found that two tests had low equivalency, what would that indicate?

Internal Consistency

Internal Consistency Items within a test are highly correlated to each other

As the name implies, **internal consistency** relates to the consistency of a single test. The test scores should be consistent when the test is taken again during the same day (called same day test–retest), or if different test items or trials are compared to others within the same test (called split-half). Let's say a researcher has developed a motor skills test designed to provide a "clumsiness" quotient based on 6 different items that includes two fine motor skills, two gross motor skills, and two balance skills. If the test has internal consistency based on the same day test–retest technique, then a high correlation will exist in scores obtained on two tests within the same day. Several problems may exist in establishing internal consistency this way. First, if participants can learn how to take the test better by taking the test (a practice effect), then internal consistency would be artificially high. On the other hand, if participants experience fatigue that limits their ability to repeat the test, then internal consistency would be artificially low. Therefore, the split-half technique provides an alternative way to determine this type of reliability. In this technique, the test is split in half, and the two halves are correlated. In our example, the researcher could split the skills into two sets containing one fine motor skill, one gross motor skill, and one balance skill in each and correlate them. A high correlation would indicate internal consistency of the test.

OBJECTIVITY OR INTERRATER RELIABILITY

Imagine a situation where researchers want to determine the impact of a physical education curriculum on children's motor skills. Two elementary schools are involved in the study; one serves as a control group, and the other is administered the curriculum throughout the school year. Several hundred children will be pre- and posttested on the Test of Gross Motor Development (TGMD 2)[9] by teams of research assistants at the schools. It is critical that both teams of research assistants establish that they score the TGMD in the same way. If differences exist, they could wash out or inflate the effect of the intervention. Therefore, prior to any testing, the researchers must establish **objectivity**, or interrater reliability, to show that they score the same participants the same way on the TGMD.

To calculate objectivity, two raters score the same participants on the same test, and those scores are correlated. Another measure that can be calculated is interobserver agreement. In this technique, the number of times the two

> **Objectivity** Two independent raters provide the same scores when observing the same performance

SPECIAL INTEREST BOX 14.2

Establishing Interobserver Agreement

If two raters have low interobserver agreement, they are not doomed to disagree forever. Like any skill, novice researchers can practice their observation skills. One way to improve interobserver agreement is for the raters to train with an expert, who has substantial experience using the particular observational tool or test, and points out key aspects of the test for the novices to focus on.

To use the Test of Gross Motor Development as an example, raters can watch video clips of children who perform the different test items (e.g., hopping, running, catching, dribbling) with an expert who has reliably used the instrument before. The expert can provide feedback, training, and advice on scoring, then allow the raters to score sample data, and point out where errors were made. For example, one of the locomotor items is the skill "run." This has four performance criteria that are scored as either present (1) or absent (0), which are

1. Arms move in opposition to legs and elbows bent

2. Brief period where both feet are off the ground

3. Narrow foot placement landing on heel or toe

4. Nonsupport leg bent approximately 90 degrees

The expert can show the novices how to detect a 90-degree angle and what is meant by "narrow foot placement." After a period of training, the expert randomly selects a percentage of trials from each test item (10% of the total number of trials is appropriate), and both the expert and the novice raters score them independently. These are compared using the formula described above, comparing each rater to the expert and to each other. If scores are in less than 90% agreement, the training process is repeated. Once the raters reach a 90% agreement rate, they can be satisfied they are consistently scoring the TGMD the same way.

raters agree on a score (called agreements) is divided by the total number of scores, and this number is multiplied by 100 to get a percentage of agreement. A certain representative number of trials should be observed, such as 10% of the total number of trials—these should be selected randomly from the entire sample and should represent the different sections in the test (see Special Interest Box 14.22).

✔ Check Your Knowledge

1. Why is internal consistency important in tests or questionnaires?
2. What can two researchers do if they have low interobserver objectivity?

STANDARD SCORES

Oftentimes, researchers are required to compare measures that have no basis for comparison. For example, a motor test used to determine motor deficiencies in children is called the Movement Assessment Battery for Children (MABC II)[10]; researchers may want to compare how well their participants did on the MABC II against the TGMD 2. However, each test provides a unique raw score that is not directly comparable. The MABC II is a validated, norm-referenced, and product-oriented motor assessment that quantitatively assesses motor competence in three subtests in children between the ages of 3 and 16 years. The TGMD 2 is a validated, criterion-, and norm-referenced process-oriented assessment that qualitatively assesses fundamental motor skill performance of children between the ages of 3 and 10 years.[8] In order to compare these tests, the scores have to be converted to some sort of standard score. This can be useful in many different contexts, particularly when comparing tests that include different types of test items, and systems of scoring. A commonly used standard score is called the **Z score**. Z scores relate a score to its mean and standard deviation in order to standardize it for comparison. The equation for a Z score is

Z Score A standard score that relates means to standard deviations

$$Z = X - M/s \hspace{3cm} \text{Equation 14.1}$$

where M = mean of all scores, X is the observed score, and s is the standard deviation of the distribution.

Z scores can be used to compare scores on a test to published norms. For example, Pope, Lui, and Getchell[11] wanted to compare items from the Object Control subtest of the TGMD (which includes catching, throwing, kicking, rolling, dribbling, and striking) taken from a group of Hispanic preschoolers enrolled in a Head Start program to the age norms, in order to determine if developmental delays exist in this group. In order to make this comparison, they had to convert the raw Object Control scores into Z scores and then performed a MANOVA on the data. The results indicated that the Head Start group scored significantly lower that age norms on the Object Control test.

✔ Check Your Knowledge

1. What is a standard score?
2. How is a Z score calculated?

RATING SCALES

To this point in the chapter, we have described concepts in measurement with examples such as physical function or motor skills tests or with educational, written tests. However, some researchers in the health sciences and kinesiology require an entirely different sort of measurement technique in order to measure their variables of interest, which are emotions, feelings, and sentiments, or affective behaviors. Researchers in biobehavioral health may want to know how likely individuals are to exercise in a local park. Nursing researchers may investigate the impact of phone support on feelings of engagement in a nutritional program for diabetics. A classic

Standard scores allow you to compares tests that are different in form and content.

SPECIAL INTEREST BOX 14.3

Developing an Accurate Rating Scale: Exercise, Physical Activity, and Breast Cancer Survivors

For novice researchers, accurately measuring behaviors such as exercise may seem relatively simple. However, what the novice researcher assumes to be true may not necessarily translate well for the test respondent. This true story illustrates this point rather well.

As a summer project, a group of undergraduate students at a mid-Atlantic university developed a questionnaire to examine what factors facilitated and impeded exercise and physical activity for breast cancer survivors state-wide. The students first surveyed a group of survivors and then used that survey to guide their questionnaire, which they hoped to distribute statewide. The first section of the questionnaire was designed to examine current exercise characteristics such as frequency, intensity, time, and type as compared to before diagnosis. The students developed the following series of questions:

1. How frequently do you exercise now?

Not at all	1–2 days a week	3–4 days a week	5–6 days a week	Every day

This question was designed to establish exercise frequency and was followed by a question designed to establish the types of physical activities the respondent was involved in. This question was in the form of a checklist, with 20 selections that could be made.

2. What types of physical activity are you involved in? Check all that apply:

The group of students agreed that these two questions would tell them what the respondents were doing and how often they were doing it. However, what the group assumed was that individuals outside the field of exercise science would equate the terms "exercise" and "physical activity."

They administered the questionnaire to their first respondent, who seemed to be taking a long time to answer a 15-item questionnaire. Finally, the respondent asked a simple question: How do you define "exercise"? She did not consider herself to be a person who exercised, because she did not run, bike, play sports, go to a gym, etc. However, she was physically active every day, with walking to the store, gardening, yard work, and the like. In fact, she was physically fit without ever exercising, to her knowledge. For her, the two questions were at odds with each other because they related to different constructs. The students assumed that exercise and physical activity would be perceived as equivalent in the eyes of the respondents. With a little rewording and some help from a biobehavioral health scientist, new items were developed to better define and describe exercise and physical activity.

example used by many physiologist and exercise specialists is Borg's rating of perceived exertion,[12] in which an individual engaged in physical activity provides a measure of how hard they feel they are exercising. Many other types of research use rating scales to measure how individuals feel about some aspect of health.

By their nature, affective behaviors are subjective, yet they can still be measured and compared in to each other in a standardized way by creating a rating scale. What is of paramount importance is that the rating scales accurately reflect the range of the behavior in question, and that these are placed on a continuum with specific levels that make sense to the individuals being evaluated. Therefore, the rating scale must provide specific criteria at each level, with care spent on determining the intervals between are equivalent. In Chapter 7, we introduced the topic of rating scales when we discussed Likert scales in questionnaires. Examine the example provided on page 9. Notice that there are actually two continuums within the test item. First, the questions related to outdoor activities are scaled from light (walking) to strenuous (far right column), to reflect the different types of activities in which an individual may engage in a park. This accounts for different types of activities. Within each row, individuals can select the degree to which air pollution affects each level of physical activity. Note that the descriptors range from not at all to completely, and the levels in between are calibrated so that each number in the Likert scale represents an approximately equal unit of measure.

While developing a rating scale, researchers must spend significant time determining that the scale is both valid and reliable. It is not sufficient to place a target behavior on a continuum from 1 to 5 and assume that it accurately measures the behavior.

✔ Check Your Understanding

1. When creating a Likert scale, what are some of the important considerations?
2. How do you space items on a rating scale?

CHAPTER SUMMARY

- If a test, instrument, or variable accurately measures what it is supposed to measure, it is valid.
- Just because a measure seems valid does not mean it is valid.
- Content validity can be used to ensure that tests or measures accurately reflect content.
- When a variable is measured against the gold standard for that measure, the correlation of the result is used to establish criterion validity.
- The degree to which a test or variable reflects a hypothetical construct is a measure of its construct validity.
- To be reliable, an instrument should measure the same phenomena in a consistent way.
- There are different ways to establish reliability, such as comparing the scores of a test from one time to another (stability).
- Equivalence or alternate forms reliability should be established if two different tests are being used in a pre- and posttest.
- If two halves of a test or questionnaire are highly correlated, it has internal consistency.
- When researchers use observational rating scales, they must establish that they are rating in an objective manner.
- Standard scores provide a means by which two different types of tests or scores can be compared.
- When developing rating scales, researchers must carefully calibrate their values so they are equivalently spaced.

REFERENCES

1. Resnick B, Zimmerman SI, Orwig D, et al. Outcome expectations for exercise scale: utility and psychometrics. *J Gerontol B Psychol Sci Soc Sci* 2000;55B:S352–S356.

2. Gutin B, Litaker M, Islam S, et al. Body composition measurement in 9-11 year old children by dual energy x-ray absorptiometry, skinfold thickness measures and bioimpedance analysis. *Am J Clin Nutr* 1996;63:287–292.

3. Jackson AS, Pollock ML. Generalized equations for predicting body density of men. *Br J Nutr* 1978;40: 497–504.

4. Jackson AS, Pollock ML, Ward A. Generalized equations for predicting body density of women. *Med Sci Sports Exerc* 1980;12:175–182.

5. Lyons BD, Hoffman BJ, Michel JW, et al. On the predictive efficiency of past performance and physical ability: the case of the National Football League. *Hum Perform* 2011;24:158–172.

6. Jones CJ, Rikli RE, Beam WC. A 30-second chair stand test as a reliable and valid measure of lower body strength in older adults. *Res Q Exerc Sport* 1999;70:113–119.

7. Broglio SP, Ferrara MS, Macciocchi SN, et al. Test-retest reliability of computerized concussion assessment programs. *J Athl Train* 2007;42(4):509–514.

8. Benedict RH, Duquin JA, Jurgensen S, et al. Repeated assessment of neuropsychological deficits in multiple sclerosis using the Symbol Digit Modalities Test and the MS Neuropsychological Screening Questionnaire. *Mult Scler J* 2008;14:940–946.

9. Ulrich DA. *Test of Gross Motor Development–2*. Austin, TX: Pro–Ed, 2000.

10. Henderson SE, Sugden DA, Barnett AL. *Movement Assessment Battery for Children–2*. London: Harcourt Assessment, 2007.

11. Pope M, Lui T, Getchell, N. Object control skills in Hispanic preschool children enrolled in Head Start. *Percept Mot Skills* 2011;112:1–8.

12. Borg G. *Physical Performance and Perceived Exertion. Studia Psychologica et Paedagogica. Series altera, Investigationes XI.)* Lund, Sweden: Gleerup, 1962.

RELATED ASSIGNMENTS

1. **Do an Internet search using the terms "concurrent validity" plus a specialty in health sciences (e.g., exercise science, nutrition, sports psychology). Select at least four distinct studies that interest you. Create an annotated bibliography of these studies.**

2. **Do an Internet search using the terms "standard score" plus a specialty in health sciences (e.g., exercise science, nutrition, sports psychology). Select at least four distinct studies that interest you. Create an annotated bibliography of these studies.**

IN-CLASS GROUP EXERCISES

1. **Break into four groups. Each group will determine the measurement pros and cons of a particular instrument used to calculate the same construct. Groups will need to investigate the instrument carefully using the Internet or other resources. As a class, debate what instrument should be used for data collection for each construct.**

   a. Body composition (skinfold, BMI, BOD POD, bioelectrical impedance)
   b. Cardiovascular fitness (VO_2max test, Rockport 1-mile walk test, step test, Cooper test)
   c. Strength (class determines different instruments)

15

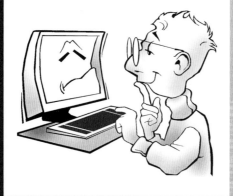

Selecting Statistical Tests within Research Designs

"I checked it very thoroughly," said the computer, "and that quite definitely is the answer. I think the problem, to be quite honest with you, is that you've never actually known what the question is."—Douglas Adams, The Hitchhiker's Guide to the Galaxy (1979)

CHAPTER OBJECTIVES

After studying this chapter, you will be able to:

1. Explain the importance of incorporating an appropriate statistical test into the design of a research study.
2. Discuss the pitfalls of not selecting the statistical procedures prior to data collection.
3. Describe the criteria to use in selecting statistical tests for descriptive research.
4. Explain how different versions of ANOVA, ANCOVA, and MANOVA are similar and different.
5. Describe the purposes of commonly used nonparametric tests.
6. Differentiate between appropriate uses of statistical tests based on numbers of independent and dependent variables, number of data collections per participant, and the underlying purpose of the study.

■ As suggested by the chapter opening figure caption, asking the right question is of paramount importance. This is especially true within the realm of research. There is a vast difference, for example, in asking whether two data sets are significantly correlated and whether they are significantly different. The first question asks about degree of sameness and the second about degree of difference. We could run statistical tests for both correlation and difference on the same data set. However, only one of these tests is likely to be useful in assessing the results of the study and determining the answer to the original research question.

With any study, the research design and included statistical procedures should be those that best shed light on the purpose of the study. Given the importance of selecting statistical methods that best fit the research design, we have dedicated this chapter to presenting strategies for doing just that. Given that we have already discussed individual statistical tests in the preceding chapters, the approach in this chapter will be a cursory review of the commonly used statistical procedures with emphasis on choosing the best statistical test to match the purpose of the study and the structure of the research design. Because of the close interrelationships between research design and statistics, understanding the matches between designs and statistics will also improve your understanding of the research process.

THE INTERRELATIONSHIPS BETWEEN DESIGNS AND STATISTICS

The research design for a study is the plan for collecting and analyzing data such that the results will best shed light on the research question or problem. The design process includes making decisions about factors such as how many groups of participants are needed, what experimental treatments will be included, how many times data will be collected, and how the data will be statistically analyzed. These decisions should be based on how to best address the research question as well as practical considerations such as participant availability, time requirements, and data collection costs.

As discussed in the previous chapters in this section, appropriate selection of statistical tests is a vitally important part of the research design process. Proper planning of a study should encompass determination of the pattern and process of data collection, as well as the related statistical methods. Serious flaws in the design of a study can result in the inability to legitimately show the kinds of comparisons or differences necessary to either confirm or refute the study's hypotheses. Design flaws can also produce a data set that is not a fit for analysis using a conventional statistical approach. An equally serious mistake would be to select a familiar statistical test and artificially design the collection of data such that they can be analyzed using that test. It is therefore essential that the determination of both the data collection design and the statistical procedures to be used for analysis of the data be made before the data are collected. There should be a clear plan for generating a data set that can be analyzed using known statistical procedures and with the results enabling confirmation or rejection of the study's hypotheses.

The Pitfalls of Not Planning the Statistical Analysis in Advance

It is not uncommon for well-meaning individuals not trained in research to launch a massive collection of data with only a vague sense of purpose with the thought that after the data are collected, a statistician can surely analyze them. Unfortunately, this is not always the case. Two such examples come to mind: certain physicians and certain teachers. Of course, there are both physicians and teachers with good knowledge of research design who would never do such a thing. The examples we present here are about the exceptions.

Day-to-day work in some professions involves the routine collection of data. Physicians, for example, collect health-related data on their patients on a daily basis. At minimum, a record of each patient appointment includes information such as age, gender, height, weight, and reason for the visit.

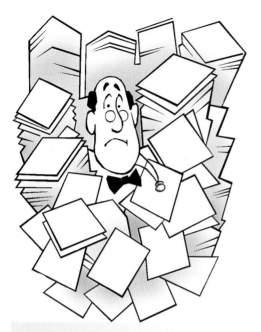

I know I can publish a paper about something.

Similarly, physical education teachers may keep records of student scores on fitness tests or skill tests. Given only the information described, there is no statistical test that can be applied to answer a question such as "What is the health status of my patients?" or "What is the fitness level of my students?" Although these individuals may develop questions after the fact, chances are they missed the opportunity to collect a useful dependent variable along the way.

With some preplanning and identification of a research design, however, a physician might randomly select a large, equal number of patients in their 20s, 30s, 40s, 50s, and 60s and do a frequency count of those presenting with flu-like symptoms. Using the nonparametric Kruskal–Wallis test, she could then determine if patients representing any decade evidenced significantly more flu symptoms than those in other decades. If the flu is a topic of interest, however, the physician might have also had her patients report additional information such as severity and duration of flu symptoms. Including this additional information in the data set could make for a much more informational study.

With preplanning, a physical education teacher could investigate the efficacy of different instructional activities on student fitness test scores if he systematically used different instructional approaches for different classes of students and then used repeated measures analysis of variance (ANOVA) to statistically analyze any differences in the fitness test scores across different classes. Additional information he might have collected to make his data set more useful includes things such as each student's fitness scores at both the beginning and end of the instructional period, each student's prior physical activity history, and other physical activities the students were engaging in outside of class.

The Pitfalls of Choosing an Inappropriate Statistical Analysis

Suppose a researcher wanted to investigate whether there is a difference in quadriceps strength gains among sedentary college women following 6 weeks of training with two different strength training protocols. A well-planned study might include the following:

- A power analysis to determine the number of participants needed in order to legitimately find a difference
- Random selection of participants meeting the study inclusion criteria
- Random division of participants into two groups
- A pretest of quadriceps strength to ensure that the two groups were equal on that measure at the beginning of the study
- Careful supervision of the participants following the two exercise protocols
- Instructions to the participants to not engage in other quadriceps exercise during the study period
- A test to assess quadriceps strength at the end of each week during the 6 weeks of the study

A graph of what the week-by-week results might look like is shown in Figure 15.1. Given the scenario described, what statistical test should the researcher choose in order to answer the research question? Reasoning that if the strength scores from the two groups are shown to have a low correlation that they must be different, suppose the researcher chooses Pearson Product Moment Correlation and comes up with an r value of 0.62. Further reasoning that this is not a very strong correlation, he

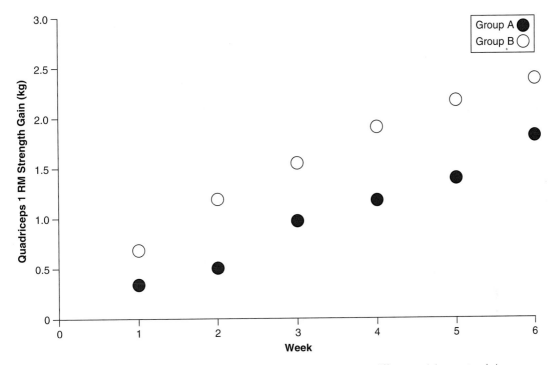

FIGURE 15.1 Graph showing gains in quadriceps strength for two groups on different training protocols in a hypothetical 6-week study.

proposes that the results of the statistical analysis show that protocol A has produced greater strength gains than protocol B. The problem here is that tests of correlation, such as the Pearson test, are designed to demonstrate the degree to which two sets of measures are the same. Pearson is not a test for difference. Having a low degree of sameness does not necessarily translate into being statistically different. To assess whether these sets of scores are statistically different, we would need to use a repeated measures ANOVA. ANOVA is the classic test for differences between groups, and the repeated measures version is appropriate here because each participant was tested a total of seven times.

If you are confused about whether a test for correlation or a test for difference is called for, take a close look at the research question or problem statement. If the word *relationship* appears in the problem statement, the appropriate test is for a correlation. If the study is to examine the *effects* of the independent variable on dependent variables, to show any effect, you would need to show a difference.

Selecting an Appropriate Statistical Test

There are many factors to consider in selecting the statistical test that best helps to analyze data collected to address a given research question. As described in the preceding section, one choice is between tests of relationship, or correlation, and tests of difference. Different research designs can also involve different numbers of participant groups, different numbers of independent and dependent variables, and different numbers of measures per participant, with each of these differences precipitating the choice of a different statistical test. At perhaps the most basic level is the difference in parametric and nonparametric data sets, with different statistical tests for each. The checklist shown in Special Interest Box 15.1 is handy for helping identify the selection of an appropriate statistical test.

SPECIAL INTEREST BOX 15.1

Narrowing Down Selection of Statistical Test

Selection of the best statistical test for a given research study can be a daunting task for novice researchers. You have just read five different chapters covering a whole host of topics related to statistics and measurement in research. Where do you start in identifying a statistical test for your own study? The following ordered checklist includes questions that, if answered correctly, can point you in the right direction.

Questions to answer in narrowing down a choice of a statistical test are as follows:

1. Are the data parametric or nonparametric? (If nonparametric, your test is likely one discussed in Chapter 13. In either case, continue on to the next question.)

2. Are you looking for a relationship or a difference? (If unsure, look at the wording of the research question carefully. Often, the word *relationship* or the word *difference* is used. Studies examining *effects* are looking for a difference.)

3. How many independent variables are involved? (Remember that the independent variables are the factors under study, while the dependent variables are being measured during the study.)

4. How many dependent variables are involved? (More than one dependent variable being measured per subject is indicative of a multivariate test.)

5. How many times is each dependent variable measured on each subject? (More than one measurement of a given variable per subject is indicative of repeated measures.)

6. How many groups of subjects are involved? (Some tests allow comparison of only two groups.)

7. Are there two or more groups in a pretest and posttest arrangement? (This may call for analysis of covariance [ANCOVA] if one dependent variable is being measured and MANCOVA if more than one dependent variable is being measured.)

For more complicated designs, it is often useful to sketch out a diagram showing D's for each data collection and T's for each treatment or intervention. This is the system used to illustrate common experimental designs in Chapter 6. A visual diagram helps to make more clear which type of design is being followed. The following sections of this chapter drill down to enable further narrowing of the selection of the optimal statistical test within a given research design.

✔ Check Your Understanding

1. Explain how research design and statistics are related.
2. Give examples of some potential pitfalls associated with poor planning for research.

SELECTING STATISTICAL TESTS FOR DESCRIPTIVE RESEARCH

As discussed in Chapter 1, descriptive research is a form of nonexperimental research because it does not involve any manipulation of independent variables by the researchers. Descriptive research, as the name suggests, is conducted to provide a detailed, useful description of the characteristics of a population, a group, or an individual. Descriptive studies may be quantitative, qualitative, or mixed methods (a combination of both).

Descriptive Statistics

Descriptive statistics, discussed in Chapter 10, include measures of central tendency—mean, median, and mode—and measures of variability, such as standard deviation and standard error of the mean. Descriptive statistics represent the most basic form of quantitative description of the characteristics of a group or an individual. It is quite common to see descriptive statistics for means and standard deviations of participant ages, heights, and weights at the beginning of the methods section in many kinds of research papers.

Correlation

A major subset of descriptive research involves use of statistical tests of correlation techniques to quantify the degree of similarity between two or more variables. As described in Chapters 10 and 11, tests of correlation can be utilized in two different ways. First, they can document relationships between variables that are positive (both variables increase together) and negative (one variable increases as the other decreases). Knowing that two variables, such as smoking and lung cancer incidence, are positively correlated is the first step in a process of demonstrating a cause–effect relationship. Second, tests of correlation can be useful for purposes of prediction. If, for example, there is a positive relationship between study time and grades in a research methods class, this would send a strong message that students who wish to achieve good grades should put in time studying. Within the field of kinesiology, use of correlation for purposes of prediction has proven to be exceptionally valuable. If a quick, simple field test yields results that correlate well with the results of an expensive, time-consuming, or difficult laboratory test, then the field test is clearly preferred under some circumstances. Examples are the various skinfold caliper tests and walk–run tests, for which results have been correlated with the much more troublesome underwater weighing and Bruce treadmill protocols, respectively.

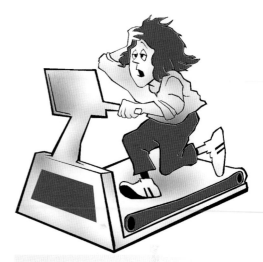

"Please come up with a test for this that I can do while painting my nails!"

Tests for Simple Correlation

Once you have determined that it is a test of correlation for purposes of description that you need to use in a given study, your selection task has been dramatically simplified. There are two commonly used tests for simple correlation between two variables: Spearman's rho is used for correlating two nonparametric data sets, and Pearson Product Moment is used for correlating two parametric data sets. Once an r value from a Spearman or Pearson test has been calculated, recall that beyond determining whether the r is significant, interpretation often involves also calculating r^2, the coefficient of determination. The coefficient of determination is an indicator of the percentage of variation in one variable that can be explained by variance in the other variable.

Tests for Regression and Multiple Regression

As discussed in Chapter 11, when the goal is use of correlation for purposes of prediction, data are plotted in an x–y-type array, with one variable on the vertical axis and the other on the horizontal

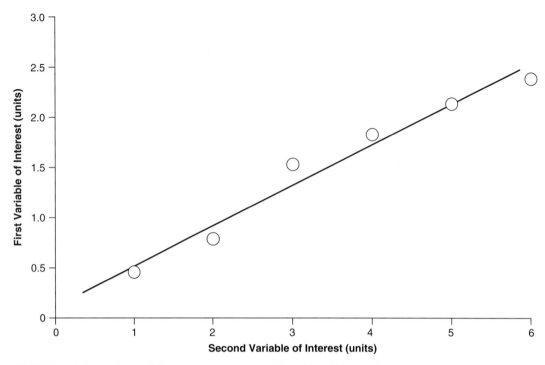

■ **FIGURE 15.2** Regression analysis involves determining a "line of best fit" to a plot of data.

axis (Fig. 15.2). Mathematical techniques enable deriving a line of best fit, which can then be used to predict a corresponding value of y when a value of x is known. Often, x is a score on a field test, such as a skinfold caliper reading, with y being body fat percentage as measured by a more sophisticated laboratory technique. The standard error of estimate then provides a quantitative value for the +/– error range associated with each prediction.

Multiple regression, also called multiple correlation, utilizes one criterion variable, or dependent variable, and two or more predictor variables, which are considered to be independent variables. Skinfold caliper assessments from multiple sites on the body can be used as the independent variables for predicting total body percentage fat using this technique. As you might expect, using more than one predictor variable generally results in greater accuracy of prediction, with smaller standard errors of estimate.

Tests for Multivariate Correlation

There are a number of procedures available for performing correlations of more than two variables simultaneously. Multiple correlation, where two or more predictor variables are correlated with a criterion variable, was just described in the preceding section. In this section, we will mention two more of the more commonly used procedures for multivariate correlation.

Canonical correlation is used to investigate the relationship between two or more independent (predictor) variables and two or more dependent (criterion) variables. For example, a researcher might conduct a study to explore which predictor variables, such as height, weight, vertical jump height, and certain strength measures, are best related to performance variables, such as speed, power, and endurance.

With factor analysis, correlations are calculated between all possible pairwise combinations of three or more measured variables that are known to be correlated. The goal is to analyze the variability among

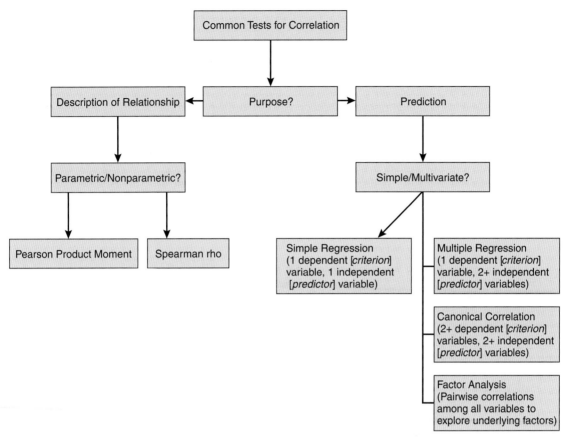

■ **FIGURE 15.3** Common tests for correlation.

these correlated variables in order to identify a smaller number of unobserved, underlying variables called factors. Figure 15.3 summarizes the common statistical tests for correlation described in this section.

Chi-Square

Chi-square is a test for use with nominal (nonparametric) data or frequency counts. It gives the researcher the ability to determine whether the number of counts for each category being observed is different from what would be expected due to either chance or a predicted number based on known information or a hypothesis. In other words, is there some reason causing the number in some observed category to be significantly different than it normally would be? Because there is no other statistical test that compares observed to expected frequency counts, it is not easy to confuse chi-square with another test. Chi-square is discussed in detail in Chapter 13.

Check Your Understanding

1. Which descriptive statistics would be important to report to characterize the academic ability of all freshman students entering a college or university?
2. What are the two purposes of correlation techniques?
3. Explain the different ways that multivariate correlations can be used.

Selecting Statistical Tests for Experimental Research

The general goal of experimental research is to ask the "why?" question, establishing or disestablishing cause–effect relationships. This typically involves investigating whether true differences exist between conditions. Sometimes, the question of interest is whether there are differences between groups, as between males and females, young and old, or trained and untrained, on some variable of interest. Another common research question is whether there are differences in a variable of interest before and after a period of time, which may include an intervention of some sort. The intervention may involve diet, training, a therapeutic drug, or a medical treatment. Some studies are designed to compare two different types of intervention, such as two different diets.

As with tests of correlation, a variety of statistical tests exist for analyzing differences. Appropriate choice of a statistical test for difference is based on whether the data are parametric or nonparametric, the numbers of independent and dependent variables, the number of different groups, the number of times each participant is tested, and the organizational pattern of interventions or treatments and periods of data collection (observations).

Univariate Tests for Differences between Two Conditions

For parametric data, the *t* test is specifically designed to test for a difference between two sets of data. There are three types of *t* test: the *t* test between a sample and a population mean, the independent *t* test between two independent samples, and the dependent or related *t* test between two sets of measures on one group of participants, typically in a pretest–posttest comparison. Within all three types of *t* test, a distinction is also made between two-tailed and one-tailed *t* tests. A one-tailed test is appropriate when it is clear before the data collection that there will be a difference between the data sets, with the only question being how large that difference will be. For example, we would expect the heights and weights of sixth grade students to be greater than those of fifth grade students. When the direction of a difference is unknown prior to analysis, the two-tailed test is selected.

When the data are nonparametric, a nonparametric test must be used in place of *t* test for analyzing a difference between two data sets. The Mann–Whitney U test is the nonparametric equivalent of the independent *t* test. The Wilcoxon test is the nonparametric version of the dependent *t* test. Figure 15.4 displays the choices to be made when selecting a test for differences between two conditions.

Univariate Tests for Differences between Two or More Conditions

ANOVA extends the purview of the *t* test to testing for differences among three or more conditions where a single dependent variable is being assessed. The term univariate implies one dependent variable. There are four different versions of ANOVA, depending on the nature of the data sets being compared.

SIMPLE ANALYSIS OF VARIANCE

Simple ANOVA can be used to evaluate differences between two or more independent sets of parametric data. It is appropriate for data sets based on one dependent variable and where only one independent variable is under study. If we wanted to look at differences in weight loss across three groups, with each group having been on a different diet for 6 months, simple ANOVA would be the test of choice. In this case, the one independent variable is diet, and the one dependent variable is weight loss. The analogous test for differences among multiple independent means with nonparametric data is the Kruskal–Wallis test.

What a simple ANOVA test yields is a single *F* value, which is then evaluated for statistical significance. Suppose the weight loss means from our weight loss study are as follows: Group A, 12 lb; Group B, 18 lb; and Group C, 22 lb (Fig. 15.5). We find that the *F* value for this comparison

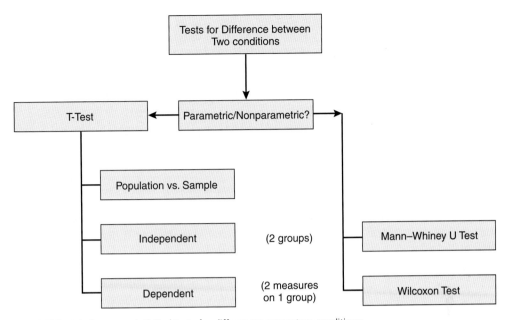

■ **FIGURE 15.4** Common statistical tests for differences across two conditions.

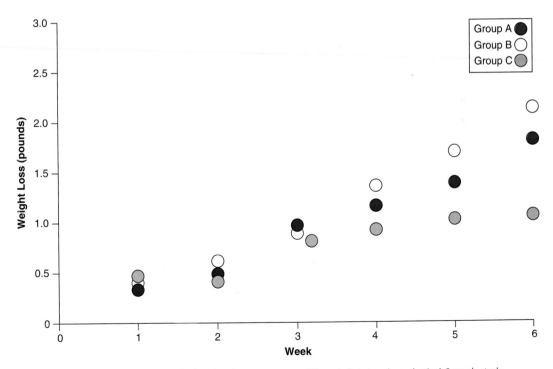

■ **FIGURE 15.5** Graph showing weight loss for three groups on different diets in a hypothetical 6-week study.

is statistically significant. This tells us that somewhere among the three group means for weight loss, there is a significant difference. We can be certain that the difference between the weight loss for Group C is greater than that for Group A, because this is the largest pairwise difference. But did Group B also lose significantly more weight than Group A? Did Group C also lose significantly more weight than Group B?

In order to answer these questions, we must run a post hoc or follow-up test. The follow-up test drills down to show exactly where all of the pairwise statistically significant differences lie. There are several commonly used post hoc tests, including Duncan, Tukey, Newman–Keuls, and Scheffé.

FACTORIAL ANALYSIS OF VARIANCE

Suppose in our study of weight loss we wanted to look at the effects of three different diets combined with the effects of a walking program as compared to no exercise. In this case, we would be studying the effects of two independent variables—diet and walking—on one dependent variable, weight loss. The appropriate statistical test for such as study is factorial analysis of variance, which enables evaluation of the effects of two or more independent variables (or factors) on one independent variable. Figure 15.6 shows the different treatments that six different groups of participants would receive. In cases such as this where there are two independent variables being simultaneously studied, the analysis is sometimes referred to as a two-way ANOVA. If there were three independent variables simultaneously under study, the analysis could be termed a three-way ANOVA.

The results of a two-way ANOVA yield three F values, including one for each independent variable and one for the interaction between the independent variables. Should the F value for diet be significant, we would once again need to use a post hoc test to determine where the differences among the three diet groups lie. In the case of exercise status, however, there are only two conditions—walking and no exercise. A significant F value for this independent variable would tell us whether there is a significant difference between these conditions or not. Should the F for interaction be significant, more follow-up tests must be run, as described in Chapter 12. The Friedman test is used for factorial ANOVA with nonparametric data.

REPEATED MEASURES ANALYSIS OF VARIANCE

For evaluation of differences involving more than one assessment per participant, repeated measures ANOVA is the test of choice. In the simplest case, pretest and posttest measures are compared on a single group of participants in a design incorporating one independent variable and one dependent variable. We could also incorporate repeated measures into our study involving three groups of dieters by measuring weigh change at the end of each month over the 6-month intervention. Any time more than two sets of measurements are being compared, a post hoc test will be necessary to further explain a significant F value. The sign test is the version of repeated measures ANOVA for nonparametric statistics.

Exercise Status	Diet		
	A	**B**	**C**
Walking	Diet A Walking	Diet B Walking	Diet C Walking
No exercise	Diet A No exercise	Diet B No exercise	Diet C No exercise

■ **FIGURE 15.6** Treatment combinations for a two-factor study with independent variables being diet and exercise status.

FACTORIAL REPEATED MEASURES ANALYSIS OF VARIANCE

When a study investigating the effects of two or more independent variables on a single dependent variable also incorporates more than one measure per participant, the required statistical test is factorial repeated measures ANOVA. If we assessed participant weight every month in our 6-month study of the combined diet and walking protocols, we would have a factorial repeated measures situation. There are a multitude of different combinations of factors and measurements for which this statistical test is appropriate. The key to analyzing the appropriate statistical test for any study involving analysis of difference on a single dependent variable, however, is that if there are two or more independent variables, the ANOVA should be factorial, and if there is more than one measurement per participant, the ANOVA should be repeated measures.

ANALYSIS OF COVARIANCE

As discussed in Chapter 12, analysis of covariance (ANCOVA) is a specialized version of ANOVA that incorporates an adjustment for a covariate. The covariate is a variable that can affect the scores on the dependent variable being assessed and, if not accounted for, skew the results. Generally, application of ANCOVA involves first making an appropriate adjustment to the data to account for the effects of the covariate and then running the appropriate version of ANOVA, be it simple, factorial, and/or repeated measures.

Multivariate Tests for Differences among Two or More Conditions

Anytime we wish to evaluate differences across two or more conditions and, in so doing, gather data on two or more dependent variables, it is likely that some version of multiple analysis of covariance (MANOVA) can be used. The four types of ANOVA and ANCOVA just discussed are all statistical analyses for data sets involving only one dependent variable. If we incorporate collection of data on two or more dependent variables, the appropriate statistical test will be the corresponding version of MANOVA. Accordingly, we have simple MANOVA, factorial MANOVA, repeated measures MANOVA, factorial repeated measures MANOVA, and all the same variations for MANCOVA.

Table 15.1 summarizes the different versions of ANOVA, ANCOVA, MANOVA, and the related nonparametric tests. Notice in Table 15.1 that when selecting a statistical test for difference, there are only a few things you need to understand about the research design. Are the data parametric or nonparametric? If the latter, you have a choice of three commonly used tests. How many independent variables are there? If only one and the data are parametric, your selection will be some version of

TABLE 15.1   Common Tests for Differences across Two or More Conditions

Characteristics	Parametric			Nonparametric
	ANOVA (1 dependent variable)	**ANCOVA (1 dependent variable, 1+ covariates)**	**MANOVA (2+ dependent variables)**	
(1 Independent variable)	Simple ANOVA	Simple ANCOVA	Simple MANOVA	Kruskal–Wallis test
(2+ Independent variables)	Factorial ANOVA	Factorial ANCOVA	Factorial MANOVA	Friedman test
(2+ Measures per participant)	Repeated measures ANOVA	Repeated measures ANCOVA	Repeated measures MANOVA	Sign test

ANOVA or ANCOVA. If there is a covariate, the selection will be a version of ANCOVA, but otherwise ANOVA. How many dependent variables are there? If more than one, your choice will be a version of MANOVA.

A special case arises when we wish to predict or discriminate across two or more levels of an independent variable based on measures of two or more dependent variables. (In our example study with diets and walking, we had three levels, or categories, of diet—A, B, and C—and two levels of exercise, walking vs. no exercise.) Discriminant analysis is the statistical test that enables discrimination between the levels of the independent variable, which is group or category membership, based on two or more dependent variables. In some countries, children with athletic ability are assessed on a variety of dependent measures such as height, weight, strength measures, quickness measures, and coordination measures to determine if they should be trained as gymnasts, track or field athletes, swimmers, etc. In this case, the independent variable might be termed athletic potential, and the levels are the different sports. Elite performers in many sports have been training since childhood.

✔ Check Your Understanding

1. Which of the statistical tests discussed in this section can be used in situations where there is one independent variable and one dependent variable?
2. Which of the statistical tests discussed in this section can be used in situations where there are two independent variables and one dependent variable?
3. Which of the statistical tests discussed in this section can be used in situations where there is one independent variable and two dependent variables?
4. Which of the statistical tests discussed in this section can be used in situations where there are more than one measurement of a dependent variable?

NAVIGATING THE SELECTION OF A STATISTICAL TEST

Selecting the appropriate statistical test is not always easy, but in this chapter, we have attempted to show that a clear understanding of the research design simplifies the task of making this decision. The sections of this chapter have focused, one at a time, on three major categories of statistical tests: tests for correlation, tests for differences in situations where there is one dependent variable, and tests for differences in situations where there are two or more dependent variables. The primary statistical tests of descriptive research are descriptive statistics and the different correlation techniques. For experimental research, there is a large array of common statistical tests depending on the numbers of independent and dependent variables, the number of repeated measures, and the experimental design. As discussed in Chapter 6, experimental design includes the ordering of treatments and observations or data collections. Table 15.2 displays the major experimental designs and associated statistical tests.

On a more basic level, selection of research design and statistical tests relate back to the original research question. As indicated in the caption to the opening figure, sometimes it's all about asking the right question. Special Interest Box 15.2 provides an example.

A good understanding of research design and statistics is rooted in understanding what might be considered the building blocks of research design:
- Levels of data (nominal, ordinal, interval, ratio)
- Independent and dependent variables
- Repeated measures
- Testing for sameness versus testing for difference
- A clear, testable research question or problem statement

TABLE 15.2 Statistical Tests Associated with Experimental Designs

Experimental Design	Arrangement	Possible Statistical Test
One shot study	T D	(none)
One group pretest–posttest	D_1 T D_2	Dependent t test
Static group comparison (two or more groups)	T D D	Independent t test
Posttest only (two or more groups)	R T D R D	ANOVA
Pretest–posttest (two or more groups)	R D_1 T_1 D_2 R D_1 D_2	Repeated measures ANOVA or ANCOVA
Solomon four group	R D_1 T D_2 R D_1 D_2 R T D R D	Factorial AONVA
Time series	D_1 D_2 D_3 D_4	Repeated measures ANOVA
Nonequivalent control group (2 or more groups)	D_1 T_1 D_2 D_1 D_2	ANCOVA
Ex post facto (T not controlled by researcher)	T_1 D T_2 D	Independent t test

Designing a Study about Performance Variables in Basketball

Suppose you are interested in better understanding some performance variables in basketball, such as practice time (PT), years playing experience (PE), free-throw shooting percentage (SP), and player height. How would you design a study and select a statistical test? As a first step, you might think about what variables are of greatest interest. Perhaps you are interested in determining what differences there are in some of these variables between skilled (varsity) and not quite so skilled (junior varsity) players. Or perhaps it would be interesting to know what differences there are between players in different positions. Recall that your research problem statement cannot be so vague as "I want to understand basketball performance." Depending on exactly what you want to determine, your research question must be specific, and it must be testable through the collection and statistical analysis of data. Here are some examples of related research questions you might ask and the associated statistical tests:

Sample Research Question/Design	Statistical Test
What is the relationship between PT and free-throw SP? (30+ subjects assessed once at end of season for PT and SP)	Pearson r
Same as above, but with 10 or fewer subjects	Spearman rho
To what extent are PT, height (H), and years PE associated with SP and playing time (YT)?	Canonical correlation
Is there a difference in SP between the varsity team and the junior varsity team?	Independent t test

SPECIAL INTEREST BOX 15.2 (*Continued*)

Is there a difference in SP between varsity players at the beginning and end of the season?	Dependent *t* test
Is there a difference in SP between three different basketball teams?	Simple ANOVA
Are there any differences in SP assessed among members of one team at pre-, mid-, and postseason?	Repeated measures ANOVA
Is there a difference in SP, PE, or H among members of one basketball team?	Simple MANOVA
Is there a difference in SP, YT, or H when these variables are assessed pre-, mid-, and postseason among members of one basketball team?	Repeated measures MANOVA
What are the effects of varsity vs. junior varsity status and forward vs. guard status on SP?	Factorial ANOVA
What are the effects of varsity vs. junior varsity status and forward vs. guard status on SP at the beginning and end of the season?	Factorial repeated measures ANOVA
What are the effects of varsity vs. junior varsity status and forward vs. guard status on SP and YT?	Factorial MANOVA
What are the effects of varsity vs. junior varsity status and forward vs. guard status on SP and YT during the first and last games of the season?	Factorial repeated measures MANOVA

The assignments and exercises at the end of this chapter are designed to review and clarify these important concepts within the context of selection of appropriate statistical tests.

✔ Check Your Understanding

1. What factors must be considered when selecting a statistical test?
2. Explain the importance of an appropriate research question or problem.
3. What are the building blocks of research design?

CHAPTER SUMMARY

- With any study, the research design and included statistical procedures should be those that best shed light on the purpose of the study.
- Appropriate selection of statistical tests is a vitally important part of the research design process.
- There are pitfalls associated with not planning the statistical analysis in advance of data collection.
- Similarly, there are pitfalls associated with choosing an inappropriate statistical analysis.
- When choosing a statistical test for descriptive research, it is important to understand whether the purpose of the study is grounded in pure description or prediction.
- When choosing a statistical test for experimental research, the choice of test is largely determined by whether the data are parametric or nonparametric, the numbers of independent and dependent variables, the number of observations per participant, and the potential presence of any confounding variables or covariates that influence the dependent measures.

- A good understanding of the building blocks of research, including levels of data, independent and dependent variables, repeated measures, and tests for sameness (correlation) versus tests for difference, is foundational for being able to select appropriate statistical tests.

RELATED ASSIGNMENTS

1. Data Levels and Statistical Tests

Directions: Identify the data level and appropriate statistical test for each of the following problem statements:

a. A researcher wishes to determine the effects of calcitonin (CA) and walking exercise (WE) on bone density in postmenopausal women. Subjects are randomly divided into four groups: CA and WE, CA only, WE only, and control. All groups are assessed for bone density at L5 after 1 year of participation in the research protocol.

Type of data (circle one):   parametric   nonparametric

Statistical test _____

b. A scientist wishes to evaluate which of the three beverages is absorbed most quickly in the stomach. A group of 60 volunteer subjects comes in to the lab on three different occasions for beverage absorption tests.

Type of data (circle one):   parametric   nonparametric

Statistical test _____

c. A physical therapist hypothesizes that female patients are more compliant with home exercise protocols than male patients. To test this hypothesis, she has each patient in her clinic over a 1-year period ($N = 172$) complete an exit survey, from which she extracts a single quantitative measure of compliance.

Type of data (circle one):   parametric   nonparametric

Statistical test _____

d. The next year, the same PT clinician/researcher decides to investigate the relationship between patient age and home exercise compliance. She uses the same compliance data extracted from the previous questionnaires along with recorded patient ages to the nearest year.

Type of data (circle one):   parametric   nonparametric

Statistical test _____

e. A PT student working in this same clinic decides that it is not meaningful to assign a quantitative score for exercise compliance. He repeats the research described in no. 10, but with all male and female patients categorized as either compliant or noncompliant, based on whether their scores were above or below 50%.

Type of data (circle one):   parametric   nonparametric

Statistical test _____

f. All graduate programs at a university evaluate undergraduate GPAs, GRE scores, and writing exam scores to determine which students to admit to each program. The English Department believes that their graduate students as a group are superior in quality to all other departments' graduate students. They use the available data to determine whether their supposition is correct.

Type of data (circle one):   parametric   nonparametric

Statistical test _____

g. An athletic training student was curious about the effects of exercise intensity and duration on increases in knee range of motion (ROM) among post–ACL reconstruction patients following a single bout of exercise. To study this, he randomly divided patients into four groups, who exercised with (a) high intensity and long duration, (b) high intensity and short duration, (c) low intensity and long duration, and (d) low intensity and short duration. All patients' knee ROMs were measured postexercise and categorized as (a) not increased, (b) slightly increased, or (c) greatly increased.

Type of data (circle one):   parametric   nonparametric

Statistical test _____

h. A clinician wishes to assess the effectiveness of exercises to improve patellar tracking in patients with chondromalacia over time. All chondromalacia patients are evaluated and categorized as having either good or poor patellar tracking during knee extension after 2, 4, 6, and 8 weeks of exercise.

Type of data (circle one):   parametric   nonparametric

Statistical test _____

i. The National Athletic Training Association decided to do a study comparing numbers academic courses required of athletic trainers, chiropractors, physical therapists, and kinesiotherapists. They surveyed a stratified sample including 10 programs of each program type to acquire this information.

Type of data (circle one):   parametric   nonparametric

Statistical test _____

j. A researcher wished to determine which of six different exercises were effective for strengthening the vastus medialis obliquus (VMO). A single group of 10 subjects performed all six exercises in random order while myoelectric activity levels in the VMO were monitored.

Type of data (circle one):   parametric   nonparametric

Statistical test _____

IN-CLASS GROUP EXERCISES

Directions: Perform each of the following exercises working within your group:

1. **Tests of Correlation and Difference for Parametric Data**

Directions: For each of the investigations described, identify (a) the independent and dependent variable(s), (b) the research design(s) employed, and (c) the appropriate statistical test to be used:

a. Researchers conduct a study to evaluate the effectiveness of Nautilus equipment as compared to free weights for the development of power in the leg muscles. They test all members of two weight training classes for vertical jump performance at the beginning of the semester. One class then trains with Nautilus equipment, while the other trains with free weights over the course of the semester. At the end of the semester, they test both classes again on vertical jump performance.

Ind. V(s). _____ Dep. V(s). _____

Design _____ Stat. Test _____

b. Ergonomists conduct a study to examine the effects of lifting speed and the amount of weight lifted during a designated lifting task. Variables measured among the ten subjects include low back muscle tension, intraabdominal pressure, and vertical ground reaction forces throughout the lifts. Three lifting speeds and three weight levels are tested, resulting in a total of nine lifting speed/weight combinations. Each subject performs nine lifts, with lifting conditions ordered randomly.

Ind. V(s). _____ Dep. V(s). _____

Design _____ Stat. Test _____

c. A researcher wishes to study the effect of training on a pogo stick on vertical jump performance. She assesses twelve subjects on vertical jump performance before and after a 10-week pogo stick training program.

Ind. V(s). _____ Dep. V(s). _____

Design _____ Stat. Test _____

d. Researchers randomly assign subjects to one of three experimental groups. Each group is administered the same amount of a different "sport beverage" at regular intervals during a controlled treadmill run. At the end of the run, subjects are assessed for subjective feelings of fatigue on a 10-point scale.

Ind. V(s). _____ Dep. V(s). _____

Design _____ Stat. Test _____

e. A researcher wishes to study the effects of a mental concentration program and free-throw practice on free-throw shooting ability in basketball. Four groups of players are randomly formed, and all players' free-throw shooting percentages are recorded. Then, during the off-season, two of the groups receive the mental concentration training (MC) program, while two groups do not (N). One MC group and one N group also practice, while the other two groups do not. The free-throw shooting percentages of the players in all four groups are then assessed over the next season.

Ind. V(s). _____ Dep. V(s). _____

Design _____ Stat. Test _____

f. A clinician wishes to assess the effectiveness of two different exercises on patellar tracking among patients with chondromalacia. Patients assigned to one physical therapist do static quad sets, and patients assigned to a second physical therapist do straight-leg raises with external femoral rotation. At the end of 3 months, all patients are evaluated and scored on a 10-point scale for proper patellar tracking during knee extension.

Ind. Var(s). _____ Dep. Var(s). _____

Design _____ Statistical Test _____

g. A purveyor of ergogenic aids wishes to compare the effects of topically applied emu oil, ostrich oil, and snake oil on muscle strength gains. He convinces the instructors of three university weight training classes to have students rub one of these oils (one oil per class) over their triceps prior to performing bench-press exercises. At the end of the semester, he assesses maximum bench-press capability across classes.

Ind. Var(s). _____ Dep. Var(s). _____

Design _____ Statistical Test _____

h. A researcher wishes to determine the effects of calcitonin (CA) and walking exercise (WE) on bone density in postmenopausal women. Subjects are randomly divided into four groups: CA and WE, CA only, WE only, and control. All groups are assessed for bone density at L5 after 1 year of participation in the research protocol.

Ind. Var(s). _____ Dep. Var(s). _____

Design _____ Statistical Test _____

i. The effect of participation in a running class on VO_2 max is studied. A group of forty subjects are matched as closely as possible on finish times for the mile run. The members of each matched pair are randomly assigned to groups. One group participates in a running class, while the other does not. Both groups' VO_2 maxs are tested at the end of the semester.

Ind. Var(s). _____ Dep. Var(s). _____

Design _____ Statistical Test _____

j. An instructor wishes to assess the relationship between time students spend studying and performance on a research methods exam. All students in a class of 12 are asked to self-report the number of hours of preparational study. These times (which are *not* normally distributed) are then correlated with scores on the exam.

Ind. Var(s). _____ Dep. Var(s). _____

Design _____ Statistical Test _____

k. A PT student was curious about the effects of exercise intensity and duration on increases in knee range of motion (ROM) among post–ACL reconstruction patients following a single bout of exercise. To study this, he randomly divided patients into four groups, who exercised with (a) high intensity and long duration, (b) high intensity and short duration, (c) low intensity and long duration, and (d) low intensity and short duration. All patients' knee ROMs were measured postexercise.

Ind. Var(s). _____ Dep. Var(s). _____

Design _____ Statistical Test _____

l. A researcher is interested in the effect of fatigue on running stride length in rats. A group of rats is run to exhaustion on rat treadmills. Every 2 minutes, a high-speed camera is turned on to enable measurement of rat stride length.

Ind. Var(s). _____ Dep. Var(s). _____

Design _____ Statistical Test _____

m. Researchers conduct a study to evaluate differences in the tension present in each of the four quadriceps during the performance of eight exercises commonly used for rehabilitation in postsurgery ACL reconstruction patients. They measure and record muscle tensions among thirty subjects, with each subject performing all eight exercises in random order.

Ind. Var(s). _____ Dep. Var(s). _____

Design _____ Statistical Test _____

2. Nonparametric Statistics

Directions: Make up an example of a research study for which use of each of the following statistical tests would be appropriate. For each example, also identify the independent and dependent variables:

a. Chi-square—test of differences in frequency data cells; can be used with one or more independent variables; Compares actual frequencies to expected frequencies

Example:

A car salesman wonders if Jeeps are more popular than Explorers, Pathfinders, or Outbacks. He stands out on the street corner by his lot 1 day for an hour and records the numbers of vehicles of each type that pass by. The expected frequency for each vehicle type would be 25% of the total if popularity levels are equal. The chi-square compares the actual frequencies with the expected frequencies to determine if Jeeps pass with significantly greater frequency. (Independent variable = vehicle popularity. Dependent variable (1) = numbers of each vehicle counted.)

Your example:

b. Spearman rank-difference correlation—test of correlation of two sets of ranked data

Example:

c. Mann–Whitney *U* test—same as the independent *t* test, but for nonparametric data

Example:

d. Wilcoxon test—used on nonparametric data in matched pairs designs

Example:

e. Kruskal–Wallis test—same as simple ANOVA, but for nonparametric data

Example:

f. Friedman test—same as factorial ANOVA, but for nonparametric data

Example:

g. Sign test—same as repeated measures ANOVA, but for nonparametric statistics

Example:

Understanding How to Effectively Propose and Report Research

Part IV

16

Preparing a Research Grant Proposal

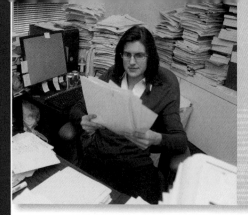

"Writing a grant application is a major undertaking."—Office of Extramural Research, National Institutes of Health

CHAPTER OUTLINE

CHAPTER OBJECTIVES

After studying this chapter, you will be able to:

1. Describe the federal organizations provide grant funding in kinesiology and health sciences.
2. Match your research to the mission of one or more of the different institutions that fund grants.
3. Differentiate between types of grant proposals requested by NIH, NSF, and DOE.
4. Compare foundation funding to federal funding agencies.
5. Create a general outline for a grant proposal
6. Develop specific aims related to a project.
7. Design a basic plan of study for a grant proposal
8. Understand the different components included in grant proposals.

■ To this point in the text, we have focused on the research process. The current chapter targets those who, by desire or necessity, want to procure grant funding. Those who plan to pursue a research career in kinesiology and the health sciences generally have to transition from mentored research to independent scholarship. At research universities, not only does this require publishing in peer-reviewed journals (see Chapter 17) but it also often includes obtaining funding in support of your research from internal and external sources. To be sure, not all research requires funding and not all researchers are required to obtain grants. Unfunded studies often serve as a foundation for future, funded projects, but can also stand alone as a high-quality research. At the same time, many academic positions request that applicants have some grant writing experience or have a fundable research line as a prerequisite for hire. Over the past decade, funding has become more competitive, which provides an additional challenge for all grant writers. However, different resources exist to help you find sources and obtain funding from grant proposals. This chapter provides an overview of different federal and foundation funding resources, along with some tips to get the novice grant writer started on writing a proposal.

Many universities have internal funding mechanisms exclusively for their own students or faculty.

Use the Internet to help locate local and regional funding sources.

IDENTIFYING A FUNDING SOURCE

A motto of many department chairs is "Any funding is good funding, particularly compared to no funding." One of the first steps in obtaining a grant is identifying the funding sources (large and small) that are appropriate for your research. Many academic institutions have internal grants of various sizes, often used as seed money to help junior faculty perform small studies that will serve as pilot work for larger grant applications. Local and regional health-related organizations fund research that serves to benefit their constituents, often targeting researchers within the state or geographic area. Different federal institutes and departments provide opportunities for financing larger-scale or more expensive projects. Many countries have federally funded granting institutions, so researchers outside the United States should check within their own countries for institutions similar to the ones listed below (see Special Interest Box 16.1 on page 8). Note that some institutions, such as the National Institutes of Health, support research grants to researchers and organizations outside of the United States.

National Institutes of Health

The most well-known funding agency within the United States for supporting research in the health sciences is the National Institutes of Health (NIH), which is a division of the U.S. Department of Health and Human Services. NIH is composed of institutes and centers (ICs), each focused on an area of research related to a specific disease or disorder (National Institute for Cancer), body system (National Eye Institute), age group (National Institute for Aging), or some other health-related characteristic (National Center for Complementary and Alternative Medicine). In all, 27 ICs exist. Each institute or center may put out a request for applications (RFAs) or researchers may submit unsolicited research applications program announcements (PAs Table 16.1 lists the different institutes and centers at the NIH. Not all of these organizations fund grant proposals all the time.)

Because several different institutes within the NIH may fit your area of research, be sure to read descriptions carefully to determine which is the most appropriate.

NIH Institutes and Centers

NIH has three different types of grant programs that are of interest to an individual researcher: the R, K, and T&F series. By far, the majority of grants provided to researchers come from the R (Research) series. R grants

NIH, while originating within the United States, frequently funds individuals and institutions from outside the country.

are organized by their purpose. For example, the R01 is the most commonly used grant mechanism and can fund longer-term, more costly grants. The R03 is the small grant program, designed for short-term projects with funding limits of $50,000 for 2 years. The R21 grant program is designed for developmental or exploratory research with high risk/high impact. The K series is designed for career development and ranges from career transition to mentored research scientist development awards. These awards can be particularly useful for new investigators and researchers interested in significantly changing their research focus at some during their careers. The T & F series is related to different fellowships and training grants. Of particular interest to students may be the Ruth L. Kirschstein National Research Service Awards (NRSA), which offers awards from undergraduate through postdoctorate levels.

The NIH does a great job of providing novice researchers with details about the grant submission process, types of funding, peer review process, and other important information. Visit the website of the Office of Extramural Research, and you will find a lot of useful information, from tips to writing the different sections to information about the peer review process. There is even a link to grants for novice investigators (see http://grants.nih.gov/grants/oer.htm for details). As we mentioned previously, NIH funds researchers both within and outside of the United States, and they note that many of their grantees have collaborators from abroad. Within the NIH, the Fogarty International Center is related to global health grants and fellowships. A variety of programs exist, ranging from pre- and postdoctoral fellowships, faculty grants, travel funding, and institutional exchanges.

TABLE 16.1   NIH Institutes and Centers

NIH Institute or Center

National Institute of Cancer (NIC)	National Institute of Biomedical Imaging and Bioengineering (NIBIB)	National Institute of Mental Health (NIMH)	John E. Fogarty International Center for Advanced Study in Health Sciences (FIC)
National Eye Institute (NEI)	Eunice Kennedy Shriver National Institute of Child Health and Human Development (NICHHD)	National Institute on Minority Health and Health Disparities (NIMHD)	National Center for Complementary and Alternative Medicine (NCCAM)
National Heart, Lung, and Blood Institute (NHLBI)	National Institute on Deafness and Other Communication Disorders (NIDCD)	National Institute of Neurological Disorders and Stroke (NINDS)	National Center for Advancing Translational Sciences (NCATS)
National Human Genome Research Institute (NHGRI)	National Institute of Diabetes and Digestive and Kidney Diseases (NIDDK)	National Institute of Nursing Research (NINR)	NIH Clinical Center (CC)
National Institute on Aging (NIA)	National Institute on Drug Abuse (NIDA)	National Library of Medicine (NLM)	
National Institute of Allergy and Infectious Disease (NIAID)	National Institute of Environmental Health Sciences (NIEHS)	Center for Information Technology (CIT)	
National Institute of Arthritis and Musculoskeletal and Skin Diseases (NIAMS)	National Institute of General Medical Sciences (NIGMS)	Center for Scientific Review (CSR)	

Department of Education

NIH is not the only federal agency that funds health-related research. Other funding agencies may not have health as their central focus but will provide funding for health-related projects that enter into their particular domain. For example, the U.S. Department of Education (DOE) provides grants for education-related projects. The Mission of the Department of Education is to "... promote student achievement and preparation for global competitiveness by fostering educational excellence and ensuring equal access." Within the DOE, some priority goals are to

- Improve outcomes for all children from birth through third grade
- Improve learning by ensuring that more students have an effective teacher
- Demonstrate progress in turning around the nation's lowest-performing schools
- Make informed decisions and improve instruction through the use of data
- Prepare all students for college and career
- Improve students' ability to afford and complete college

Within the DOE discretionary grant program, there are eight principal offices. These are included in Table 16.2

TABLE 16.2 Department of Education Offices Relevant to Kinesiology and Health Sciences

Offices	Overview of Objectives
Office of Innovation and Improvement (OII)	To support and test innovations throughout the elementary and secondary education system, in areas such as alternate routes to teaching certification, dropout prevention, and arts in education
Office of Postsecondary Education (OPE)	To improve postsecondary educational facilities and programs and to support for programs that recruit and prepare disadvantaged students for the successful completion of postsecondary education
Office of Elementary and Secondary Education (OESE)	To improve the achievement of elementary and secondary school students and to assure equal access to services leading to such improvement for all children, particularly children who are economically or educationally disadvantaged
Office of Safe and Drug-Free Schools (OSDFS)	To provide support for drug and violence prevention activities, and for projects that promote the health and well-being of students in elementary and secondary schools and institutions of higher education
Institute of Education Sciences (IES)	To support research that leads to improved academic achievement for all students and particularly for those whose education prospects are hindered by inadequate education services and conditions associated with poverty, limited English proficiency, disability, and family circumstance
Office of Special Education and Rehabilitative Services (OSERS)	To meet the needs and develop the full potential of children with disabilities through the provision of special education and early intervention programs and services
Office of English Language Acquisition, Language Enhancement, and Academic Achievement for Limited English Proficient Students (OELA)	To provide national leadership to help ensure that English language learners and immigrant students attain English proficiency and achieve academically
Office of Vocational and Adult Education (OVAE)	To improve adult education and literacy, career and technical education, and community colleges

In particular, the Office of Special Education and Rehabilitative Services (OSERS) funds projects that relate to disabilities and rehabilitation research. Some of the listings are

- Traumatic Brain Injury Model Systems
- Spinal Cord Injury Model Systems
- Disability Rehabilitation Research Projects
- Advanced Rehabilitation Research Training

More information can be found at ed.gov, which is the general website for the U.S. Department of Education, under the link for funding.

Even though you may not perform research in the area of education, you may find requests for proposals from the Department of Education that are closely aligned with your field of expertise.

Another program that has funding potential within health and physical education is Carol M. White Physical Education Program (PEP), which "… provides grants to local educational agencies, school districts, and community-based organizations to initiate, expand, or enhance PEPs that help students in kindergarten through 12th grade meet their state standards for physical education." The PEP grant program does not accept applications from students or faculty members in higher education, but frequently, community organizations or schools partner with researchers from a university in order to develop a PEP grant. Awards range from $100,000 to $750,000 per year.

National Science Foundation

The National Science Foundation (NSF) is another federal organization that funds kinesiology and health sciences research. Created in 1950, the NSF has a mission to "…promote the progress of science; [and] to advance the national health, prosperity, and welfare by supporting research and education in all fields of science and engineering" (nsf.org). With such a broad target encompassing science and engineering as well as education, researchers from many different fields can find opportunities for funding within the NSF.

The NSF has 10 different program areas, each with several different divisions. Below, Table 16.3 provides an overview of the different program areas that are most relevant to research related to health sciences.

In general, the NSF funds between 20% and 24% of the proposals it receives (e.g., in 2012, it funded 11,534 of 48,623 received). Interdisciplinary opportunities exist, as do opportunities that cross-cut different programs within NSF and a wide variety of undergraduate, graduate, and postgraduate opportunities. The NSF website can be located at nsf.gov (see Table 16.2).

Other Major Sources of Funding

Besides these major funding sources, several other well-known organizations fund research in kinesiology and health sciences. We will mention two here, although many others exist. The first is the Department of Defense (DOD), and the second is the Society for Health and Physical Education America(SHAPE America), formally American Alliance for Health, Physical Education, Recreation, and Dance (AAHPERD).

DEPARTMENT OF DEFENSE

You may be surprised to find that another substantial funding source comes from the DOD, through their Congressionally Directed Medical Research Programs (cdmrp.org). There is a broad range of programs for which funding is granted, among that are

- Autism
- Duchenne muscular dystrophy
- Lung cancer

TABLE 16.3	National Science Foundation Program Areas Related to Kinesiology and Health Sciences Research	
Program Area	**Mission**	**Divisions**
Engineering Grants	To build and strengthen a national capacity for innovation that can lead overtime to the creation of new shared wealth and a better quality of life	Chemical, Bioengineering, Environmental, and Transport Systems (CBET); Civil, Mechanical and Manufacturing Innovation (CMMI); Electrical, Communications and Cyber Systems (ECCS); Engineering Education and Centers (EEC); Emerging Frontiers in Research and Innovation (EFRI); Industrial Innovation and Partnerships (IIP)
Mathematical and Physical Sciences	To make discoveries about the Universe and the laws that govern it; to create new knowledge, materials, and instruments that promote progress across science and engineering; to prepare the next generation of scientists through research; and to share the excitement of exploring the unknown with the nation	Divisions of Astronomical Sciences, Chemistry, Materials Research, Mathematical Sciences, Physics, and the Office of Multidisciplinary Activities.
Computer and Information Science and Engineering	To develop and maintain cutting-edge national computing and information infrastructure for research and education generally and contributes to the education and training of the next generation of computer scientists and engineers	Division of Computing & Communication Foundations (CCF); the Division of Computer and Network Systems (CNS); and the Division of Information and Intelligent Systems (IIS)
Biological Sciences	To enable discoveries for understanding life. BIO-supported research advances the frontiers of biological knowledge, increases our understanding of complex systems, and provides a theoretical basis for original research in many other scientific disciplines	Biological Infrastructure (DBI); Environmental Biology (DEB); Integrative Organismal Systems (IOS); Molecular and Cellular Biosciences (MCB); Emerging Frontiers (EF)
Social, Behavioral and Economic Sciences	To build fundamental knowledge of human behavior, interaction, and social and economic systems, organizations, and institutions	Division of Behavioral and Cognitive Sciences (BCS), Division of Social and Economic Sciences (SES), and SBE Office of Multidisciplinary Activities (SMA).
Education and Human Resources	To support the development of a diverse and well-prepared workforce of scientists, technicians, engineers, mathematicians, and educators and a well-informed citizenry that has access to the ideas and tools of science and engineering. The purpose of these activities is to enhance the quality of life of all citizens and the health, prosperity, welfare, and security of the nation	Graduate Education (GE); Research on Learning in Formal and Informal Settings (DRL); Undergraduate Education (DUE); Human Resource Development (HRD)

(Continued)

TABLE 16.3	National Science Foundation Program Areas Related to Kinesiology and Health Sciences Research *(Continued)*	
Office of International Science & Engineering	To build and strengthen effective institutional partnerships throughout the global science and engineering research and education community, and it supports international collaborations in NSF's priority research areas	
Office of Cyberinfrastructure	To support the acquisition, development, and provision of state-of-the-art cyberinfrastructure resources, tools, and services essential to the conduct of the 21st century science and engineering research and education	

- Psychological health and traumatic brain injury
- Spinal cord injury
- Breast cancer

Each program area has vision and a mission. For example, the Autism program has a vision to "improve the lives of individuals with autism spectrum disorders now" and the mission to "promote innovative research that advances the understanding of autism spectrum disorders and leads to improved outcomes." This organization has made $7.08 billion in awards since 1992 (see Table 16.3).

SOCIETY FOR HEALTH AND PHYSICAL EDUCATION AMERICA (FORMALLY AMERICAN ALLIANCE FOR HEALTH, PHYSICAL EDUCATION, RECREATION, AND DANCE)

Within SHAPE America, several opportunities for funding exist. For those not familiar with this organization, their mission is to "…promote and support leadership, research, education, and best practices in the professions that support creative, healthy, and active lifestyles" (aahperd.org). There are six associations within the organization, and two of these offer funding opportunities. Note that in order to apply for these grants, individuals must be registered members of the particular associations for at least 1 year. These include the Research Consortium (RC) and the National Association for Sport and Physical Education.

The RC functions as the primary research branch of the organization. Its mission is to advance and disseminate research in physical activity and health, and its grant programs are designed to assist in the development of new scholars within these fields. The RC has two grant programs, one for early career investigators (<5 years postdoctorate) with $5,000 of funding and one for graduate students, with $3,000 of funding.

SPECIAL INTEREST BOX 16.1

Grant Funding Outside of the United States

Many different funding bodies besides the one mentioned here exist outside of the United States. Table 16.4 provides a brief list of some of these funding bodies in several different countries, with particular focus on countries that may use this textbook as a reference.

TABLE 16.4 Funding Organizations in Multiple Countries

Country	Name of the Organization	Brief Description and Link
Global	World Health Organization	Grants support a wide variety of research areas that impact global health (http://www.who.int/en/)
Australia	National Health and Medical Research Council	Grants fund development and maintenance of public and individual health standards (http://www.nhmrc.gov.au/grants)
Australia	Australia Research Council	Grants support policy and programs that advance Australian research and innovation globally and benefit the community (http://www.arc.gov.au/)
Australia	Department of Health and Aging	Grants support a variety of different health-related projects (http://www.health.gov.au)
Canada	Canadian Institutes of Health Research	Grants fund creation and translation of new scientific knowledge to improved health, more effective health services, and products (http://www.cihr-irsc.gc.ca)
Canada	Natural Sciences and Engineering Research Council of Canada: Collaborative Health Research Projects	Grants fund science and technology innovation (http://www.nserc-crsng.gc.ca)
European Union countries and collaborators	European Commission: Public Health program	Grants support activities that improve and protect human health (http://ec.europa.eu/health/programme)
New Zealand	Health Research Council	Grants fund projects to improve the health and quality of life of all New Zealanders (http://www.hrc.govt.nz/)
New Zealand	Lottery Health Research	Grants support projects that will improve the health status of New Zealanders (http://www.communitymatters.govt.nz/)
The United Kingdom	Wellcome Trust	Grants fund biomedical research and medical humanities (http://www.wellcome.ac.uk/index.htm)
The United Kingdom and Commonwealth countries	The Royal Society	Grants to recognize, promote, and support excellence in science and to encourage the development and use of science for the benefit of humanity (http://royalsociety.org/)
The United Kingdom	Medical Research Council	Grants to improve human health through world-class medical research (http://www.mrc.ac.uk/index.htm)

Since 2006, the National Association for Sport and Physical Education has a 3-year, $30,000 Research Grant Program offered once every 3 years. The purpose of this mechanism is to fund "…critical applied research issues that are related to NASPE's mission (to enhance knowledge, improve professional practice, and increase support for high-quality physical education, sport, and physical activity programs) and have the potential for significant impact on physical education, physical activity, and/or youth/school sport programs" (www.aahperd.org).

Outside the United States, there are also a considerable amount of funding opportunities. Special Interest Box 16.1 provides a short list of funding organizations in different countries.

Foundations and Other Sources of Funding

Besides funding sources from the federal government, many different foundations provide research grant related to their particular mission. Foundations are either nonprofit organizations (e.g., American Heart Association [AHA]) or charitable trusts (e.g., Robert Wood Johnson Foundation [RWJF]); both types may fund scientific or educational research (Special Interest Box 16.2). You must read through the mission of each foundation carefully, as you will need to match your research project with the philosophy, goals, and mission of the funding agency. Foundations look for proposals that support and add to their core mission and will not read proposals that are not specifically written following their overall priorities. For example, a foundation that funds research in autism spectrum disorders is the Simons Foundation Autism Research Initiative (SFARI). However, not everyone who performs research in autism fit the priorities of SFARI.

Each funding organization should have a weblink dedicated to creating a proposal in their desired format. Read these carefully and follow all instructions.

When resubmitting a grant to a new organization, remember to tailor the grant to the specifics of the new foundation.

Foundations often have very specialized missions, so write your objectives to fit their priorities.

The "SFARI's immediate priority is to drive research that benefits individuals challenged by autism spectrum disorders, but its research programs are expected to yield insights into the neural mechanisms of fundamental human capabilities, thereby complementing the foundation's work in other basic sciences" (sfari.org).

Researchers who investigate therapeutic or educational interventions would probably do better to look elsewhere for funding, as the types of grant proposals they write (and research they perform) will have more applied than basic aspects. A better foundation for potentially funding therapeutic or educational interventions would be the Organization for Autism Research (OAR), who states their priorities in the following way:

SPECIAL INTEREST BOX 16.2

Web Resources for Finding Grants and Foundations

You can search for grant funding in many different ways on the Internet. One way is to do a general search, typing in your area of research and then "grants." However, if you have tried this, you know it is not a very efficient way to search for grants, because many irrelevant Web sites will be included in the search. Fortunately, several Web sites allow you to do targeted searches and therefore are very efficient in directing you to requests for applications and proposals in your specific area of research. Here is a list of several:

1. Community of Science PIVOT (http://pivot.cos.com/)—this site may be available to you through your institution of higher education.

2. Grants.gov—this helps you navigate through the federal funding opportunities.

3. Oak Ridge Associated Universities (http://www.orau.org/)—opportunities for individuals within the 100 + Universities within the association.

4. http://foundationcenter.org/

5. Your University's Research website

By using these websites, you can quickly find information within your research area. Your own university will most likely include a place to search for grants within the website maintained by the research office. This will likely include an institutionally supported search engine like COS Pivot and other sources that faculty and students at your university frequently use.

"OAR's singular focus is in the area of applied research, which OAR defines as research that directly impacts the day-to-day quality of life of learners with autism. OAR's continuing goal is to promote practices from evidence-based research" (researchautism.org).

Some foundations have relatively vague mission statements that can be interpreted in a variety of ways. For example, RWJF (www.rwjf.org) describes their mission as follows: "Through our investments in our grantees, we seek to improve the health and health care of all Americans." As broad as this may seem, they actually accept proposals in seven specific program areas:

- Childhood Obesity
- Coverage
- Human Capital
- Pioneer
- Public Health
- Quality/Equality
- Vulnerable Populations

In other words, a grant proposal that had a well-designed study related to traumatic brain injury would not likely be funded through RWJF, because that is not one of their priorities. Examples of grant proposals that RWJF has funded in the previous year include the following:

- Improving access to affordable foods and reducing exposure to unhealthy food marketing in the Latino community to reduce childhood obesity
- Developing a culturally relevant intervention to reduce health disparities in African American women
- Examining the impact on public health outcomes of decreased spending for local health departments in North Carolina

Another important point to consider is that the written grant proposal for a foundation significantly differs from that of a federally funded proposal. Many have a preproposal process, requiring a one- to two-page letter of intent. Oftentimes, foundations will have for shorter proposals as well (three to six pages), which may focus on different aspects of the proposal than those required by DOD, DOE, NIH, or NSF. Therefore, it is not acceptable to take an unfunded grant proposal submitted elsewhere and submit it as is to a foundation; usually, substantial revisions are necessary to align the proposal with the mission of the foundation and to reformat the proposal to the specifications of the foundation.

Remember when applying for foundation grants that the granting institutions have a specific goal and will be unlikely to fund projects outside of their mission, regardless of how well written and compelling the proposed project is. With that in mind, be sure to match the proposal in clear, identifiable ways to the particulars of that mission.

Researchers should not overlook smaller grants, which can provide critical seed money to get pilot data or may be sufficient to fund an entire project. Many different sources exist, such as university-specific internal funding, discipline- or association-specific grants (e.g., Association for Applied Sport Psychology, American College of Sports Medicine), city or regional funding for specific project, or regional/state/provincial funding (2) Information about funding for graduate students can be found in Special Interest Box 16.3.

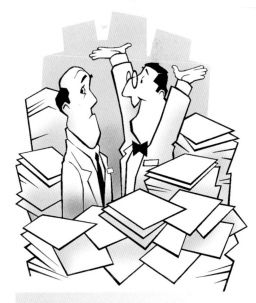

"I'm developing a grant proposal that will give me funding to write a grant proposal"

SPECIAL INTEREST BOX 16.3

Funding Opportunities for Graduate Students

In many of the organizations we have described, there are specific funding opportunities for graduate students (and even some for undergraduates). Two organizations in particular, NIH and NSF, have significant funding available specifically for graduate students.

1. NIH Ruth L. Kirschstein NRSA. There are several types of NSRA awards available. For example, the F30 award is an individual predoctoral research training fellowship designed to provide "support for promising doctoral candidates who will be performing dissertation research and training in scientific health-related fields relevant to the missions of the participating NIH Institutes and Centers (ICs) during the tenure of the award." The individual fellowship (F30) is available for MD/PhD candidates with the potential to become productive, independent, highly trained physician–scientists, and other clinician–scientists, including patient-oriented researchers in their scientific mission areas.

2. NSF Graduate Research Fellowship Program. "The program recognizes and supports outstanding graduate students who are pursuing research-based master's and doctoral degrees in fields within NSF's mission. The GRFP provides 3 years of support for the graduate education of individuals who have demonstrated their potential for significant achievements in science and engineering research."

WRITING GRANT PROPOSALS: AN OVERVIEW

The hard work begins once you have found a grant program that fits your area of research—you have to provide the funders with a compelling reason to fund your grant proposal over the hundreds of others submitted to the same place! We will provide you with an overview as well as some tips to get you started in the grant writing process; there are many different books, websites, and programs designed to help you find research funding that you should consult for more detailed information.

At the heart of a good grant proposal is a good, researchable idea for which you can make a compelling case based on the related literature, logic, and pilot data. When starting your proposal, you have several questions to which you will need to convey compelling answers, based on what reviewers want to know.[1]

- What are we going to learn as a result of the proposed project that we do not know now? (goals, aims, and outcomes)
- Why is it worth knowing? (significance)
- How will we know that the conclusions are valid? (criteria for success)
- Why are these researchers well qualified to carry out the proposed research?
- Can this research be performed in the time allotted by the researcher?

Within the body of the grant proposal, you must detail answers to these questions clearly and carefully so that the reviewers feel confident that proposed research is a good investment of research dollars.

Different granting agencies have different requirements but most have similar elements that need to be included in the grant proposal. Overall, proposals will need an abstract or summary of the project, a "specific aims" page, a plan of study, a time frame, budget and justification, and a biosketch. We will briefly go through these elements of the proposal to give some general ideas about how to approach grant writing.

Proposal Summary/Abstract

Unlike an abstract for a research paper, a grant project summary focuses not only on technical information but also on the overall impact of the grant proposal. To make matters interesting, the project summary is often restricted in length. For example, NIH stipulates that an abstract be 30 lines or less. Because of this, writing must be concise and only include the most essential elements of the proposal. Be sure to include a statement of how the proposed research fills a knowledge gap; this helps to establish the significance of the research. Also, be sure to include information about your specific aims.

Although this section comes first in the proposal order, it is often the most difficult to write. One of the issues lies in the fact that the proposal must be complete in order for a project summary to be developed. Therefore, save this section to be the last portion written before submission.

Creating Compelling Specific Aims

Given that reviewers may be reading dozens of other proposals, it is imperative that you quickly and concisely make clear the significance, innovation, and clinical relevance of your research. This occurs in a section called Specific Aims. This section is generally short (in NIH grants, this section is one page), and there are several elements that need to be clearly, concisely expressed.

First and foremost, you must grab the attention of the reviewers from the outset. The first several sentences of your proposal are critical. Remember, grant reviewers will have many proposals to read, oftentimes related to similar phenomena, so the writer must try to provide compelling data that supports the need for research and is not common knowledge. Examine this opening statement:

> "Within the United States, the number of individuals diagnosed with autism has increased at an alarming rate."

At first blush, it may appear compelling—except this information is well established in the media. Furthermore, the statement is so general, and it is unclear what the research focuses on. Contrast that with this opening statement:

> "In the United States, children with autism have almost twice the risk of obesity as their neurotypical peers."

The second statement is more compelling, in that it quickly outlines the severity of the issue (obesity in children with autism) by providing evidence of which the reviewer was likely not aware.

Arguably, the most important part of your grant is the specific aims section. This is what reviewers will read first, to get an overview of your proposal. If you do not provide a clear, compelling idea for your proposal, then they may read no further! Plan your specific aims section to be no more than one page long. Start with an introduction, which provides a rationale for the proposed research. You should provide current knowledge about the issue of interest, outline the knowledge gap that your proposed research will address, and include a statement of the clinical relevance of the research. All told, this part of the specific aims should be about a paragraph long.

Next, you need to outline the long-term goal of the research. This will indicate what your entire research agenda is for this particular issue (i.e., the big picture). Follow this with a description of your current objectives—what you want to accomplish with this specific research proposal. These are your "specific aims" for this research. Bullet point your aims, and for each specific aim, you must provide a research hypothesis. Your aims should be short, strong declarative statements, and your hypotheses should be specific. Finally, you end this section with a short discussion of

Remember the three C's of the specifics aims page: Concise, compelling, and clinically relevant.

The first one to two sentences of a grant proposal can make or break the proposal.

expected outcomes and the positive impact from the project. Again, these should reflect the clinical relevance of the research.

Because this point is so important, we will repeat it here: Write your specific aims as though that is the only page your reviewers will read. If you cannot capture their attention within that first page, you will not capture their attention at all. Have knowledgeable individuals such as professors or graduate students read your specific aims to see if your points are compelling.

Developing a Plan of Study

When you develop a plan of study, you outline the rationale for experimental procedures and provide justification for the strategies you will use as well as description of experimental controls. To begin to develop your plan of study, you need to start with the specific aims.

Within your plan of study, you must convince the reviewers that you can perform the research.

For each aim, you need to establish what you are going to accomplish. You should include an objective, the working hypothesis, rationale, and outcomes for this specific aim. This serves as an introduction to the aim. Follow this with your research design. When you write up your design, it is not possible to include all of the technical detail that you would when developing a thesis or dissertation. More importantly, include detail that is meaningful, such as the approach, critical equipment, participant numbers (with method of calculation), statistical analyses, controls within the study, and how the results will be interpreted. Further, each aim should have a section devoted to expected outcomes, and the outcomes from all of the aims should be tied together to highlight how these will contribute to the overall objectives of the research grant proposal. The final piece of the plan of study is identifying the potential problems that could occur during the study and then the alternative strategies you would take if one of these problems occurs.

One aspect of the plan of study that is important is to link what you propose to do with what you have already done in pilot studies, providing evidence that you are well qualified to complete the research. As discussed in earlier chapters, pilot studies are preliminary investigations typically conducted with a small number of participants that allow you to test your hypotheses. By providing pilot study data within a grant proposal, you demonstrate that you have the ability and means by which to complete the proposed research. Based on pilot study data, you will also be able to calculate an effect size (which will make for a more solid estimation of needed participant numbers for your proposed study). The pilot study also enables trying out your procedures, equipment and data collection techniques, and setting up your data files for statistical analysis. All of these make for better research besides making your proposal more fundable.

To help you develop a plan of study, we recommend that you visit the Research Consortium's Web site (http://www.aahperd.org/rc/toolkit/), which contains a Researcher's toolkit. Within the tool kit, you will find different e-lectures, multimedia presentations, and interactive activities designed to make your research both better and more fundable. The e-lectures have been designed by scholars within the Research Consortium who have extensive experience developing and reviewing research proposals (see Special Interest Box 16.3).

Developing a Time Frame

Your time frame is an important piece of the grant proposal puzzle. If the proposed research has an excellent rationale and methodology, but cannot be completed in the time frame set by the funding agency, then the proposal will not be funded. Within the time frame, provide different benchmarks or phases to be completed by a particular date or point in time. For example, most studies include a start-up phase, for acquisition of and training on new equipment, participant recruitment, and general

SPECIAL INTEREST BOX 16.4

Resources to Help You Develop Your Grant Proposal

Many resources exist that will help you develop a successful grant proposal. You can find resources on the internet, and many of them not only are free but come from reputable sources. For example, the NIH has an entire webpage devoted to writing NIH grant proposals (http://grants.nih.gov/grants/grants_process.htm). This provides a three-step process of planning, writing, and submitting, each with its own links containing detailed descriptions of what to do at that stage of grant proposal writing. The NIH website even has tips from experts for each section as well as a timetable for completion. NSF also has a website for preparing NSF proposals (https://www.nsf.gov/funding/preparing/).

There is practically limitless information compiled by others about the grant writing process. Most universities will have a section of their research website devoted to preparing successful grant proposals—if your university does not, you can easily check out one from another university. You should cull through this plethora of tips to find only those that inform you how to prepare grant proposals within your own interest area. Resources include webinars, e-presentations, PowerPoint presentations, and white papers, among others.

If you want a more hands on experience, you can take one of a growing number of classes or seminars designed to help you create successful grant proposals. An example of an organization that provides these and other related resources is the Grant Writers' Seminars and Workshops (http://www.grantcentral.com/), which markets books, workshops, and seminars on how to write successful NIH proposals. Similar organizations are the Grant Training Center (http://granttrainingcenter.com) and the American's Grant Writers Association (http://www.agwa.us/grantwritingworkshop).

preparation for the proposed research. The next phase is data acquisition; depending on the type of research performed, this can last a short time or throughout the entire grant period. Data reduction and analysis occur next, followed by some sort of written progress report. These phases should be reported across the time period permitted for the grant. Be sure to include any prescribed benchmarks or progress reports required by the funding agency.

Pilot studies strengthen grant proposals.

Because many grants have restrictive page limits, it is better not to write out details in sentence form but to use a table to represent progress across the time period. Two examples of time frame tables are represented in Figure 16.1A and B.

Budget and Budget Justification

Developing a budget can be a time-consuming process, because all expenses must be detailed and justified. There are generally several subsections of the budget. These include personnel (both key and other), equipment, and supplies. Different funding agencies may have different ways in which to set up the budget and justification. NIH has modular form, in which researchers can key in specific information. In general, you need to identify the expenses that are both necessary and reasonable related to your proposal.

Developing your budget will require that you gather information you may not be familiar with, particularly in relation to personnel. You may not understand the difference between indirect and direct

A

Month	1	2	3	4	5	6	7	8	9	10	11	12
Write computer code	X	X										
Create Marker Grids		X		X		X		X		X		
Intervention Training	X	X	X									
Subject Recruitment		X	X	X	X	X	X	X	X	X		
Data Collection			X	X	X	X	X	X	X	X	X	
Alogrithm Refinement				X	X	X	X	X	X	X	X	
Analysis/Reporting						X					X	X

B

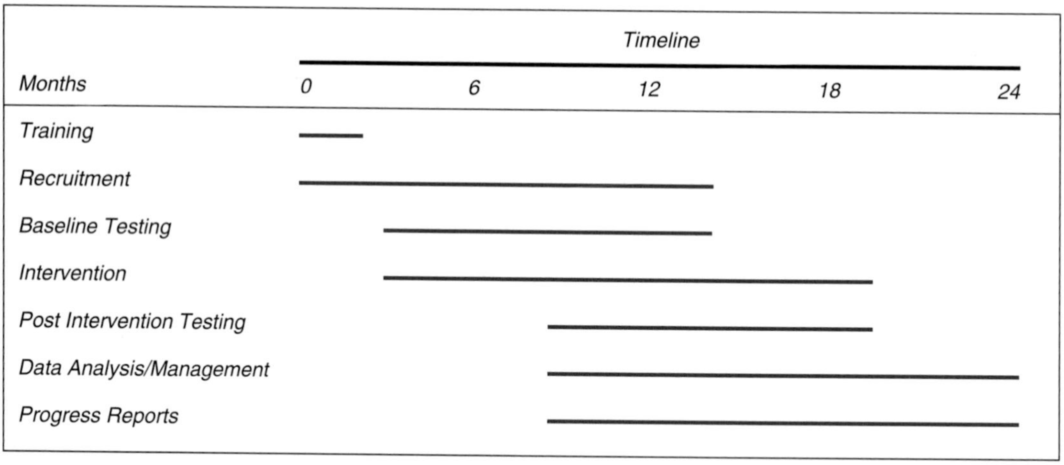

■ FIGURE 16.1 **A, B.** Two different ways of presenting a timeline.

costs or how to derive a figure for salary, including fringe benefits for a research assistant. Fortunately, most universities have resources to help both at the university and individual unit levels. A great place to start is by looking at the NIH website, which has a section on budget development (http://grants.nih.gov/grants/developing_budget.htm).

CHAPTER SUMMARY

- The first step in developing a grant proposal is identifying a funding source.
- Match the content of your research idea with the mission of specific funding organizations.
- Within the NIH, 25 different divisions exist that provide funding for health-related research.
- Different types of funding mechanisms exist within the NIH, from fellowships through different types of research grants.

- The DOE has eight different offices that fund a variety of different types of research.
- The mission of the NSF is to promote the advancement of science and to improve the nation's health. Eight of the program areas are applicable to health sciences research.
- Both the DOD and SHAPE America have research awards at a variety of funding levels.
- Private foundations offer alternatives to federal funding.
- With foundation grants, the proposal must closely match the goals and mission of the foundation.
- When developing a proposal, writers must prepare compelling specific aims.
- The specific aims section should include a rationale for study, long- and short-term goals, and specific hypotheses.
- The plan of study outlines the researchers approach in addressing the specific aims.
- When developing a plan of study, researchers should focus on meaningful rather than overly technical details.

REFERENCES

1. Przeworski A, Salomon F. *Some Candid Suggestions for Applicants to Social Science Research Council Competitions.* In: *The Art of Writing Proposals.* New York, NY: Social Science Research Council, 2004.

RELATED ASSIGNMENTS

1. **Go to the internet and type in key words related to your area of interest, followed by the word "grants." What results do you find?**

2. **Repeat this process using one of the internet search engines provided in Special Interest Box 16.2.**

3. **Go to your college or university website. Find the webpage of Research Office. What resources are available to you there?**

4. **Locate a funding source for undergraduate and/or graduate students within the DOE, NIH, or NSF.**

17

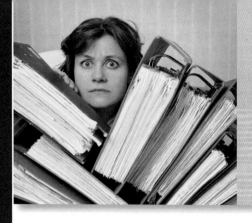

Disseminating Research Findings

"The prevailing pragmatism forced upon the academic group is that one must write something and get it into print. Situational imperatives dictate a 'publish or perish' credo within the ranks"
—L. Wilson, in the 1942 book The Academic Man: A Study in the Sociology of a Profession

CHAPTER OBJECTIVES

After studying this chapter, you will be able to:

1. Determine the scopes of different professional journals.
2. Create a list of target journals to which you might submit research manuscripts.
3. Reformat a dissertation or thesis into a journal manuscript.
4. Identify the different sections of a journal manuscript.
5. Prepare a poster presentation for a conference.
6. Prepare and present an oral presentation.

■ THE research process demands a certain level of skill in a wide variety of areas. Perhaps one of the more daunting areas is that of writing up research into a manuscript for submission to a journal. This requires that students, as authors, interpret the statistical findings and then discuss what exactly these results mean in the bigger context of the topical area. If the results

Check the scope of a journal to be sure your research fits prior to submitting your manuscript.

were unexpected, authors may have to reimmerse themselves into the literature to find explanations or debate why one explanation works better than another does. Finally, the authors must structure the entire study into a cohesive, detailed "story" within the parameters set out by the journal publisher. Publishing papers in scientific journals can be an extended process, but in the end, it is rewarding to see the fruits of many months of labor recognized as worthy by peers.

PUBLISHING PAPERS IN RESEARCH JOURNALS

Identifying an Appropriate Target Journal

Many strategies exist for identifying the most appropriate target journal for your work. One of the most important first steps is to classify the type of research you have done. Journals have a specific research focus or scope, usually detailed somewhere in the journal or on the journal's Web site, in a section labeled "Scope" or "About This Journal." You should develop a list of journals that focus on your area of research as potential targets for your manuscript. The initial step is to determine if your research fits within the scope of a specific journal; if it does not, there is no point in submitting your article there.

Let's look at an example. Suki Student's research involves a comparison of motor skills and physical activity between a group of typically developing children and children with cerebral palsy while they play outside during recess. She wants to publish the results and has heard that the journal *Medicine and Science in Sports and Exercise* has a high impact factor. She checks the Web site under "About This Journal" and reads the following:

> Medicine & Science in Sports & Exercise®features *original investigations, clinical studies, and comprehensive reviews on current topics in sports medicine and exercise science. With this leading multidisciplinary journal, exercise physiologists, physiatrists, physical therapists, team physicians, and athletic trainers get a vital exchange of information from basic and applied science, medicine, education, and allied health fields.*

The scope of the journal is broad, and Suki feels that her research *might* fit, but it is not necessarily a close fit to her research on motor skills. In fact, motor skills aren't even mentioned directly. For comparisons sake, she compares this to another journal, *Perceptual and Motor Skills*.

> ***Perceptual and Motor Skills:*** *experimental and theoretical articles dealing with perception or motor skills, especially as affected by experience; articles on general methodology; special reviews.*

Based on the described scopes of these journals, Suki decides that "Perceptual and Motor Skills" is a better fit for her work.

After formulating a list of target journals for your submission, you need to narrow your choices and ultimately decide on one. Almost all journals will require you to state that you have not concomitantly submitted your manuscript elsewhere. Be sure to discuss the choice of journals with all of your coauthors. They may be concerned with the impact factor of the journal (discussed in Chapter 3).[1] Further, they may have knowledge or experiences with a certain journal that will make it more or less desirable as an outlet for your research.

Reformatting a Thesis to Become a Manuscript

For those who have gone through the thesis or dissertation process, no doubt, it is a happy day when the final version of the work is handed off to the proper administrator, where it will be bound into a book and placed in the library. The traditional thesis format generally consists of five chapters: introduction, literature review, methodology, results, and discussion (which include conclusions); this format is lengthy, with some redundancies across chapters. Many higher education institutions have moved from the traditional format to a manuscript-type format, which more closely resembles one or more manuscripts to be submitted to a journal. In either case, the thesis process, from the initial research question through the writing up of results, with countless edits and revisions in between, can be long and grueling, and students may be tempted to put it in a drawer and forget about it. While we understand this feeling (having been through it several times ourselves), we would like to suggest an alternative: revise the thesis into a manuscript, and disseminate the information as quickly as possible.

There are several reasons why students should go through the publication process soon after finishing their tomes. First and most obviously, finishing the thesis provides momentum to write. All the time reworking different sections of the thesis is well spent—the author knows all the pieces and how they fit together. In addition, the student has culled through the extant literature, so is aware of the most current research findings in the area. If the author waits very long before preparing the manuscript, then a thorough review of literature will be required again. Furthermore, the longer the author waits to publish findings, the more likely it is that someone else will have performed a similar study and published the results, lowering the impact (and the likelihood of acceptance) of the original research. Many a good thesis has languished on the library bookshelf, never to be published. Yet, when a thesis has been approved, a good portion of the work necessary for creating a manuscript has already been completed. In fact, if the thesis originally was created in manuscript format, then the need for revision may be substantially reduced.

Do not wait too long to publish your thesis or dissertation; work on it while everything is fresh in your mind.

Manuscript writing requires efficiency of expression.

There are several steps necessary for reformatting a thesis or dissertation to be a manuscript. The primary difference between student research and that published in journals is the scale of the document. Professors often require detailed rationales for the methodology and development of hypotheses and want the student to demonstrate expertise in the topic area within the thesis. The result is bulk: theses are often more than 50 pages, and dissertations may top 100 pages. Journals, on the other hand, often limit the number of written pages to around 20 for a manuscript submission, with additional pages for figures and tables. This means that information from the theses or dissertation must be scaled back and concisely written to meet the page limits of the journal. In fact, dissertations may include more than one (and often multiple) study, which may or may not be appropriate for individual manuscripts. Typically, the authors scale back the literature review considerably, so that it includes only the most relevant and directly related literature as part of the rationale for the study in the introduction. The methodology should be concise but contain enough detail to provide an overview of the participants, procedure, instrumentation, and statistical methods. Authors may be able to describe participants succinctly using demographic tables. If instruments or procedures have been used in other publications, the author may be able to refer to that publication rather than redescribing it. Results may be used in their entirety, as long

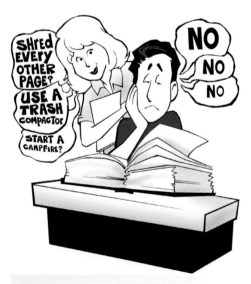

Alternative ways of making a dissertation more compact for publication.

as extraneous detail (such as a discussion of the results) is removed. Be sure to limit the discussion to exploring explanations for the results from the literature, rather than a lengthy recap of the results. In short, cut back wherever possible! However, cutting is easier than creating original works, so do not hesitate to submit the newly remastered product for publication in a journal.

Writing Specific Sections of the Manuscript

The specific sections of a manuscript most often include an abstract, introduction, methodology, results, discussion, and conclusions. We have discussed how to create a literature review (which will result in the bulk of the introduction) as well as developing a methodology earlier in this text. We will cover these sections briefly here starting with the introduction. We will focus more deeply on how to report and interpret results for publication—these come in different forms in the abstract, results, discussion, and conclusions.

INTRODUCTION

The introduction provides rationale for the research study as well as a logical lead up to the statement of the problem and research hypothesis. The first two to three sentences are critical for engaging a reader. The first sentence introduces the topical area. Then, the next one to two sentences should compellingly introduce the problem/question area. The remainder of the introduction fleshes out the rationale and leads the reader down the path to understanding exactly why it is important that this particular study was conducted within the context of the problem area. The rationale often explains how the study may address a gap in the literature, replicate another body of research using a different population, or extend an existing line of research. All of this is written using the most recent or supportive literature in the field. The introduction should end with a statement of the research problem or question, followed by one or more specific research hypotheses.

METHODOLOGY

We refer you back to Chapter 4, where we discussed how to develop and write methods in greater detail. There are several important features of writing a methodology that journal reviewers will carefully consider. First, the methodology should be specific enough so that another researcher can successfully replicate the study with little difficulty. This means that as many pertinent details as possible should be included. This could include photos or schematics of devices, test items, and instrumentation details among other details (these are highly field dependent). Second, this section should provide a holistic overview of the entire research process, without glossing over important details.

Generally, the methodology opens with a "participants" section. Be sure to specifically state that all of your participants signed an informed consent/assent and that your institution's IRB approved your research. In doing so, be sure to maintain your participants' anonymity, so do not disclose information that could provide readers with any more than a general knowledge of where they were recruited, their demographics, etc. Provide important group demographics, particularly information that will influence the interpretation of your findings. For example, researchers often report the number of participants of each gender, height, weight, age, and other pertinent information.

The rest of the sections within the methodology may vary, depending on the research field. What is important within all methods sections is that authors establish that valid, reliable equipment, instruments, or tests were used; values for validity

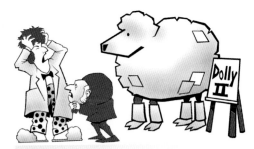

"I said 'Replicate', not 'Replicant'!"

and reliability should be reported where possible. In addition, a clear description of the experimental design and research protocol should be provided. Finally, a detailed description of the statistical analysis is necessary. This should include important details such as the statistical tests used, alpha levels, or any other relevant details.

RESULTS

The results section reflects the hard work you put into your research and represents what you have added to the existing literature in your area of study. All other sections may be compelling, but ultimately, the value of your research comes down to the results. Anyone who has acted as a reviewer of manuscripts can tell you that the results section can make or break a submission. It is therefore surprising that authors often appear to spend little thought on the organization and presentation of the results. Approach this section carefully, with an eye toward making it effectively communicate your findings in a concise manner.

There is no single way to organize the results section, so you will need to consider how to best organize the presentation of results for clarity. You may want to discuss the outcomes in terms of dependent measures, particularly if you have more than one. If the most important aspect of the study is a comparison of groups who have different characteristics, then present the results to highlight that. You may also want to discuss the results as a function of the different independent variables. For example, if the purpose of the research was to examine the stability of gait before and after training in individuals

A researcher reading the methodology should be able to replicate the study.

with mild and moderate cerebral palsy, the results could be structured in several ways. The first could be to describe differences in pre- and posttests in both of the groups, with section headers of *pretest gait stability* and *posttest gait stability*. Another way to structure the results would be to focus on the groups, so that the section headers would be *changes in mild CP group* and *changes in moderate CP group*. The first headers emphasize intervention changes and the second emphasize differences between the groups.

In experimental research, most results sections start by presenting the statistically significant results of the research. These are presented using the specific rules adopted by the specific editorial style (see Chapter 2 for more information on editorial styles). The results should provide information about the statistic used and its value, along with the p value. Table 17.1 provides some examples of unacceptable result reports and acceptable alternatives. Be sure to take note of any special characteristics of statistical copy, such as italicizing or underlying the statistic.

TABLE 17.1 Acceptable and unacceptable descriptions of results

Unacceptable	Acceptable
"The experimental group significantly differed from the control group in VO_2max"	"The experimental group had a significantly higher VO_2max ($F (1, 28) = 4.39, p = 0.002$"
"There was a significant main effect and a significant interaction"	"There was a significant main effect for group ($p = 0.003$), and one significant interaction between group and trial number (0.024)"
"The correlation was very significant at $r = 0.89$"	"There was a significant positive correlation between strength and training time ($r = 0.89, p < 0.05$)"

DISCUSSION AND CONCLUSIONS

The discussion section is deceptively difficult to write. It is difficult in one sense, because there is no formula for writing a discussion section. Your results may confirm the results of previously published research or not. You may have anticipated your results, based on the original research hypotheses, or your results may have surprised you. Notably, some of the most significant, landmark studies are among those that have resulted in surprising findings. In all cases, it is here in the Discussion section that the authors have the ability to make a case for why their findings are important in some way and at minimum, to hypothesize as to why their results turned out as they did.

While an abstract should provide an accurate synopsis of the manuscript, it should not be a "cut-and-paste" job from the text.

One of the frequent reasons that reviewers reject manuscripts for publication is that the discussion and conclusions overreach the scope of the study. That is, the authors over generalize the results of the study to a larger population beyond the scope of the study participants or overstate the impact of the research (given a small sample or effect size). That is, the study may lack the external validity that the researchers assert. It is usually a mistake to try to describe far-reaching implications for treatment, teaching, or training based on the results of a single study. Authors need to refrain from excessive speculation, and stick to what the data say.

The results section should reflect the overall hypotheses of the research.

This is a good segue for the next section within the discussion, which is "limitations of the research." Every experiment has limitations. As an author, you can identify your limitations or you can wait for the reviewers to do it for you. We recommend the former strategy, as it shows that authors have reflected on the results and can identify the real impact that their work has, given the inherent shortcomings of research. Finally, the last piece of information that fits into the discussion is an overview of suggestions for future research on the study topic. Suggested future research should build on the evidence provided in the current study. Authors should outline future studies in detail rather than with vague phrases such as "more research on the topic is necessary." The future directions may include new studies that avoid or overcome the limitations of the current research. Many novice researchers use this section to restate the finding of the study, which is not the purpose of the discussion. You may begin with a brief recap of the outcomes of the study, but only as they pertain to the hypothesis; in other words, indicate if the results supported the hypothesis or not. The bulk of the discussion should go beyond the current study and explore how the results fit into the extant literature. It is common to read about how the results of the study either confirm or refute the results of similar previous studies. If your results are different from those of similar studies, the discussion section is the place to point this out and offer some proposed explanation. Discuss the results in relation to relevant worldviews, perspectives, or theories. Do the results support or refute contemporary theory? Surprising results that go against hypotheses should be considered from alternative theoretical points of view. Support for the hypotheses should be discussed in terms of their implications for theory or practice.

Be careful not to over reach the results when making your conclusions.

Following the discussion is a short section titled "conclusions." Many students seem to think that conclusions and summary are synonymous. In fact, they are not! Conclusions are concise statements of the "take-home" information that may be extracted directly from the results of the study and applied only to the population from which the study sample was extracted. Conclusions should include only the data-based findings of the study and should not include any speculation.

ABSTRACT

An abstract is a succinct summary of the contents of the manuscript and is located at the beginning of the manuscript. As counterintuitive as it may initially seem, authors should write the abstract last even though it comes first in a journal. In order to summarize a manuscript accurately, you have to write the manuscript first! Although different journals have different formatting requirements for abstracts, all successful abstracts should have several characteristics. First, they concisely encompass the total manuscript. This means that there is an introduction, methods, results, and discussion (some journals require these labels). Second, they should not be cut and pasted directly from the manuscript text but restructured with a paucity of words. Third, they should include the most important statistical results, with *p* values. Do not structure the results into general phrases (e.g., "some significant results were found") that convey no meaning about outcomes. Finally, the discussion can be less detailed but should not over reach the data by being too vague.

Be aware that many journals have restrictive character or word limits on their abstracts, so approach each word carefully. The abstract is the point at which many readers begin to interface with a research article. Many databases provide abstracts with the results of key word searchers; readers can quickly scan the abstract to see if the article is interesting and appropriate for their needs. Researchers can write terrific articles that will never be read or cited because the abstract presents the experiment poorly. So, be sure to approach the abstract as an important entity unto itself, rather than an afterthought to completed research.

Submitting the Manuscript

Most journals require electronic submission of manuscripts (gone are the days of creating three to five hard copies of the manuscript and sending a gigantic packet off to the journal editor). In some ways, the ease of electronic submission can lead to laziness on the part of the author, since submission is just a click away. But, manuscripts that do not follow the journal's guidelines for format or have excessive numbers of spelling and/or grammatical errors may be rejected before anyone besides the editor ever reads them. In addition, editors can quickly pick out manuscripts submitted (and presumably rejected) elsewhere and "flipped" to another journal without reformatting to the new journal's specifications. Thus, be sure to read and follow the instructions for authors provided on journals' websites. Most journals will require several specific submission elements, including a cover letter, a blinded manuscript, and figures.

Journals often require specific information within the cover letter.

THE COVER LETTER

The cover letter should provide basic information about the manuscript that will allow the editor to determine if the manuscript fits the scope of the journal. Each journal editor asks for specific information within the cover letter. Be sure to include all of that information. Generally, this will include the title of the manuscript, identification of the section to which it is submitted (e.g., brief report, original research, research review), a description of length (written pages, figures, total length), a statement of ethical treatment of participants, a statement that the manuscript is not currently under review elsewhere, and contact information for the corresponding author (See Special Interest Box 17.1). For example, Research Quarterly for Exercise and Sport requires the following in a cover letter:

Authors must

- Include the statement: "This manuscript represents results of original work that have not been published elsewhere (except as an abstract in conference proceedings). This manuscript has not and will not be submitted for publication elsewhere until a decision is made regarding its acceptability for publication in *Research Quarterly for Exercise and Sport*. If accepted for publication, it will not be published elsewhere. Furthermore, if there are any perceived financial conflicts of interest related to the research reported in the manuscript, I/we (the author/s) have disclosed it in the Author's Notes."
- Include the statement: "All authors acknowledge ethical responsibility for the content of the manuscript and will accept the consequences of any ethical violation."
- Include the statement: "This research is not part of a larger study." If it is, then authors must follow the guidelines specified on pp. 13–15 of the *APA* publications manual (6th ed.).
- Indicate the section in which they want the manuscript to be reviewed. Interdisciplinary manuscripts are encouraged, and authors should indicate the sections that overlap the manuscript content.

SPECIAL INTEREST BOX 17.1

Sample Cover Letter for Submitting a Manuscript

Department of Kinesiology and Applied Physiology
My University
City, State zip code
Week day, Month day, Year

Dr. Will Accept, Editor
Name of Journal
Street Address
City, State zip code

Dear Dr. Accept:

Please find enclosed a manuscript entitled: *"Title"* which I am submitting for consideration of publication as an article in *Name of Journal*.

 The paper demonstrates significant finding and its significance. As such, this paper should be of interest to a broad readership including those interested in what kinds of research, topics, and techniques—should be those targeted by the journal. This manuscript is not under review elsewhere at this time. All research describes were approved by My University's institutional review board.

 Knowledgeable referees for this paper might include

- Ike Canreed (what is his/her technical expertise relevant to the paper) (e-mail)

- I.C. Noble (what is his/her technical expertise relevant to the paper) (e-mail)

Thank you for your consideration of my work. Please address all correspondence concerning this manuscript to me at My University and feel free to correspond with me by e-mail (my@emailaddress).

Sincerely,
Your Name
Title

COMMON PITFALLS

The first time that a novice researcher submits a manuscript for peer review can often provide a jolting surprise. While researchers may deem their manuscripts as ground breaking, reviewers may see that same work as verbose, ill conceived, and poorly written. It is always a shock to see that a manuscript has been rejected with a long list of concerns from the reviewers. At least some of these concerns can be addressed simply by carefully reviewing your own work before hitting the "send" button.

Do not rely on spell check for spelling! Go over each page carefully.

1. *Spelling and grammatical errors.* In an era of computer-driven word processing programs, spell check is both a blessing and a curse. Just because a word-processing program indicates that there are no spelling errors, it does not mean that there *are* no spelling errors! Authors must carefully check spelling and grammar prior to submitting the manuscript for review; nothing irritates a reviewer more than having to sort through bad spelling and grammar to determine the content of the experiment. In fact, reviewers may return a manuscript unread, requiring the authors to rewrite it before they provide a substantial review.

2. *Incorrect formatting.* Some journals provide very specific directions in how they want submissions to be formatted. These may include sections to include (with headers), font style and size, manuscript length, margins, key words, and special features, among others. Certainly, it is frustrating to modify format once the manuscript is written, so authors may be tempted to submit a manuscript "as is" with the notion of fixing it if accepted. However, these guidelines are provided with a purpose in mind. One of the surest ways to avoid publication is to ignore these formatting guidelines.

3. *Incorrect citation style.* Each journal will provide specific citation styles that they want you to use, such as APA, MLA, and Chicago (see Chapter 2 for information on specific citation styles). Because each style has its own distinct elements, one cannot be substituted for another. Therefore, be sure to carefully modify citations and references into the style required by the specific journal. This is an arduous task when taken on by hand. Therefore, we recommend that researchers use tools such as Endnote and Refworks when gathering literature. These help users generate a reference list more easily and also provide a simple means by which citation style can be changed.

4. *Self-plagiarism.* As researchers write more and more manuscripts based on a certain line of research or using a specific experimental procedure, they may find that introductions, methodologies, and discussions begin to look similar. There may be a temptation to cut and paste a section from one manuscript into the next. However, this is a special case of plagiarism termed self-plagiarism. Self-plagiarism occurs when authors reuse some or all of their own previously published works in a new manuscript without citation or reference to the previous work.[2] The American Psychological Association[3] distinguishes plagiarism from self-plagiarism in the following way: "Whereas plagiarism refers to the practice of claiming credit for the words, ideas, and concepts of others, self-plagiarism refers to the practice of presenting one's own previously published work as though it were new" (p. 170).

A key issue with self-plagiarism is copyright. Prior to publication of a manuscript, authors must often sign a copyright agreement, which states that the manuscript has not been published elsewhere. Further, authors sign the rights to the manuscript over to the journal. Thus, even though authors have written the original manuscript, they no longer "own" it after publication. The safest way to avoid self-plagiarism is to always write manuscripts as unique entities. Also, in situations where similarities exist between a manuscript and previously published research, be sure to cite that research.

5. *Incorrect figures/tables.* Several common mistakes exist in relation to figures and tables. These can be avoided by taking the following steps. First, each should have a caption that provides an overview of what is displayed within. Figure captions should have a greater degree of detail and should clearly present to describe the content of the figure. Table captions are often only one line but clearly convey the content of the table. Second, each figure and table should be organized in a manner that highlights pertinent details such as statistical significance. Third, the wording within the figures and tables should match the wording in the manuscript text (in other words, don't change acronyms).

Even though you are the author of a published work, you most likely do not own the copyright.

Know before you go: Learn the time and length restrictions of presentations before developing them.

6. *Not "blinding" the entire document.* Blinding a document means removing any information that indicates who the author is or where they are from. Authors often remember to black out their names and institutions on the front page. However, there may be additional information in the methodology related to specific universities, or places where data were collected. Additionally, authors often forget to blind their acknowledgments section. Any place where author identification is possible should be blinded.

FINDING RESOURCES TO HELP WITH DISSEMINATION OF RESEARCH

Besides funding opportunities (e.g., Chapter 16), the Research Consortium (RC) provides a researchers' toolkit on its Web site, which is an excellent resource for researchers at all levels.[4] The RC describes this toolkit as "… a series of e-lectures, multimedia case studies, interactive assessment activities and online reference links aimed at providing faculty, early career researchers and students with information and resources on various topics related to planning, conducting and disseminating research in physical activity and health."

PREPARING AND DELIVERING RESEARCH PRESENTATIONS

Some individuals have a natural knack for public speaking. For them, standing up in front of a group of scholars and presenting their own research does not represent a particularly difficult obstacle. For the rest of us, however, just the thought of delivering a research presentation causes stress. Yet, we all must present our research at some point in time, and the best way to approach these presentations is to use the old Boy Scout motto of "Be Prepared." In the next section, we will provide some strategies on how novice scholars can approach presentations in way that will allow them to be prepared. The Research Consortium has developed an e-lecture entitled "Preparing Effective Research Presentations" as part of their Researchers' Toolkit and that is the basis for much of what we present here.[4]

In order to create an effective presentation, researchers must convey who, what, where, when, and how of their studies in a way that captures the interest of their audience. If people cannot follow the information presented on a poster or within a talk, they will lose interest, regardless of how important that research presented may be. Fortunately, effective presentations of research have several key elements; if novice presenters include these elements, they will have a foundation from which they can develop presentation skills.

At the center of any good presentation is the research itself. As we have discussed throughout this textbook, you must carefully plan and conduct research in order to have both internally and externally valid studies: Audiences appreciate these types of research projects. Studies with many limitations or that do not extent our knowledge base in any way will not make for interesting presentations. Remember that professional presentations provide you with an opportunity to inform and impress audience members who may one day be your future colleagues. Students looking for academic employment should consider any presentation as a potential job interview!

What to Know Prior to Creating a Presentation

When presenting research, researchers need to effectively communicate with their audience. This requires matching the structure and content of the presentation to the audience's level of understanding. At discipline specific, professional meetings, this is not a difficult task, as many people share a certain level of knowledge and expertise. However, researchers making a presentation for a lay audience, such as a local civic organization or a group of prospective students and their families at a university student recruitment event, must adapt their content so that a wider audience can understand their meaning. The bottom line is "know your audience" before you begin.

When preparing an oral presentation, keep in mind the exact time limit allowed for the presentation. Most professional conferences have a 10- to 15-minute time allocation for oral presentations of research studies. Such a short time slot requires brevity on the part of the presenter, since an introduction, methods, results, and discussion must all be crammed into that time. Both novice and experienced presenters can have issues with overrunning their time slot, which is why many professional conferences have moderators with stop watches to cut long presentations off. With this in mind, prepare a presentation that fills but does not exceed the time limitations, and practice it until the timing is correct.

With poster presentations, a similar issue exists. Presenters must place a large amount of information in a relatively small space and do so in a manner that does not overwhelm the audience. Before developing a professional poster, researchers should know the exact dimensions of the display area of the poster. Overall, the plan is to fill that area with just enough information to accurately express the main points of the research. A word of caution: be sure that you understand the appropriate length and height requirements correctly. Do not assume these if not explicitly identified. Nothing is worse than having a carefully constructed poster fit incorrectly on the poster board!

Organization of the Presentation

For many professional presentations, the organization of a presentation should resemble that of a research paper. Research papers start with an introduction that provides a rationale for the study; similarly, presentations begin with an introduction designed to catch the audience's attention. Just as with research papers, the introduction should end with a clearly stated purpose of the study, which should appear in text on a slide or at the end of the introduction section of the poster. The methodology follows the introduction. This should provide enough detail to provide a basic understanding of participants, procedures, and the like, but not an excessive amount of technical detail.

Use diagrams or figures with brief text descriptions where appropriate. The results section follows the methodology. Unlike in a research paper, presenters may need to limit these to their most important results, in the interest of time or space. An effective way to present results is through well-labeled figures or graphs, which enable the audience to grasp the essence of the findings more easily than tables or text. Use colored lines or shapes to highlight important points on a graph, so the audience can focus on it. Finally, present the discussion and conclusions. Within the discussion, highlight how the results compare to those of similar studies as well as the importance of the results. A space-/time-saving strategy is to combine results and discussion. You can accomplish this by providing a graphic of a result, explaining the graphic, then discussing it. Lastly, succinctly state the conclusion in several sentences. It is not necessary to provide a summary at the end and nor are you likely to have time for that. If you received funding for the research, be sure to acknowledge the funding source at the end of the presentation.

Oral and poster presentations are organized similarly, except posters usually include an abstract at the beginning. Posters normally include more text than is practical to use in a slide presentation, but graphs and figures should still be liberally incorporated to promote understanding of the study, as well as to add interest.

Preparing and Delivering Poster Presentations

In recent years, many professional organizations have increased the number of poster presentations in relation to oral presentations. This achieves two positive outcomes. First, it allows for the dissemination of a larger number of research studies overall. In addition, poster sessions get more researchers to conferences. Many of those who attend conferences are required to make a presentation in order to obtain funding from their institutions. Since conferences often occur in 2 or 3 days, the number of slots for oral presentations is limited, so to increase participation, conference organizers often have several poster sessions with a hundred or more posters per session. With that many posters within a session, many conference attendees will view your poster quickly, without taking the time to ask for any interpretation. Therefore, your poster must provide an accurate and succinct representation of your research. Universities often have print shops that will manufacture the poster on one large sheet of paper, for a nominal cost. Another alternative is to have the poster printed on a lightweight fabric, so it can be folded into a suitcase. Both options make transportation and storage relatively simple (see Special Interest Box 17.2).

Tips for Preparing a Poster Presentation

Tips for creating a poster presentation The Research Consortium has developed the following checklist with important tips for preparation of a good research presentation poster.

1. Begin with a diagrammatic overview or blueprint for text and figures by content area (introduction, methods, results, etc.) within the area of your poster. It can save a considerable amount of time if you are modifying the layout of a previously used research poster rather than starting from scratch.

2. Use a consistent background and color scheme throughout the poster.

3. Use contrasting text and background colors. A light background with dark text displays best under all lighting conditions. A white background provides maximal flexibility for selection of text and figure colors. Beware of using text and background colors of the same color intensity! (The text will wash out and be virtually impossible to read.) Also, avoid use of too many or distracting colors.

4. Use a common text font such as Arial or Times New Roman throughout the poster. Unusual fonts can be difficult to read.

5. Use a consistent font size for text that is readable from at least three feet away (title slide text can be larger and citation text can be smaller).

6. Cite references on slides appropriately and provide citations for graphic material copied from other sources.

7. Avoid overuse of text. Figures and graphs can serve as valuable aids to understanding, as well as adding interest to the poster presentation.

8. If displaying a table, highlight the numbers you wish to stand out.

9. Avoid large blank spaces on the poster; use as much of the display area as possible.

10. Proofread your poster carefully for typos and other errors. Ask a colleague with an eye for detail to do the same.

Most conferences divide poster presentations into thematic sessions that can last for 1 to 2 hours, during which time you must stand by your poster to respond to questions. It is important to fulfill your responsibilities for the presentation by hanging and removing your poster at the designated times and by being available to answer questions during the designated period. Be prepared to answer all questions about the poster and respond to all questions in a professional manner, and don't engage in long conversations that do not relate to your research in some way—this may inhibit an interested conference attendee from asking questions.

Some conferences have "Thematic Poster" sessions, in which an audience gathers and focuses attention on one poster at a time within the thematic grouping. In this format, the presenter makes a short, 5- to 7-minute presentation focusing on research highlights, followed by questions from the audience. When preparing for such a session, practice the brief presentation a number of times to ensure you do not over or undershoot your allocated time. It is also important to be especially well prepared to answer questions.

Preparing and Delivering Oral Presentations

With few exceptions, most presenters use Power Point or some similar type of slide show program to provide visual information during an oral presentation. Well-prepared slides provide the foundation for a strong oral presentation of research. Therefore, be sure to take the time to develop a set of slides that provide the audience with an appropriate amount of information in a clearly visible and understandable format, including the sections described above.

In this age of high-density computer graphics, presenters may be fooled into believing that their slides have sufficient contrast or appropriate font size because they look so good on the computer screen. However, be sure to check that you can actually read the slides once projected onto a screen. Slides that look good on a computer display may not have sufficient color contrast or text font size to be clearly readable when projected. The following checklist, provided by the Research Consortium, identifies the "Do's and Don'ts" of preparing slides for a research presentation.

1. Begin with a list of slide descriptions, so you have a plan for how many slides you will develop and what each one will communicate to the audience. With the exception of title and acknowledgment slides, plan on no more than approximately one slide per minute of presentation.
2. Spend the time to develop interesting, well-designed slides. Once you have planned the content of each slide, if you do not seem to have an eye for slide design, seek the help of someone who does. Many universities have individuals trained in graphic arts available in an IT department.
3. Use a consistent background and color scheme throughout the presentation slides.
4. Limit the amount of text displayed on each slide. Summarize main points rather than writing sentences. Bulleted phrases can convey an adequate amount of information to the audience and also remind you of the main points you wish to make when speaking about the slide. The audience does not want to read your entire presentation from your slides!
5. Use contrasting text and background colors. A light background with dark text displays best under all lighting conditions. A white background provides maximal flexibility for selection of text and figure colors. Beware of using text and background colors of the same color intensity! (The text will wash out and be virtually impossible to read.)
6. Use a common text font such as Arial or Times New Roman. Unusual fonts can be difficult to read. Particularly beware of using less common fonts if your slides will be projected from a computer that is not your own. A different version of the slide software can cause your text to be reformatted, with surprising and undesired results!
7. Use a consistent font size for text (title slide text can be larger and citation and caption text can be smaller) and make sure that when projected, the text will be readable in the back row of your audience. A 24- to 32-point font generally works well for slide text.
8. Cite references on slides appropriately and provide citations for graphic material copied from other sources.
9. Incorporate figures, graphics, or even appropriate clip art into your slides. Slides composed of nothing but text are generally *boring*!
10. Audiences can digest graphs much more rapidly than tables, so use figures or graphs rather than tables on slides when possible. If displaying a table, highlight the numbers you wish to stand out.
11. Avoid large blank spaces on slides; use as much of the display area as possible.
12. Do not use the sound feature of PowerPoint, unless showing a video/audio clip relevant to your presentation.
13. Do not get carried away with overuse of animation effects on slides. (Your goal is not to make the audience dizzy!)
14. Proofread your slides carefully for typos and other errors. Ask a colleague with an eye for detail to do the same.

Although you may feel that you know the information on your slides well (since you did all that research and also developed the slides), you should practice your presentation at least several times before presenting in to an audience. The more you practice, the more natural and confident you will sound when delivering the presentation.

SPECIAL INTEREST BOX 17.3

Tips for Delivering an Oral Presentation

The following checklist provides tips for delivery of your presentation. It is a good idea to follow as many of these tips as possible when practicing.

1. Dress professionally for your presentation.
2. Speak from your slides, which are your visual aids, referring to specific things on the slides and explaining each slide. Do not assume that the audience will be able to interpret the slides for themselves.
3. However, do not stare at your slides the whole time. Your presentation should be delivered facing the audience and you should establish some level of eye contact with the audience.
4. If you use a laser pointer, use it judiciously to point to selected items you wish to draw the audience's attention to and then put it down or turn it off. Do not use the laser pointer on every slide and do not use it to move down a line of text you are reading. Under no circumstances should you wave or jiggle a laser pointer around rapidly over a slide.
5. Remember that there may be members of your audience for whom English is not the first language, so speak more slowly and distinctly than you normally would. This will be appreciated by those for whom English is the first language, as well!
6. Do not read your presentation.
7. Stand erect and do not lean on the podium.
8. Do not speak about something that has nothing to do with the slide in front of the audience.
9. Make sure that your presentation is finished within the designated time limit.
10. Be prepared to answer questions about your presentation.

PowerPoint and similar programs allow you to make notes to use as prompts for each slide. By the time you deliver the "real" presentation you should be sufficiently practiced that you do not need the notes. In the unhappy case of failed technology, you may need to be prepared to give the presentation without slides. The best presenters do not appear to be checking notes; they know the information so well that the presentation is like a conversation. Finally, remember to relax! (See Special Interest Box 17.3.)

CHAPTER SUMMARY

- One of the positive outcomes of research is publishing it in a journal.
- Select a journal that has a scope that matches your type of research.
- When reformatting a thesis or dissertation to be a manuscript, cut extraneous content wherever possible in order to get to the journal's target length.
- Manuscripts generally include an abstract, introduction, methodology, results, discussion, and conclusions.
- Abstracts must concisely provide an overview of the entire study.
- Research hypotheses should come at the end of the introduction.

- When writing the methodology, include enough detail so that the study could be replicated by another researcher.
- Organize results to reflect the central questions answered by the research.
- The discussion should go beyond a recapitulation of the results.
- Be sure to blind the entire manuscript prior to submitting it.
- When writing a cover letter, address all the specific points required by your target journal.
- Learn to avoid the common pitfalls that lead to manuscript rejection, like poor spelling and incorrect formatting.
- Whether a presentation is oral or poster, several common, preparatory steps should be taken prior to creating it, such as time or length restrictions.
- Poster presentations must provide an overview of the research study in an organized, visually appealing way.
- Practice an oral presentation several times until you can perform it without notes.

REFERENCES

1. Hopkins WG. The impact-factor Olympics for journals in sport and exercise science and medicine. *Sport Sci* 2012;16:17–19, www.sportsci.org/2012/wghif.htm.
2. Roig M. Avoiding plagiarism, self-plagiarism, and other questionable writing practices: a guide to ethical writing. Retrieved from http://facpub.stjohns.edu/~roigm/plagiarism.doc
3. American Psychological Association. *The Publication Manual of the American Psychological Association.* 6th ed. Washington, DC: American Psychological Association, 2010.
4. Research Consortiums Researchers' toolkit: http://www.aahperd.org/rc/toolkit/

RELATED ASSIGNMENTS

1. **Find the impact factors for five different field-specific journals where you could potentially publish your research. Compare and contrast these. What does the impact factor indicate about the journal?**

2. **Go the Web sites of the journals you have listed above. Write down the scope of each journal. Compare and contrast these. Which do you think would be the most appropriate journal for your type of research?**

Index

Note: Page numbers in *italics* indicate figure; page numbers followed by b indicate box; those followed by t indicate table.